Health and Preventive Strategies in Order to Protect Pregnancy

Health and Preventive Strategies in Order to Protect Pregnancy

Editors

Claudio Costantino
Antonio Maiorana

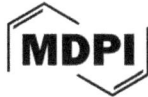

Basel • Beijing • Wuhan • Barcelona • Belgrade • Novi Sad • Cluj • Manchester

Editors
Claudio Costantino
University of Palermo
Palermo, Italy

Antonio Maiorana
ARNAS (Center of National
Relevance and of High
Specialization) Civic Hospital
of Palermo
Palermo, Italy

Editorial Office
MDPI
St. Alban-Anlage 66
4052 Basel, Switzerland

This is a reprint of articles from the Special Issue published online in the open access journal *Women* (ISSN 2673-4184) (available at: https://www.mdpi.com/journal/women/special_issues/protect_pregnancy).

For citation purposes, cite each article independently as indicated on the article page online and as indicated below:

Lastname, A.A.; Lastname, B.B. Article Title. *Journal Name* **Year**, *Volume Number*, Page Range.

ISBN 978-3-0365-9578-8 (Hbk)
ISBN 978-3-0365-9579-5 (PDF)
doi.org/10.3390/books978-3-0365-9579-5

© 2023 by the authors. Articles in this book are Open Access and distributed under the Creative Commons Attribution (CC BY) license. The book as a whole is distributed by MDPI under the terms and conditions of the Creative Commons Attribution-NonCommercial-NoDerivs (CC BY-NC-ND) license.

Contents

About the Editors vii

Preface ix

Matteo Riccò, Pietro Ferraro, Silvia Corrado, Alessandro Zaniboni, Elia Satta and Silvia Ranzieri
Respiratory Syncytial Virus in Pregnant Women: Systematic Review and Meta-Analysis
Reprinted from: *Women* **2022**, 2, 16, doi:10.3390/women2020016 1

Vincenza Gianfredi, Alessandro Berti, Marilena D'Amico, Viola De Lorenzo and Silvana Castaldi
Knowledge, Attitudes, Behavior, Acceptance, and Hesitancy in Relation to the COVID-19 Vaccine among Pregnant and Breastfeeding Women: A Systematic Review Protocol
Reprinted from: *Women* **2023**, 3, 6, doi:10.3390/women3010006 15

Putunywa Zandrina Nxiweni, Kelechi Elizabeth Oladimeji, Mirabel Nanjoh, Lucas Banda, Felix Emeka Anyiam, Francis Leonard Mpotte Hyera, et al.
Factors Influencing the Utilization of Antenatal Services among Women of Childbearing Age in South Africa
Reprinted from: *Women* **2022**, 2, 27, doi:10.3390/women2030027 25

Patricia Anafi and Wisdom Kwadwo Mprah
Knowledge and Perception of Risk in Pregnancy and Childbirth among Women in Low-Income Communities in Accra
Reprinted from: *Women* **2022**, 2, 35, doi:10.3390/women2040035 45

Ritsuko Shirabe, Tsuyoshi Okuhara, Hiroko Okada, Eiko Goto and Takahiro Kiuchi
Support Needs for Anxiety among Pregnant Women in Japan: A Qualitative Pilot Study
Reprinted from: *Women* **2023**, 3, 8, doi:10.3390/women3010008 57

Maria Rita Infurna, Eleonora Bevacqua, Giulia Costanzo, Giorgio Falgares and Francesca Giannone
Psychosocial Risk Factors and Psychopathological Outcomes: Preliminary Findings in Italian Pregnant Women
Reprinted from: *Women* **2023**, 3, 10, doi:10.3390/women3010010 69

Osaretin Christabel Okonji, Chimezie Igwegbe Nzoputam, Michael Ekholuenetale, Emeka Francis Okonji, Anthony Ike Wegbom and Clement Kevin Edet
Differentials in Maternal Mortality Pattern in Sub-Saharan Africa Countries: Evidence from Demographic and Health Survey Data
Reprinted from: *Women* **2023**, 3, 14, doi:10.3390/women3010014 81

Matteo Riccò, Antonio Baldassarre, Milena Pia Cerviere and Federico Marchesi
Vaccine Hesitancy in Women of Childbearing Age and Occupational Physicians: Results from a Cross-Sectional Study (Italy, 2022)
Reprinted from: *Women* **2023**, 3, 19, doi:10.3390/women3020019 95

Tam Anh Nguyen, Mohammed Mohsin, Batool Moussa, Jane Fisher, Nawal Nadar, Fatima Hassoun, et al.
Determinants of Antenatal Education and Breastfeeding Uptake in Refugee-Background and Australian-Born Women
Reprinted from: *Women* **2023**, 3, 20, doi:10.3390/women3020020 121

Praise Ebimaye Tangbe, Mary Shaw-Ridley, Gerri Cannon-Smith, Sheila McKinney, Nelson Atehortua and Russell Bennett
Prenatal, Delivery and Postpartum Care Experiences among Black Women in Mississippi during COVID-19 Pandemic 2020–2021
Reprinted from: *Women* **2023**, *3*, 22, doi:10.3390/women3020022 . . . . **139**

Kgaladi Mpule Mohlala, Livhuwani Muthelo, Mpho Gift Mathebula, Masenyani Oupa Mbombi, Tshepo Albert Ntho and Thabo Arthur Phukubye
Clinical Equipment as a Potential Impediment to Optimal Intrapartum Monitoring and Delivery for Pregnant Women in South Africa
Reprinted from: *Women* **2023**, *3*, 25, doi:10.3390/women3020025 . . . . **155**

Cristina Genovese, Carmela Alessia Biondo, Caterina Rizzo, Rosaria Cortese, Isabella La Spina, Paola Tripodi, et al.
Knowledge, Propensity and Hesitancy among Pregnant Women in the Post-Pandemic Phase Regarding COVID-19 Vaccination: A Prevalence Survey in Southern Italy
Reprinted from: *Women* **2023**, *3*, 28, doi:10.3390/women3030028 . . . . **169**

About the Editors

Claudio Costantino

Prof. Claudio Costantino (MD, PhD, and MPH) is an Associate Professor of Preventive Medicine, Public Health, and Epidemiology at the University of Palermo and Medical Officer at the Clinical Epidemiology with Tumor Registry Unit at the University Hospital of Palermo. CC has been a Medical Specialist in Preventive Medicine and Public Health since 2014 and she has a PhD in Clinical Medicine and Behavioral Sciences since 2017. She is also a Vaccination Unit Coordinator at the University Hospital of Palermo since 2018 and has been a member of the Sicilian Region Task Force for COVID-19 Vaccinations since 2020. Since 2020, she has been a collaborating expert for COVID-19 vaccine communication and outreach for the European Medicines Agency and a member of the National Ministry of Health Technical Table for the renewal of the National Immunization Plan 2023–2025. She is also a member of the National Comitee of VaccinarSi.org and Scientific Referent and Coordinator of VaccinarSiinsicilia.org websites since 2017 and the incoming President of the Sicilian Section of the Italian Society of Hygiene, Preventive Medicine, and Public Health (S.It.I.) for 2024–2026.

Antonio Maiorana

Dr. Antonio Maiorana is an MD and Director of the Complex Operative Unit of Obstetrics and Gynecology in Palermo "Civico" Hospital. Additionally, she is the Director of the Regional Excellence Center of Endometriosis and Selected Membre of AAGL (American Association of Gynecologic Laparoscopist). Furthermore, she is a member of the Italian Society of Gynecologic Endoscopy.

Preface

The topics that were handled in the SI "Health and Preventive Strategies in Order to Protect Pregnancy" of Women were quite various in order to guarantee the best health status during pregnancy.

From factors influencing antenatal birth in South Africa to the knowledge and perceptions of risks during pregnancy and childbirth in Ghana and the support needs againt anxiety in pregnancy in Japan.

The psychosocial risk factors and psychopathological outcomes were analyzed among Italian pregnant women, and the differentials in maternal mortality patterns in Sub-Saharan African countries were an interesting topic.

Vaccine hesitancy among Italian pregnant women was analyzed in two different papers (one dedicated to COVID-19 vaccination in pregnancy), and the impact of the COVID-19 pandemic on the experiences of pregnant women in Mississipi (during prenatal, delivery, and postpartum care) was also analyzed.

Finally, the determinants of antenatal education and breastfeeding uptake from women of a refugee background, Australian-born women, and the impact of clinical equipment on optimal intrapartum monitoring in South Africa were analyzed in depth.

In the systematic review, the impact of respiratory syncytial virus on pregnant women was evaluated, and a protocol for vaccine hesitancy evaluation among pregnant and breastfeeding women was also published.

Claudio Costantino and Antonio Maiorana
Editors

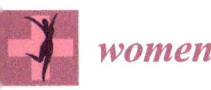

Systematic Review

Respiratory Syncytial Virus in Pregnant Women: Systematic Review and Meta-Analysis

Matteo Riccò [1,*], Pietro Ferraro [2], Silvia Corrado [3], Alessandro Zaniboni [4], Elia Satta [4] and Silvia Ranzieri [4]

1. AUSL–IRCCS di Reggio Emilia, Servizio di Prevenzione e Sicurezza Negli Ambienti di Lavoro (SPSAL), Local Health Unit of Reggio Emilia, Via Amendola n. 2, I-42122 Reggio Emilia, Italy
2. Occupational Medicine Unit, Direzione Sanità, Italian Railways' Infrastructure Division, RFI SpA, Piazza della Croce Rossa n. 1, I-00161 Rome, Italy; dott.pietro.ferraro@gmail.com
3. Department of Medicine DAME, Division of Pediatrics, University of Udine, Via delle Scienze, n. 206, I-33100 Udine, Italy; silviacorrado90@gmail.com
4. Department of Medicine and Surgery, University of Parma, Via Gramsci 14, I-43126 Parma, Italy; alessandro.zaniboni@unipr.it (A.Z.); elia.satta@unipr.it (E.S.); silvia.ranzieri@unipr.it (S.R.)
* Correspondence: matteo.ricco@ausl.re.it or mricco2000@gmail.com; Tel.: +39-339-2994343 or +39-522-837587

Abstract: Human Respiratory Syncytial Virus (RSV) is a highly contagious viral pathogen. In infants, it is usually listed among the main causes of medical referrals and hospitalizations, particularly among newborns. While waiting for the results of early randomized controlled trials on maternal vaccination against RSV, the present systematic review and meta-analysis aimed to collect available evidence on maternal RSV infections. According to the PRISMA statement, Pubmed, Embase, and pre-print archive medRxiv.og were searched for eligible studies published up to 1 April 2022. Raw data included the incidence of RSV infection among sampled pregnant women, and the occurrence of complications. Data were then pooled in a random-effects model. Heterogeneity was assessed using the I^2 measure, while reporting bias was assessed by means of funnel plots and regression analysis. A total of 5 studies for 282,918 pregnancies were retrieved, with a pooled prevalence of 0.2 per 100 pregnancies and 2.5 per 100 pregnancies with respiratory tract infections. Neither maternal deaths nor miscarriages were reported. Even though detailed data were available only for 6309 pregnancies and 33 RSV cases, infant outcomes such as low birth weight and preterm delivery were rare (in both cases 0.04%), but up to 9.1% in cases where RSV diagnosis was confirmed. No substantially increased risk for preterm delivery (RR 1.395; 95%CI 0.566 to 3.434) and giving birth to a low-birth-weight infant (RR 0.509; 95%CI 0.134 to 1.924) was eventually identified. *Conclusions*. Although RSV is uncommonly detected among pregnant women, incident cases were associated with a relatively high share of complications. However, heterogeneous design and the quality of retrieved reports stress the need for specifically designed studies.

Keywords: respiratory syncytial virus; respiratory tract infections; vaccine; pregnancy; epidemiology

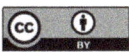

1. Introduction

Since its first description in 1956 [1], human Respiratory Syncytial Virus (RSV) (genus orthopneumovirus, family of Pneumoviridae) [2–8] has emerged as a highly contagious viral pathogen. According to available figures, RSV represents the main cause of hospitalization among infants < 1 year of age in western countries, and a leading cause of lower respiratory tract infections (RTI) in children in their first year of life [4,9–12], with a well-defined seasonal trend [4,8].

Likewise, other viral agents of RTI do not elicit a long-lasting immunity, and adults are constantly re-infected throughout their lives, with annual rates ranging from 2 to 12% [13,14]. Until recently, the only available therapeutic option has been represented by supportive care (i.e., respiratory support and the management of volume depletion) [7,15], and preventive interventions have been limited to monoclonal antibodies (mAb) [16–18].

Even though real-world evidence has shown that mAb are rather effective in reducing hospitalizations and preventing lower RTI in some high-risk groups (i.e., prematurely born infants under 6 months of age, and children with certain comorbidities under 2 years of age during the RSV season) [19–24], mAb are affected by several shortcomings. Firstly, they must be injected once each month during the RSV season, for a total of five subsequent weight-dependent doses (i.e., 15 mg/kg), with obvious logistic issues and costs ranging between $1661 and $2584 per dose [25]. As a consequence, alternative strategies including long-acting mAb [26–29] and new, effective vaccines have been more recently explored [2,4,19,30,31].

In this regard, maternal vaccination strategies appear particularly attractive [32–35], as transplacental transfer of neutralizing antibodies is well-documented even in RSV infections, and high titers of maternal antibodies have been shown able to reduce the risk of infant RSV infections, particularly in the first 30 days of life [36–39].

Despite the potential analogies with other maternal vaccination programs, such as influenza and pertussis vaccination programs [40–42], some significant ethical issues still remain to be addressed. More precisely, while there is consolidated evidence that pregnant women are at increased risk of serious illness and mortality due to influenza virus infection [43], giving some further rationale to their vaccination, more limited information is available on RSV infections. On the one hand, RSV usually does not cause significant disease in healthy adults. On the other hand, some earlier reports have suggested that RSV infection in pregnancy may increase the risk of early delivery by cesarean section [44–46], as well as higher rates of adverse pregnancy outcomes [44,47,48]. While we are waiting for the results of the earlier large randomized controlled trials on maternal vaccination [49,50], an updated synthesis of the literature is therefore needed to ascertain (1) whether RSV infection may be acknowledged or not as a rare occurrence in pregnant women; (2) whether available evidence confirms that RSV infections in pregnancy are associated with more severe outcomes for mothers and children or not.

2. Results

As shown in Figure 1, a total pool of 970 entries (i.e., 505 from PubMed; 132 from MedRxiv; 333 from EMBASE) were initially retrieved. After duplicates were removed (No. 299), the resulting 671 articles were screened by title and abstract. Of them, 271 entries were removed after the title and abstract screening. Twenty-eight articles were then assessed and reviewed via full-text screening. Finally, five papers were included in the qualitative and quantitative analysis.

A detailed description of individual studies is available in Table 1, and their corresponding risk of bias (ROB) assessment is summarized in Figure 2.

Table 1. Summary description of individual studies.

Reference	Year	Settings	Study Design	Target Population	RSV Sampling
Chaw et al. [51]	2016	Mongolia 2013–2015	Prospective study on influenza-like illnesses (ILI) and severe acute respiratory infections (sARI) in the semirural district of Baganuur. Periodic follow-up (1 call every 2 to 5 days) in order to catch ILI episodes.	Pregnant women with ILI and sARI	Reported ILI and sARI
Chu et al. [52]	2016	Nepal 2011–2014	Prospective study performed during a randomized controlled trial on maternal influenza immunization.	Pregnant women in the second trimester of pregnancy.	Reported or measured fever (>38 °C) with at least one symptom among cough, myalgia, sore throat, or rhinorrhea.

Table 1. Cont.

Reference	Year	Settings	Study Design	Target Population	RSV Sampling
Hause et al. [53]	2019	USA (Texas) 2015–2016	Cross-sectional surveillance study.	Outpatients from an outpatient obstetric and gynecologic clinic. Pregnant women in 2nd or 3rd trimester with diagnosis of sARI in the 7 days before the visit.	Reported sARI
Hause et al. [46]	2021	USA (California) 2010–2017	Case series, retrospective study.	Pregnant women having live births outcomes at Kaiser Permanente in Southern California.	Unclear rationale.
Madhi et al. [54]	2018	South Africa 2011–2012	Retrospective study on three cohorts of pregnant women: 2 HIV-uninfected and 1 HIV-infected that were initially defined for a randomized controlled trial on maternal influenza immunization.	Women developing any respiratory symptoms during the follow-up.	Women complaining symptoms compatible with the diagnosis of ILI (i.e., presence of fever ($\geq$38 °C on oral measurements) or chills/rigors or feeling feverish in past <7 days, and one of the following for <7 days duration: (i) cough/sore throat/pharyngitis, or (ii) muscle aches/joint aches/headaches, or (iii) chest pain while breathing/feeling short of breath/difficulty breathing)

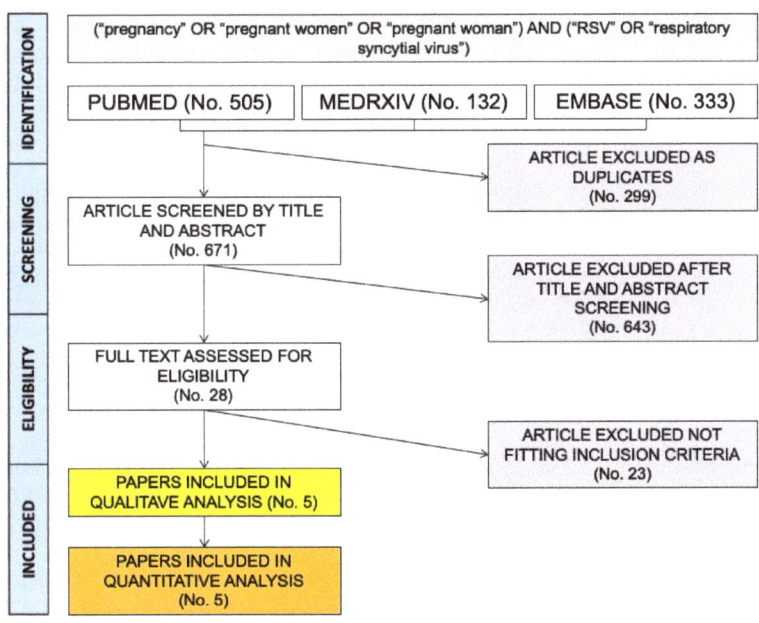

Figure 1. Flow chart for studies included in the systematic review and meta-analysis.

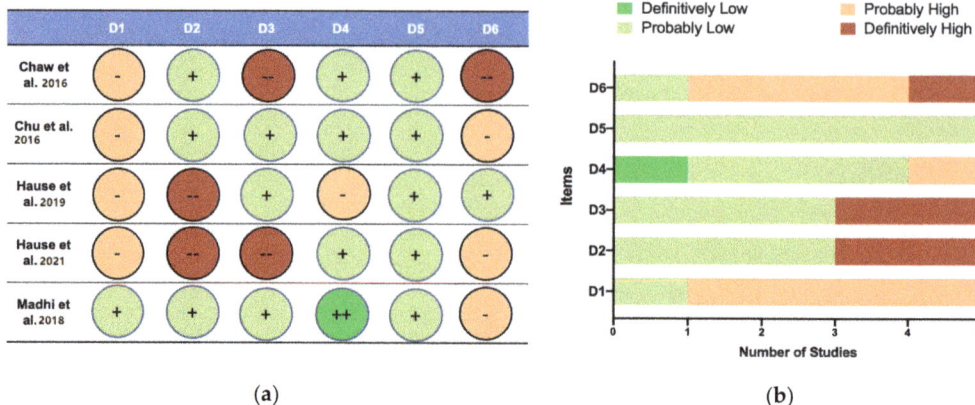

Figure 2. Summary of risk of bias assessment (Note: D1: Possibility of selection bias; D2: Exposure assessment; D3: Outcome assessment; D4: Confounding; D5: Reporting bias; D6: Other bias). (**a**) detailed report by single study [46,51–54], (**b**) summary report.

When dealing with selection bias, four out of five studies were reasonably affected by possible selection bias, as enrollment required registration with local providers [46,51–53] in areas affected by limited access to healthcare services, or specific healthcare plans of infrastructures [46,53]. Exposure assessment was affected by a definitively high risk of bias in two studies [46,53] where the clinical criteria for RSV testing were not strictly defined. The ROB for the outcome assessment was likely low in three of the reported studies, as both maternal and offspring clinical features were reported [46,52–54], while one study did not include significant information about the mother [51], and another study only reported hospitalized women giving live births [46]. Confounding factors were accurately taken into account by one study only [54], but the remaining studies considered differences among the sampled individuals for stratification, with a likely low risk of bias. Similarly, reporting bias (i.e., selective inclusion of outcomes in the publication of the study on the basis of the results) was likely low in all studies. However, in two reports [46,51], the study design presumptively impaired the proper identification of complications, while other reports lacked the proper assessment of pregnancies occurring during the RSV season or outside the RSV season [46,51,52]. Both issues were properly addressed by only one report [53].

As shown in Table 2, a total of 282,918 pregnancies were included, with the majority of them (97.3%) from a study retrieving data on women at Kaiser Permanente Southern California, whose pregnancies ended in a live birth between 1 July 2010 and 30 April 2017. A further study by Regan et al. was, in turn, excluded as reported estimates on RSV infections were only available in hospitalized women [47].

Overall, 2942 cases of RTI were documented, including a total of 62 RSV infections. In sampled pregnancies, the occurrence of RTI ranged between 0.4 and 44.0% (Figure 3a), with a corresponding share of RSV infections over RTI cases ranging between 1.0% and 12.3%, for a pooled RSV prevalence of 0.221 (95%CI 0.045 to 1.081) per 100 pregnancies, and 2.532 (95%CI 1.218 to 5.189) per 100 episodes of RTI (Figure 3b). In both cases, heterogeneity was substantial ($I^2 = 99\%$ and $I^2 = 86\%$, respectively). In total, only 11 cases required hospitalization (i.e., 0.003% of all pregnancies, 0.4% of all RTIE, and 2.5% of all RSV cases).

Table 2. Characteristics of the studies included in the quantitative analysis (Note: RSV = Respiratory Syncytial Virus; RTI = Respiratory Tract Infection).

Reference	Pregnancies (No.)	RTI (No./Total, %)	RSV (No./RTI, %)	Hospitalizations (No./RSV, %)	Pneumonia (No./RSV, %)	Miscarriage (No./RSV, %)	Preterm (No./RSV, %)	Low Birth Weight (No./RSV, %)
Chaw et al. [51]	1260	160, 12.7%	4, 2.5%	NA	NA	NA	NA	NA
Chu et al. [52]	3693	733, 19.8%	7, 1.0%	0, -	0, -	0, -	1, 14.3%	2, 28.6%
Hause et al. [53]	500	65, 13.0%	8, 12.3%	1, 12.5%	0, -	0, -	0, -	0, -
Hause et al. [46]	27,5349	1057, 0.4%	25, 2.4%	10, 40.0%	4, 16.0%	0, -	1, 4.0%	1, 4.0%
Madhi et al. [54]	2116	932, 44.0%	18, 1.9%	0, -	2, 11.1%	0, -	2, 11.1%	1, 5.6%

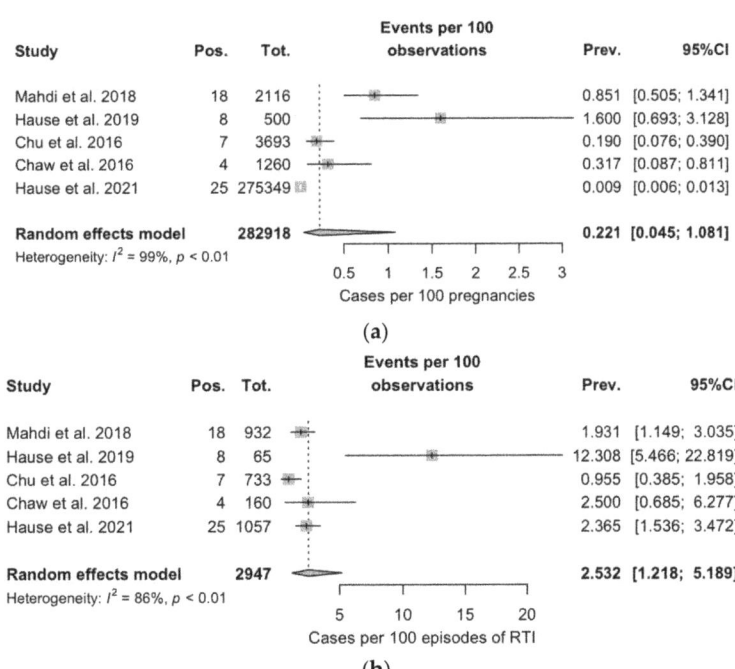

Figure 3. Incidence of RSV infections (**a**) among sampled pregnancies and (**b**) among cases of respiratory tract infections (RTI) in sampled pregnancies. A pooled incidence of 0.221 cases per 100 pregnancies (95%CI 0.045 to 1.081) and 2.532 per 100 RTI episodes (95%CI 1.218 to 5.189) was identified. In both cases, estimates were affected by substantial heterogeneity ($I^2 = 99\%$ and $I^2 = 86\%$, respectively).

Clinical characteristics of the pregnancies were reported by four studies [46,52–54], but one of them only included clinical data on hospitalized women (i.e., 10 out of 25 cases) [46]. Of them, four episodes evolved into pneumonia and two into sepsis. However, as no detailed information on other patients (i.e., 15/25 RSV positive cases) is provided, summary estimates were calculated in three studies, for a total of 33 RSV cases over 6309 pregnancies (i.e., 2% of the total sample), and are reported in Table 3 [51,53,54].

Overall, 6.1% of RSV episodes developed maternal pneumonia, but no maternal deaths were reported. On the contrary, complications in the infant were reported in approximately 1 out of 10 pregnancies, as 9.1% of RSV pregnancies resulted in preterm delivery and/or in a low-birth-weight infant.

Comparisons between RSV cases and normal pregnancies were limited to the estimates from two studies by the heterogeneity of data reporting on non-RSV cases. A pooled Risk Ratio (RR) of 1.193 was reported, 95%CI 0.076 to 18.681 ($p = 0.900$) for miscarriage, with an RR of 1.395 (95%CI 0.566 to 3.434; p = 0.479) for preterm delivery, and an RR of 0.509 (95%CI 0.134 to 1.924) for giving birth to a low-birth-weight infant (p = 0.289).

Table 3. Summary of collected outcomes of RSV cases in pregnancies. Data on studies reporting on maternal episodes in both hospitalized and non-hospitalized women were summarized [51,53,54].

Outcome	No.	% (No./6309 Pregnancies)	% (No./33 RSV Cases)
Pneumonia in mother	2	0.03%	6.1%
Deaths in mother	0	-	-
Miscarriage	0	-	-
Preterm delivery	3	0.04%	9.1%
Low Birth Weight	3	0.04%	9.1%

The presence of publication bias was evaluated using funnel plots and regression tests for funnel plot asymmetry. In the funnel plot, studies' effect sizes are plotted against their standard errors; each point represents a separate study, and their asymmetrical distribution upon visual inspection is suggestive of publication bias (i.e., publication depending not just on the quality of the research, but also on the hypothesis tested, and the significance and direction of detected effects), as in Figure 4a. Such subjective evidence from the funnel plot was only partially confirmed after the regression test. In fact, the Egger test ruled out publication bias (i.e., t = 1.07, df = 4, p-value = 0.361). On the other hand, in radial plots (Figure 4b), estimates were substantially scattered across the regression line, suggesting no significant small-study effect.

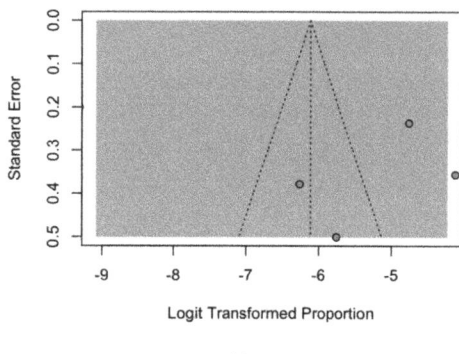
(a)

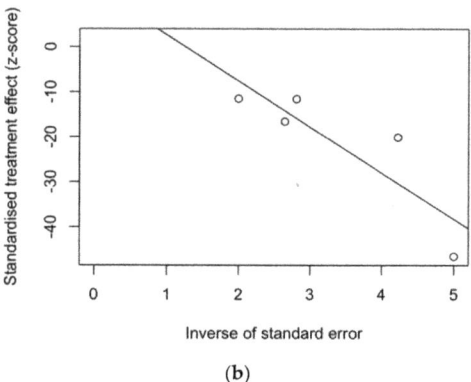
(b)

Figure 4. Funnel plots for studies included in the meta-analysis (**a**). Despite the reduced number of included studies, visual inspection suggested substantial evidence of publication bias for both subgroups, but this was substantially rejected by Egger test (1.07, df = 4, p-value = 0.361). On the other hand, in radial plots (**b**), the studies were substantially scattered across the regression line, suggesting no substantial small-study effect.

3. Discussion

Recent studies have suggested that the occurrence of RSV infections in adults has been substantially underscored [13,14,55–58], but limited data exist on the clinical characteristics of infections in pregnant women [45,47]. For instance, in a previous case series from the USA, two out of three cases eventually developed respiratory distress, requiring mechanical ventilation, suggesting that RSV infections in pregnancy may represent a clinically significant event [45].

However, as RSV is uncommonly tested among women with RTI, particularly during influenza season, substantial uncertainties about the actual prevalence of RSV infections still remain [47,59]. In fact, the interest in maternal infections and complications has been only recently raised by the ongoing RCT on RSV immunization in pregnant women, a strategy that is specifically designed in order to protect the newborns during their first months of life [32,49,50]. On the one hand, future health technology assessments on maternal vaccination strategies will require a preventive, detailed definition of the burden of disease and potential outcomes of RSV infection in pregnant women [60–62]. On the other hand, studies on maternal influenza strategies have stressed how difficult reaching targeted vaccination rates could be for a pathogen whose actual relevance in adults is irregularly acknowledged by the general population [43,63–66]. Unfortunately, RSV is an often "forgotten" pathogen, and medical professionals may also fail to acknowledge the potentially dismal consequences of RSV infection in infants and adults [67–69]. Therefore, recommending a medical intervention to otherwise healthy individuals with a low risk of complications may elicit substantial ethical issues as well as unmotivated concerns [68,69] that could be mitigated only through the characterization of a direct advantage for the pregnant women themselves [54].

In our systematic review and meta-analysis, we were able to retrieve data on a total of 282,918 pregnancies, with 58 incident cases of RSV infection, for an attack rate of 0.2%. Such estimates reasonably represent an underestimation of the actual figures, as only women with signs and symptoms of RTI were regularly tested for RSV [46,48,51–53], and in healthy adults, RSV infections are often limited to indolent mucosal infections [56,70]. For example, in family studies, RSV infections have been associated with fever in 5 to 27% of cases [56]. Not coincidentally, in a previous report on hospitalization for RTI in California, Israel, Ontario, and Western Australia, a total of 21 women out of 846 episodes of RTI were eventually positive for RSV [47], for an attack rate of around 2.5%. Even though it is reasonable that most cases of RSV in pregnant women may have occurred unnoticed, we cannot conversely rule out the potential oversampling of RSV cases. As RSV follows a clear and well-known seasonal trend [71–75], studies that mostly include "in-season" pregnancies may have over-reported cases of RSV infections compared to studies including a larger share of pregnancies outside the RSV season. In this regard, only two papers properly took into account the background viral activity [46,53]. Not surprisingly, most cases did cluster between the 44th and 52nd calendar weeks (i.e., the conventional RSV season for Southern USA).

In other words, RSV infections in pregnant women do occur, but the incidence of severe infections (i.e., those cases that have a better chance to be accurately detected, tracked, and reported) is quite rare. Corresponding figures are hardly comparable to available estimates for other respiratory tract pathogens, likewise with seasonal influenza, whose attack rates usually range between 9% and 11% [76–78], with a 0.7 to 0.9% risk for influenza infection per month [79]. On the other hand, even though both maternal and infant deaths were recorded, the occurrence of complications in incident cases was far from being inconspicuous. Not only 11 out of the 58 sampled cases (19.0%) required hospitalization [46,53], but focusing the analyses on studies that reported both hospitalized and non-hospitalized cases (No. = 33), the incidence of pneumonia was noticeable (6.1%) [51,53,54]. Similarly, the burden of infant complications was relatively high, with 9.1% of infants born preterm and/or with low birth weight. When dealing with these figures, however, a somewhat precautionary approach is forcibly required.

Firstly, the two largest studies [52,54] were based on populations affected by poverty, gender inequalities, malnutrition, and high occurrences of infectious diseases such as HIV/AIDS and tuberculosis. In other words, these infant outcomes may be rather associated with baseline conditions of the sampled population than with RSV infections. Nonetheless, no substantially increased risk for preterm delivery (RR 1.395; 95%CI 0.566 to 3.434) and giving birth to a low-birth-weight infant (RR 0.509; 95%CI 0.134 to 1.924) was eventually identified. On the contrary, as milder cases of RSV likely failed to be sampled for the pathogen being deprived of noticeable signs and symptoms, original studies may have failed to properly assess the association between RSV infection and infant outcomes [52].

Limitations. Despite the potential interest, our study is affected by several limitations. Firstly, we had to deal with the implicit limitations of all meta-analyses, being highly dependent on the quality and heterogeneity of the original studies [80,81]. From this point of view, not only the number of studies we were able to retrieve was limited, but also their quality was highly heterogeneous. In fact, as the actual burden of RSV in adults has been only recently acknowledged, the potential impact on pregnant women has been mostly ignored until the case series from Wheeler et al. [45]. Even in subsequent studies, maternal outcomes have been only rarely addressed, with the limited evidence we were able to summarize in the present review. Likewise, the comparison of prevalence rates across various studies and different sampling strategies is particularly complicated. For example, the study from Hause et al. [46] mostly focused on hospitalized cases tested for RSV, the very same case definition and sampling strategy in other collected studies were quite heterogeneous [51,53,54,82]. Moreover, two out of the five studies were performed in countries (i.e., Nepal and Mongolia) with limited access to maternal and newborn care [4,51,52,82], and the overall figures may have been substantially biased through the oversampling of cases characterized by a more severe outcome, particularly when compared to the aforementioned studies from Texas and California [46,53,59]. Not coincidentally, the reported attack rates had a very large actual range, from 0.955% to 12.308% on total RTI.

Eventually, all the reported studies were performed before the SARS-CoV-2 pandemic. The implementation and the subsequent lifting of non-pharmaceutical interventions (NPI, i.e., public health measures that aim to prevent and/or control SARS-CoV-2 transmission in the community) have resulted in a sudden and earlier-than-expected end of the RSV epidemic season, with substantially no cases detected in the following months [83–87]. NPI blocked the normal transmission of RSV to susceptible individuals at the community level [85,86,88–92], generating a larger RSV-vulnerable population, and preserving susceptibility to the pathogen during the subsequent seasons [2,88–90,93]. To date, the impact of lockdown measures has been mainly assessed on infants, but updated figures during the reemergent RSV epidemics in 2021–2022 are needed to guarantee a better cost-effectiveness estimate of potential preventive interventions.

4. Materials and Methods

This systematic review and meta-analysis of the literature were conducted following the "Preferred Reporting Items for Systematic Reviews and Meta-Analysis" (PRISMA) guidelines [94], and research concepts were preliminarily defined according to the "PICO" (Patient/Population/Problem; Intervention; Control/Comparator; Outcome) strategy (Table 4). The review was registered with PROSPERO (CRD42022330471).

Table 4. PICO worksheet (note: RSV = respiratory syncytial virus).

Item	Definition
Population of interest	Pregnant women
Investigated result	Prevalence of RSV infections
Control	Pregnancies negative for RSV infections
Outcome	Complications for mother and infant

Two scholarly databases (i.e., PubMed/MEDLINE and EMBASE) and the pre-print server medrxiv.org were searched for relevant studies from inception up to 1 April 2022, without applying any backward chronological restrictions. In order to collect the most evidence available, we opted for a broad search strategy that resulted from the combination of the following keywords (free text and Medical Subject Heading [MeSH] terms, where appropriate): ("pregnancy" OR "pregnant women" OR "pregnant woman") AND ("RSV OR "respiratory syncytial virus"). Articles eligible for review were original research publications available online or through inter-library loans. A language filter was applied, by retaining articles written in Italian, English, German, French, or Spanish, the languages spoken by the investigators.

Records whose title and abstract appeared pertinent to the search strategy were initially handled using references management software (Mendeley Desktop Version 1.19.5,

Mendeley Ltd., London, UK, 2019), being subsequently reviewed and screened by two independent authors (E.S. and A.Z.) against eligibility criteria. More precisely, retrieved studies were included if they met the following inclusion criteria:

1. Reporting a crude number of assessed pregnancies.
2. Reporting the number of RSV cases diagnosed.
3. Diagnosis of RSV infection by means of either polymerase chain reaction or point-of-care tests.

In order to avoid the risk of oversampling more severe cases, studies were excluded if the diagnosis of RSV infection was limited to hospitalized women. Only articles reporting original results were retained. Therefore, review articles, meta-analyses, case reports, case series, meeting reports, and conference abstracts were excluded from both qualitative and quantitative analysis. All articles meeting all of the inclusion criteria were retained for the full-text review. The investigators independently read full-text versions of eligible articles. Disagreements were resolved by consensus between the two reviewers; when it was not possible to reach a consensus, input from a third investigator (M.R.) was searched and obtained. Data extracted included:

1. Settings of the study.
2. Number of included pregnancies cases.
3. Number of RTI assessed (if available).
4. Number of RSV episodes.
5. Outcome of RSV episodes, and more precisely, episodes of pneumonia, maternal deaths, miscarriages, giving birth preterm, and/or giving birth to a low-birth-weight infant.

After data extraction, studies were rated on the potential risk of bias by means of the National Toxicology Program (NTP)'s Office of Health Assessment and Translation (OHAT) handbook and respective risk of bias (ROB) tool [95,96]. The ROB tool evaluates the internal validity of a given study in order to assess whether the study's design and conduct have compromised the credibility of the link between the exposure and the outcome or not. The OHAT ROB tool covers six possible sources of bias (i.e., participant selection, confounding, attrition/exclusion, detection, selective reporting, and other sources) with potential answers ranging from "definitely low," "probably low," "probably high," to "definitely high". Interestingly, the OHAT ROB tool does not apply an overall rating for each study, and the OHAT handbook also recommends that even studies with "probably high" or "definitely high" ratings should not be removed from consideration of the overall body of evidence.

Initially, a descriptive analysis was performed by calculating the crude prevalence figure per 100 pregnancies: If a study did not include raw data, either as the number of prevalent cases or a referent population, such figures were reverse-calculated from available data. In order to cope with the presumptive heterogeneity in the study design, we opted for a random-effect model. The amount of inconsistency between included studies was estimated by means of the I^2 statistic (i.e., the percentage of total variation across studies that is due to heterogeneity rather than chance), assuming the following categorization: For I^2 estimates ranging from 0 to 25%, low heterogeneity was assumed; for I^2 ranging between 26% and 50%, moderate heterogeneity; for $I^2 \geq 50\%$, the heterogeneity was acknowledged as substantial. To investigate publication bias, contour-enhanced funnel plots representing the Egger test for quantitative publication bias analysis (at a 5% of significance level) were generated. Radial plots were then calculated and visually inspected to rule out small study bias. All analyses were performed by means of "meta" and "metafor" packages with R (version 4.0.3) and RStudio (version 1.1.463) software. The meta package is an open-source add-on for conducting meta-analyses.

5. Conclusions

RSV was uncommonly detected among pregnant women, but incident cases were associated with a relatively high share of complications. In other words, RSV infections in pregnancy are a rare event that may result in severe infections, with a relatively benign outcome. However, because of the inconsistent testing strategies, it is reasonable that a substantial share of cases may have been lost from the parent estimates, eventually impairing the reliability of our estimates. Therefore, the information presented here can hardly be considered definitive, and stress the opportunity for additional studies that, through a more consistent case definition and testing strategy, would help to identify the true burden of severe RSV infections for mother and child, eventually contributing to a better definition of potential costs and benefits of upcoming maternal vaccination strategies.

Author Contributions: Conceptualization, M.R.; data curation, S.C. and S.R.; formal analysis, M.R. and A.Z.; funding acquisition, S.C.; investigation, M.R., P.F., E.S. and S.R.; methodology, S.R.; resources, P.F.; software, M.R., S.C., A.Z. and E.S.; validation, E.S.; visualization, P.F., S.C. and A.Z.; writing—original draft, M.R. and S.C. All authors have read and agreed to the published version of the manuscript.

Funding: This research received no external funding.

Institutional Review Board Statement: Not applicable.

Informed Consent Statement: Not applicable.

Data Availability Statement: Data are available on request to the corresponding author.

Acknowledgments: The authors would like to thank. Francesca DE NARD for their valuable support during the design and writing of the present paper.

Conflicts of Interest: The authors declare no conflict of interest.

References

1. Morris, J.A.; Blount, R.E.; Smadel, J.E. Recovery of Cytopathogenic Agent from Chimpanzees with Coryza. *Proc. Soc. Exp. Biol. Med.* **1956**, *92*, 544–549. [CrossRef] [PubMed]
2. Azzari, C.; Baraldi, E.; Bonanni, P.; Bozzola, E.; Coscia, A.; Lanari, M.; Manzoni, P.; Mazzone, T.; Sandri, F.; Checcucci Lisi, G.; et al. Epidemiology and Prevention of Respiratory Syncytial Virus Infections in Children in Italy. *Ital. J. Pediatr.* **2021**, *47*, 198. [CrossRef] [PubMed]
3. Pellegrinelli, L.; Galli, C.; Bubba, L.; Cereda, D.; Anselmi, G.; Binda, S.; Gramegna, M.; Pariani, E. Respiratory Syncytial Virus in Influenza-like Illness Cases: Epidemiology and Molecular Analyses of Four Consecutive Winter Seasons (2014–2015/2017–2018) in Lombardy (Northern Italy). *J. Med. Virol.* **2020**, *92*, 2999–3006. [CrossRef]
4. Shi, T.; Denouel, A.; Tietjen, A.K.; Campbell, I.; Moran, E.; Li, X.; Campbell, H.; Demont, C.; Nyawanda, B.O.; Chu, H.Y.; et al. Global Disease Burden Estimates of Respiratory Syncytial Virus-Associated Acute Respiratory Infection in Older Adults in 2015: A Systematic Review and Meta-Analysis. *J. Infect. Dis.* **2021**, *222*, S577–S583. [CrossRef]
5. Openshaw, P.J.M.; Chiu, C.; Culley, F.J.; Johansson, C. Protective and Harmful Immunity to RSV Infection. *Annu. Rev. Immunol.* **2017**, *35*, 501–532. [CrossRef] [PubMed]
6. Andeweg, S.P.; Schepp, R.M.; van de Kasteele, J.; Mollema, L.; Berbers, G.A.M.; van Boven, M. Population-Based Serology Reveals Risk Factors for RSV Infection in Children Younger than 5 Years. *Sci. Rep.* **2021**, *11*, 8953. [CrossRef] [PubMed]
7. Mazur, N.I.; Martinón-Torres, F.; Baraldi, E.; Fauroux, B.; Greenough, A.; Heikkinen, T.; Manzoni, P.; Mejias, A.; Nair, H.; Papadopoulos, N.G.; et al. Lower Respiratory Tract Infection Caused by Respiratory Syncytial Virus: Current Management and New Therapeutics. *Lancet Respir. Med.* **2015**, *3*, 888–900. [CrossRef]
8. Nair, H.; Theodoratou, E.; Rudan, I.; Nokes, D.J.; Ngama HND, M.; Munywoki, P.K.; Dherani, M.; Nair, H.; James Nokes, D.; Gessner, B.D.; et al. Global Burden of Acute Lower Respiratory Infections Due to Respiratory Syncytial Virus in Young Children: A Systematic Review and Meta-Analysis. *Lancet* **2010**, *375*, 1545–1555. [CrossRef]
9. Leader, S.; Kohlhase, K. Respiratory Syncytial Virus-Coded Pediatric Hospitalizations, 1997 to 1999. *Pediatr. Infect. Dis. J.* **2002**, *21*, 629–661. [CrossRef]
10. Leader, S.; Kohlhase, K.; Pearlman, M.H.; Williams, J.V.; Engle, W.A. Recent Trends in Severe Respiratory Syncytial Virus (RSV) among US Infants, 1997 to 2000. *J. Pediatr.* **2003**, *143*, S127–S132. [CrossRef]
11. Palmer, L.; Hall, C.B.; Katkin, J.P.; Shi, N.; Masaquel, A.S.; McLaurin, K.K.; Mahadevia, P.J. Healthcare Costs within a Year of Respiratory Syncytial Virus among Medicaid Infants. *Pediatr. Pulmonol.* **2010**, *45*, 772–781. [CrossRef] [PubMed]
12. Shi, T.; McAllister, D.A.; O'Brien, K.L.; Simoes, E.A.F.; Madhi, S.A.; Gessner, B.D.; Polack, F.P.; Balsells, E.; Acacio, S.; Aguayo, C.; et al. Global, Regional, and National Disease Burden Estimates of Acute Lower Respiratory Infections Due to Respiratory Syncytial Virus in Young Children in 2015: A Systematic Review and Modelling Study. *Lancet* **2017**, *390*, 946–958. [CrossRef]
13. Falsey, A.R.; Hennessey, P.A.; Formica, M.A.; Cox, C.; Walsh, E.E. Respiratory syncytial virus infection in elderly and high-risk adults. *N. Engl. J. Med.* **2005**, *352*, 1749–1759. [CrossRef]

14. Shi, T.; Arnott, A.; Semogas, I.; Falsey, A.R.; Openshaw, P.; Wedzicha, J.A.; Campbell, H.; Nair, H. The Etiological Role of Common Respiratory Viruses in Acute Respiratory Infections in Older Adults: A Systematic Review and Meta-Analysis. *J. Infect. Dis.* **2020**, *222*, S563–S569. [CrossRef] [PubMed]
15. Mosalli, R.; Alqarni, S.A.; Khayyat, W.W.; Alsaidi, S.T.; Almatrafi, A.S.; Bawakid, A.S.; Paes, B. Respiratory Syncytial Virus Nosocomial Outbreak in Neonatal Intensive Care: A Review of the Incidence, Management, and Outcomes. *Am. J. Infect. Control*, 2021; *epub ahead of print*. [CrossRef]
16. Nourbakhsh, S.; Shoukat, A.; Zhang, K.; Poliquin, G.; Halperin, D.; Sheffield, H.; Halperin, S.A.; Langley, J.M.; Moghadas, S.M. Effectiveness and Cost-Effectiveness of RSV Infant and Maternal Immunization Programs: A Case Study of Nunavik, Canada. *EClinicalMedicine* **2021**, *41*, 101141. [CrossRef]
17. Paes, B.A.; Frcpc, M.; Mitchell, I.; Mb Frcpc, M.A.; Banerji, A.; Mph, M.D.; Lanctôt, K.L.; Langley, J.M.; Bosco, D.; Paes, A. A decade of respiratory syncytial virus epidemiology and prophylaxis: Translating evidence into everyday clinical practice case presentation. *Can. Respir. J.* **2011**, *18*, e10–e19. [CrossRef] [PubMed]
18. Arriola, C.S.; Kim, L.; Langley, G.; Anderson, E.J.; Openo, K.; Martin, A.M.; Lynfield, R.; Bye, E.; Como-Sabetti, K.; Reingold, A.; et al. Estimated Burden of Community-Onset Respiratory Syncytial Virus-Associated Hospitalizations among Children Aged < 2 Years in the United States, 2014–2015. *J. Pediatr. Infect. Dis. Soc.* **2020**, *9*, 587–595. [CrossRef]
19. Griffiths, C.; Drews, S.J.; Marchant, D.J. Respiratory Syncytial Virus: Infection, Detection, and New Options for Prevention and Treatment. *Clin. Microbiol. Rev.* **2017**, *30*, 277–319. [CrossRef]
20. Mitchell, I.; Li, A.; Bjornson, C.L.; Lanctot, K.L.; Paes, B.A. Respiratory Syncytial Virus Immunoprophylaxis with Palivizumab: 12-Year Observational Study of Usage and Outcomes in Canada. *Am. J. Perinatol.* 2021, *online ahead of print*. [CrossRef]
21. Viguria, N.; Navascués, A.; Juanbeltz, R.; Echeverría, A.; Ezpeleta, C.; Castilla, J. Effectiveness of Palivizumab in Preventing Respiratory Syncytial Virus Infection in High-Risk Children. *Hum. Vaccines Immunother.* **2021**, *17*, 1867–1872. [CrossRef]
22. Chida-Nagai, A.; Sato, H.; Sato, I.; Shiraishi, M.; Sasaki, D.; Izumi, G.; Yamazawa, H.; Cho, K.; Manabe, A.; Takeda, A. Risk Factors for Hospitalisation Due to Respiratory Syncytial Virus Infection in Children Receiving Prophylactic Palivizumab. *Eur. J. Pediatr.* **2022**, *181*, 539–547. [CrossRef]
23. Zylbersztejn, A.; Almossawi, O.; Gudka, N.; Tompsett, D.; de Stavola, B.; Standing, J.F.; Smyth, R.; Hardelid, P. Access to Palivizumab among Children at High Risk of Respiratory Syncytial Virus Complications in English Hospitals. *Br. J. Clin. Pharmacol.* **2022**, *88*, 1246–1257. [CrossRef]
24. Batista, J.D.L.; Ferreira, M.A.P.; Xavier, C.D.S.; de Souza, I.T.A.; Cruz, L.N.; Polanczyk, C.A. A Post-Incorporation Study on the Use of Palivizumab in the Brazilian Public Health System. *Rev. Inst. Med. Trop. Sao Paulo* **2021**, *63*, 1–8. [CrossRef] [PubMed]
25. Hampp, C.; Kauf, T.L.; Saidi, A.S.; Winterstein, A.G. Cost-Effectiveness of Respiratory Syncytial Virus Prophylaxis in Various Indications. *Arch. Pediatr. Adolesc. Med.* **2011**, *165*, 498–505. [CrossRef] [PubMed]
26. Griffin, M.P.; Yuan, Y.; Takas, T.; Domachowske, J.B.; Madhi, S.A.; Manzoni, P.; Simões, E.A.F.; Esser, M.T.; Khan, A.A.; Dubovsky, F.; et al. Single-Dose Nirsevimab for Prevention of RSV in Preterm Infants. *N. Engl. J. Med.* **2020**, *383*, 415–425. [CrossRef] [PubMed]
27. Hammitt, L.L.; Dagan, R.; Yuan, Y.; Baca Cots, M.; Bosheva, M.; Madhi, S.A.; Muller, W.J.; Zar, H.J.; Brooks, D.; Grenham, A.; et al. Nirsevimab for Prevention of RSV in Healthy Late-Preterm and Term Infants. *N. Engl. J. Med.* **2022**, *386*, 837–846. [CrossRef] [PubMed]
28. Domachowske, J.; Madhi, S.A.; Simões, E.A.F.; Atanasova, V.; Cabañas, F.; Furuno, K.; Garcia-Garcia, M.L.; Grantina, I.; Nguyen, K.A.; Brooks, D.; et al. Safety of Nirsevimab for RSV in Infants with Heart or Lung Disease or Prematurity. *N. Engl. J. Med.* **2022**, *386*, 892–894. [CrossRef] [PubMed]
29. Voirin, N.; Virlogeux, V.; Demont, C.; Kieffer, A. Potential Impact of Nirsevimab on RSV Transmission and Medically Attended Lower Respiratory Tract Illness Caused by RSV: A Disease Transmission Model. *Infect. Dis. Ther.* **2021**, *11*, 277–292. [CrossRef]
30. Debes, S.; Haug, J.B.; de Blasio, B.F.; Jonassen, C.M.; Dudman, S.G. Etiology of Viral Respiratory Tract Infections in Hospitalized Adults, and Evidence of the High Frequency of Prehospitalization Antibiotic Treatment in Norway. *Health Sci. Rep.* **2021**, *4*, e403. [CrossRef]
31. Obolski, U.; Kassem, E.; Na'amnih, W.; Tannous, S.; Kagan, V.; Muhsen, K. Unnecessary Antibiotic Treatment of Children Hospitalized with RSV-Bronchiolitis: Risk Factors and Prescription Patterns. *J. Glob. Antimicrob. Resist.* **2021**, *27*, 303–308. [CrossRef]
32. Madhi, S.A.; Polack, F.P.; Piedra, P.A.; Munoz, F.M.; Trenholme, A.A.; Simões, E.A.F.; Swamy, G.K.; Agrawal, S.; Ahmed, K.; August, A.; et al. Respiratory Syncytial Virus Vaccination during Pregnancy and Effects in Infants. *N. Engl. J. Med.* **2020**, *383*, 426–439. [CrossRef]
33. Phijffer, E.W.E.M.; Bont, L.J. Are We Ready for Maternal Respiratory Syncytial Virus Vaccination? *J. Infect. Dis.* **2021**, jiab613. [CrossRef] [PubMed]
34. Walsh, E.E.; Falsey, A.R.; Scott, D.A.; Gurtman, A.; Zareba, A.M.; Jansen, K.U.; Gruber, W.C.; Dormitzer, P.R.; Swanson, K.A.; Radley, D.; et al. A Randomized Phase 1/2 Study of a Respiratory Syncytial Virus Prefusion F Vaccine. *J. Infect. Dis.* **2021**. [CrossRef] [PubMed]
35. Scheltema, N.M.; Kavelaars, X.M.; Thorburn, K.; Hennus, M.P.; van Woensel, J.B.; van der Ent, C.K.; Borghans, J.A.M.; Bont, L.J.; Drylewicz, J. Potential Impact of Maternal Vaccination on Life-Threatening Respiratory Syncytial Virus Infection during Infancy. *Vaccine* **2018**, *36*, 4693–4700. [CrossRef]

36. Buchwald, A.G.; Graham, B.S.; Traore, A.; Haidara, F.C.; Chen, M.; Morabito, K.; Lin, B.C.; Sow, S.O.; Levine, M.M.; Pasetti, M.F.; et al. Respiratory Syncytial Virus (RSV) Neutralizing Antibodies at Birth Predict Protection from RSV Illness in Infants in the First 3 Months of Life. *Clin. Infect. Dis.* **2021**, *73*, e4421–e4427. [CrossRef] [PubMed]
37. Walsh, E.E.; Wang, L.; Falsey, A.R.; Qiu, X.; Corbett, A.; Holden-Wiltse, J.; Mariani, T.J.; Topham, D.J.; Caserta, M.T. Virus-Specific Antibody, Viral Load, and Disease Severity in Respiratory Syncytial Virus Infection. *J. Infect. Dis.* **2018**, *218*, 208–217. [CrossRef]
38. Groothuis, J.R.; Simoes, E.A.; Levin, M.J.; Hall, C.B.; Long, C.E.; Rodriguez, W.J.; Arrobio, J.; Meissner, H.C.; Fulton, D.R.; Welliver, R.C.; et al. Prophylactic Administration of Respiratory Syncytial Virus Immune Globulin to High-Risk Infants and Young Children. *N. Eng. J. Med.* **1993**, *329*, 1524–1530. [CrossRef]
39. Glezen, P.W.; Paredes, A.; Allison, J.E.; Taber, L.H.; Frank, A.L. Risk of Respiratory Syncytial Virus Infection for Infants from Low-Income Families in Relationship to Age, Sex, Ethnic Group, and Maternal Antibody Level. *J. Pediatr.* **1981**, *98*, 708–715. [CrossRef]
40. Amirthalingam, G.; Andrews, N.; Campbell, H.; Ribeiro, S.; Kara, E.; Donegan, K.; Fry, N.K.; Miller, E.; Ramsay, M. Effectiveness of Maternal Pertussis Vaccination in England: An Observational Study. *Lancet* **2014**, *384*, 1521–1528. [CrossRef]
41. Gkentzi, D.; Katsakiori, P.; Marangos, M.; Hsia, Y.; Amirthalingam, G.; Heath, P.T.; Ladhani, S. Maternal Vaccination against Pertussis: A Systematic Review of the Recent Literature. *Arch. Dis. Child. Fetal Neonatal Ed.* **2017**, *102*, F456–F463. [CrossRef]
42. Fell, D.B.; Bhutta, Z.A.; Hutcheon, J.A.; Karron, R.A.; Knight, M.; Kramer, M.S.; Monto, A.S.; Swamy, G.K.; Ortiz, J.R.; Savitz, D.A. Report of the WHO Technical Consultation on the Effect of Maternal Influenza and Influenza Vaccination on the Developing Fetus: Montreal, Canada, September 30–October 1, 2015. *Vaccine* **2017**, *35*, 2279–2287. [CrossRef]
43. Buchy, P.; Badur, S.; Kassianos, G.; Preiss, S.; Tam, J.S. Vaccinating Pregnant Women against Influenza Needs to Be a Priority for All Countries: An Expert Commentary. *Int. J. Infect. Dis.* **2020**, *92*, 1–12. [CrossRef] [PubMed]
44. Gunatilaka, A.; Giles, M.L. Maternal RSV Vaccine Development. Where to from Here? *Hum. Vaccines Immunother.* **2021**, *17*, 4542–4548. [CrossRef] [PubMed]
45. Wheeler, S.M.; Dotters-Katz, S.; Heine, R.P.; Grotegut, C.A.; Swamy, G.K. Maternal Effects of Respiratory Syncytial Virus Infection during Pregnancy. *Emerg. Infect. Dis.* **2015**, *21*, 1951–1955. [CrossRef] [PubMed]
46. Hause, A.M.; Panagiotakopoulos, L.; Weintraub, E.S.; Sy, L.S.; Glenn, S.C.; Tseng, H.F.; McNeil, M.M. Adverse Outcomes in Pregnant Women Hospitalized with Respiratory Syncytial Virus Infection: A Case Series. *Clin. Infect. Dis.* **2021**, *72*, 138–140. [CrossRef]
47. Regan, A.K.; Klein, N.P.; Langley, G.; Drews, S.J.; Buchan, S.; Ball, S.; Kwong, J.C.; Naleway, A.; Thompson, M.; Wyant, B.E.; et al. Respiratory Syncytial Virus Hospitalization during Pregnancy in 4 High-Income Countries, 2010–2016. *Clin. Infect. Dis.* **2018**, *67*, 1915–1918. [CrossRef]
48. Manti, S.; Leonardi, S.; Rezaee, F.; Harford, T.; Perez, M.K.; Piedimonte, G.; Nunes, M.C. Effects of Vertical Transmission of Respiratory Viruses to the Offspring. *Front. Immunol.* **2022**, *13*, 853009. [CrossRef]
49. ClinicalTrials.gov. *A Trial to Evaluate the Efficacy and Safety of RSVpreF in Infants Born to Women Vaccinated During Pregnancy*; The United States National Library of Medicine: Bethesda, MD, USA, 2022.
50. ClinicalTrials.gov. *A Phase III Double-Blind Study to Assess Safety and Efficacy of an RSV Maternal Unadjuvanted Vaccine, in Pregnant Women and Infants Born to Vaccinated Mothers (GRACE)*; The United States National Library of Medicine: Bethesda, MD, USA, 2022.
51. Chaw, L.; Kamigaki, T.; Burmaa, A.; Urtnasan, C.; Od, I.; Nyamaa, G.; Nymadawa, P.; Oshitani, H. Burden of Influenza and Respiratory Syncytial Virus Infection in Pregnant Women and Infants under 6 Months in Mongolia: A Prospective Cohort Study. *PLoS ONE* **2016**, *11*, e0148421. [CrossRef]
52. Chu, H.Y.; Katz, J.; Tielsch, J.; Khatry, S.K.; Shrestha, L.; LeClerq, S.C.; Magaret, A.; Kuypers, J.; Steinhoff, M.C.; Englund, J.A. Clinical Presentation and Birth Outcomes Associated with Respiratory Syncytial Virus Infection in Pregnancy. *PLoS ONE* **2016**, *11*, e0152015. [CrossRef]
53. Hause, A.M.; Avadhanula, V.; Maccato, M.L.; Pinell, P.M.; Bond, N.; Santarcangelo, P.; Ferlic-Stark, L.; Ye, X.; Iwuchukwu, O.; Maurer, L.; et al. Clinical Characteristics and Outcomes of Respiratory Syncytial Virus Infection in Pregnant Women. *Vaccine* **2019**, *37*, 3464–3471. [CrossRef]
54. Madhi, S.A.; Cutland, C.L.; Downs, S.; Jones, S.; van Niekerk, N.; Simoes, E.A.F.; Nunes, M.C. Burden of Respiratory Syncytial Virus Infection in South African Human Immunodeficiency Virus (HIV)-Infected and HIV-Uninfected Pregnant and Postpartum Women: A Longitudinal Cohort Study. *Clin. Infect. Dis.* **2018**, *66*, 1658–1665. [CrossRef]
55. Hurley, L.P.; Allison, M.A.; Kim, L.; O'Leary, S.T.; Crane, L.A.; Brtnikova, M.; Beaty, B.L.; Allen, K.E.; Poser, S.; Lindley, M.C.; et al. Primary Care Physicians' Perspectives on Respiratory Syncytial Virus (RSV) Disease in Adults and a Potential RSV Vaccine for Adults. *Vaccine* **2019**, *37*, 565–570. [CrossRef] [PubMed]
56. Hall, C.B.; Long, C.E.; Schnabel, K.C. Respiratory Syncytial Virus Infections in Previously Healthy Working Adults. *Clin. Infect. Dis.* **2001**, *33*, 792–796. [CrossRef] [PubMed]
57. Pastula, S.T.; Hackett, J.; Coalson, J.; Jiang, X.; Villafana, T.; Ambrose, C.; Fryzek, J. Hospitalizations for Respiratory Syncytial Virus Among Adults in the United States, 1997–2012. *Open Forum Infect. Dis.* **2017**, *4*, ofw270. [CrossRef] [PubMed]
58. Choi, Y.; Hill-Ricciuti, A.; Branche, A.R.; Sieling, W.D.; Saiman, L.; Walsh, E.E.; Phillips, M.; Falsey, A.R.; Finelli, L. Cost Determinants among Adults Hospitalized with Respiratory Syncytial Virus in the United States, 2017–2019. *Influenza Other Respir. Viruses* **2021**, *16*, 151–158. [CrossRef] [PubMed]

59. Hause, A.M.; Avadhanula, V.; Maccato, M.L.; Pinell, P.M.; Bond, N.; Santarcangelo, P.; Ferlic-Stark, L.; Munoz, F.M.; Piedra, P.A. A Cross-Sectional Surveillance Study of the Frequency and Etiology of Acute Respiratory Illness Among Pregnant Women. *J. Infect. Dis.* **2018**, *218*, 528–535. [CrossRef]
60. Li, X.; Bilcke, J.; Vázquez Fernández, L.; Bont, L.; Willem, L.; Wisløff, T.; Jit, M.; Beutels, P.; Beutels, P.; Bont, L.; et al. Cost-Effectiveness of Respiratory Syncytial Virus Disease Prevention Strategies: Maternal Vaccine Versus Seasonal or Year-Round Monoclonal Antibody Program in Norwegian Children. *J. Infect. Dis.* **2022**, jiac064. [CrossRef]
61. Hodgson, D.; Pebody, R.; Panovska-Griffiths, J.; Baguelin, M.; Atkins, K.E. Evaluating the next Generation of RSV Intervention Strategies: A Mathematical Modelling Study and Cost-Effectiveness Analysis. *BMC Med.* **2020**, *18*, 348. [CrossRef]
62. Laufer, R.S.; Driscoll, A.J.; Baral, R.; Buchwald, A.G.; Campbell, J.D.; Coulibaly, F.; Diallo, F.; Doumbia, M.; Galvani, A.P.; Haidara, F.C.; et al. Cost-Effectiveness of Infant Respiratory Syncytial Virus Preventive Interventions in Mali: A Modeling Study to Inform Policy and Investment Decisions. *Vaccine* **2021**, *39*, 5037–5045. [CrossRef]
63. Sperling, R.S.; Riley, L.E. Immunization and Emerging Infections Expert Work Group Influenza Vaccination, Pregnancy Safety, and Risk of Early Pregnancy Loss. *Obstet. Gynecol.* **2018**, *131*, 799–802. [CrossRef]
64. Fell, D.B.; Azziz-Baumgartner, E.; Baker, M.G.; Batra, M.; Beauté, J.; Beutels, P.; Bhat, N.; Bhutta, Z.A.; Cohen, C.; de Mucio, B.; et al. Influenza Epidemiology and Immunization during Pregnancy: Final Report of a World Health Organization Working Group. *Vaccine* **2017**, *35*, 5738–5750. [CrossRef]
65. Karlsson, E.A.; Marcelin, G.; Webby, R.J.; Schultz-Cherry, S. Review on the Impact of Pregnancy and Obesity on Influenza Virus Infection. *Influenza Other Respir. Viruses* **2012**, *6*, 449–460. [CrossRef] [PubMed]
66. Riccò, M.; Vezzosi, L.; Gualerzi, G.; Balzarini, F.; Capozzi, V.A.; Volpi, L. Knowledge, Attitudes, Beliefs and Practices of Obstetrics-Gynecologists on Seasonal Influenza and Pertussis Immunizations in Pregnant Women: Preliminary Results from North-Western Italy. *Minerva Ginecol.* **2019**, *71*, 288–297. [CrossRef] [PubMed]
67. Riccò, M.; Ferraro, P.; Peruzzi, S.; Zaniboni, A.; Ranzieri, S. Respiratory Syncytial Virus: Knowledge, Attitudes and Beliefs of General Practitioners from North-Eastern Italy (2021). *Pediatr. Rep.* **2022**, *14*, 147–165. [CrossRef] [PubMed]
68. Giles, M.L.; Buttery, J.; Davey, M.A.; Wallace, E. Pregnant Women's Knowledge and Attitude to Maternal Vaccination Including Group B Streptococcus and Respiratory Syncytial Virus Vaccines. *Vaccine* **2019**, *37*, 6743–6749. [CrossRef] [PubMed]
69. Wilcox, C.R.; Calvert, A.; Metz, J.; Kilich, E.; Macleod, R.; Beadon, K.; Heath, P.T.; Khalil, A.; Finn, A.; Snape, M.D.; et al. Attitudes of Pregnant Women and Healthcare Professionals Toward Clinical Trials and Routine Implementation of Antenatal Vaccination Against Respiratory Syncytial Virus: A Multicenter Questionnaire Study. *Pediatr. Infect. Dis. J.* **2019**, *38*, 944–951. [CrossRef] [PubMed]
70. Auvinen, R.; Syrjänen, R.; Ollgren, J.; Nohynek, H.; Skogberg, K. Clinical Characteristics and Population-Based Attack Rates of Respiratory Syncytial Virus versus Influenza Hospitalizations among Adults—An Observational Study. *Influenza Other Respir. Viruses* **2021**, online ahead of print. [CrossRef]
71. Rose, E.B.; Wheatley, A.; Langley, G.; Gerber, S.; Haynes, A. Amber Morbidity and Mortality Weekly Report Respiratory Syncytial Virus Seasonality-United States, 2014–2017. *Morb. Mortal. Wkly. Rep.* **2018**, *67*, 71–76. [CrossRef]
72. Janet, S.; Broad, J.; Snape, M.D. Respiratory Syncytial Virus Seasonality and Its Implications on Prevention Strategies. *Hum. Vaccines Immunother.* **2018**, *14*, 234–244. [CrossRef]
73. Yassine, H.M.; Sohail, M.U.; Younes, N.; Nasrallah, G.K. Systematic Review of the Respiratory Syncytial Virus (RSV) Prevalence, Genotype Distribution, and Seasonality in Children from the Middle East and North Africa (MENA) Region. *Microorganisms* **2020**, *8*, 713. [CrossRef]
74. Barbati, F.; Moriondo, M.; Pisano, L.; Calistri, E.; Lodi, L.; Ricci, S.; Giovannini, M.; Canessa, C.; Indolfi, G.; Azzari, C. Epidemiology of Respiratory Syncytial Virus-Related Hospitalization over a 5-Year Period in Italy: Evaluation of Seasonality and Age Distribution before Vaccine Introduction. *Vaccines* **2020**, *8*, 15. [CrossRef]
75. Tramuto, F.; Maida, C.M.; di Naro, D.; Randazzo, G.; Vitale, F.; Restivo, V.; Costantino, C.; Amodio, E.; Casuccio, A.; Graziano, G.; et al. Respiratory Syncytial Virus: New Challenges for Molecular Epidemiology Surveillance and Vaccination Strategy in Patients with ILI/SARI. *Vaccines* **2021**, *9*, 1334. [CrossRef]
76. Atamna, A.; Babich, T.; Froimovici, D.; Yahav, D.; Sorek, N.; Ben-Zvi, H.; Leibovici, L.; Bishara, J.; Avni, T. Morbidity and Mortality of Respiratory Syncytial Virus Infection in Hospitalized Adults: Comparison with Seasonal Influenza. *Int. J. Infect. Dis.* **2021**, *103*, 489–493. [CrossRef] [PubMed]
77. Irving, W.L.; James, D.K.; Stephenson, T.; Laing, P.; Jameson, C.; Oxford, J.S.; Chakraverty, P.; Brown, D.W.; Coon, A.C.; Zambon, M.C. Influenza Virus Infection in the Second and Third Trimesters of Pregnancy a Clinical and Seroepidemiological Study. *BJOG Int. J. Obstet. Gynaecol.* **2000**, *107*, 1282–1289. [CrossRef] [PubMed]
78. Frieden, T.R.; Director Harold Jaffe, M.W.; Stephens, J.W.; Thacker, S.B.; Spriggs Terraye M Starr, S.R.; Doan, Q.M.; Phyllis King, M.H.; Roper, W.L.; Holtzman, D.; John Iglehart, G.K.; et al. Prevention and Control of Influenza with Vaccines Recommendations of the Advisory Committee on Immunization Practices (ACIP), 2010. *MMWR Morb. Mortal. Wkly. Rep.* **2009**, *59*, 1–62.
79. Dawood, F.S.; Kittikraisak, W.; Patel, A.; Rentz Hunt, D.; Suntarattiwong, P.; Wesley, M.G.; Thompson, M.G.; Soto, G.; Mundhada, S.; Arriola, C.S.; et al. Incidence of Influenza during Pregnancy and Association with Pregnancy and Perinatal Outcomes in Three Middle-Income Countries: A Multisite Prospective Longitudinal Cohort Study. *Lancet Infect. Dis.* **2021**, *21*, 97–106. [CrossRef]
80. Esterhuizen, T.M.; Thabane, L. Con: Meta-Analysis: Some Key Limitations and Potential Solutions. *Nephrol. Dial. Transplant.* **2016**, *31*, 882–885. [CrossRef]

81. Imrey, P.B. Limitations of Meta-Analyses of Studies with High Heterogeneity. *JAMA Netw. Open* **2020**, *3*, e1919325. [CrossRef]
82. Chu, H.Y.; Tielsch, J.; Katz, J.; Magaret, A.S.; Khatry, S.; LeClerq, S.C.; Shrestha, L.; Kuypers, J.; Steinhoff, M.C.; Englund, J.A. Transplacental Transfer of Maternal Respiratory Syncytial Virus (RSV) Antibody and Protection against RSV Disease in Infants in Rural Nepal. *J. Clin. Virol.* **2017**, *95*, 90–95. [CrossRef]
83. Calderaro, A.; de Conto, F.; Buttrini, M.; Piccolo, G.; Montecchini, S.; Maccari, C.; Martinelli, M.; di Maio, A.; Ferraglia, F.; Pinardi, F.; et al. Human Respiratory Viruses, Including SARS-CoV-2, Circulating in the Winter Season 2019–2020 in Parma, Northern Italy. *Int. J. Infect. Dis.* **2021**, *102*, 79–84. [CrossRef]
84. Sherman, A.C.; Babiker, A.; Sieben, A.J.; Pyden, A.; Steinberg, J.; Kraft, C.S.; Koelle, K.; Kanjilal, S. The Effect of Severe Acute Respiratory Syndrome Coronavirus 2 (SARS-CoV-2) Mitigation Strategies on Seasonal Respiratory Viruses: A Tale of 2 Large Metropolitan Centers in the United States. *Clin. Infect. Dis.* **2021**, *72*, E154–E157. [CrossRef]
85. Kuitunen, I.; Artama, M.; Mäkelä, L.; Backman, K.; Heiskanen-Kosma, T.; Renko, M. Effect of Social Distancing Due to the COVID-19 Pandemic on the Incidence of Viral Respiratory Tract Infections in Children in Finland during Early 2020. *Pediatr. Infect. Dis. J.* **2020**, *39*, E423–E427. [CrossRef]
86. van Brusselen, D.; de Troeyer, K.; ter Haar, E.; vander Auwera, A.; Poschet, K.; van Nuijs, S.; Bael, A.; Stobbelaar, K.; Verhulst, S.; van Herendael, B.; et al. Bronchiolitis in COVID-19 Times: A Nearly Absent Disease? *Eur. J. Pediatr.* **2021**, *180*, 1969–1973. [CrossRef] [PubMed]
87. Britton, P.N.; Hu, N.; Saravanos, G.; Shrapnel, J.; Davis, J.; Snelling, T.; Dalby-Payne, J.; Kesson, A.M.; Wood, N.; Macartney, K.; et al. COVID-19 Public Health Measures and Respiratory Syncytial Virus. *Lancet Child Adolesc. Health* **2020**, *4*, e42–e43. [CrossRef]
88. Hatter, L.; Eathorne, A.; Hills, T.; Bruce, P.; Beasley, R. Respiratory Syncytial Virus: Paying the Immunity Debt with Interest. *Lancet Child Adolesc. Health* **2021**, *5*, e44–e45. [CrossRef]
89. Foley, D.A.; Yeoh, D.K.; Minney-Smith, C.A.; Martin, A.C.; Mace, A.O.; Sikazwe, C.T.; Le, H.; Levy, A.; Moore, H.C.; Blyth, C.C. The Interseasonal Resurgence of Respiratory Syncytial Virus in Australian Children Following the Reduction of Coronavirus Disease 2019-Related Public Health Measures. *Clin. Infect. Dis.* **2021**, *73*, E2829–E2830. [CrossRef]
90. Foley, D.A.; Phuong, L.K.; Peplinski, J.; Lim, S.M.; Lee, W.H.; Farhat, A.; Minney-Smith, C.A.; Martin, A.C.; Mace, A.O.; Sikazwe, C.T.; et al. Examining the Interseasonal Resurgence of Respiratory Syncytial Virus in Western Australia. *Arch. Dis. Child.* **2021**, *107*, e1–e7. [CrossRef]
91. Varela, F.H.; Scotta, M.C.; Polese-Bonatto, M.; Sartor, I.T.S.; Ferreira, C.F.; Fernandes, I.R.; Zavaglia, G.O.; de Almeida, W.A.F.; Arakaki-Sanchez, D.; Pinto, L.A.; et al. Absence of Detection of RSV and Influenza during the COVID-19 Pandemic in a Brazilian Cohort: Likely Role of Lower Transmission in the Community. *J. Glob. Health* **2021**, *11*, 05007. [CrossRef]
92. Ippolito, G.; la Vecchia, A.; Umbrello, G.; di Pietro, G.; Bono, P.; Scalia, S.; Pinzani, R.; Tagliabue, C.; Bosis, S.; Agostoni, C.; et al. Disappearance of Seasonal Respiratory Viruses in Children Under Two Years Old During COVID-19 Pandemic: A Monocentric Retrospective Study in Milan, Italy. *Front. Pediatr.* **2021**, *9*, 721005. [CrossRef]
93. Ujiie, M.; Tsuzuki, S.; Nakamoto, T.; Iwamoto, N.; Ujiie, M. Resurgence of Respiratory Syncytial Virus Infections during Covid-19 Pandemic, Tokyo, Japan. *Emerg. Infect. Dis.* **2021**, *27*, 2969–2970. [CrossRef]
94. Moher, D.; Liberati, A.; Tetzlaff, J.; Altman, D.G.; Altman, D.; Antes, G.; Atkins, D.; Barbour, V.; Barrowman, N.; Berlin, J.A.; et al. Preferred Reporting Items for Systematic Reviews and Meta-Analyses: The PRISMA Statement. *PLoS Med.* **2009**, *6*, e1000097. [CrossRef]
95. *Handbook for Conducting a Literature-Based Health Assessment Using OHAT Approach for Systematic Review and Evidence Integration*; U.S. Department of Health and Human Services: Washington, DC, USA, 2019.
96. Eick, S.M.; Goin, D.E.; Chartres, N.; Lam, J.; Woodruff, T.J. Assessing Risk of Bias in Human Environmental Epidemiology Studies Using Three Tools: Different Conclusions from Different Tools. *Syst. Rev.* **2020**, *9*, 249. [CrossRef]

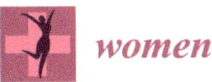

Protocol

Knowledge, Attitudes, Behavior, Acceptance, and Hesitancy in Relation to the COVID-19 Vaccine among Pregnant and Breastfeeding Women: A Systematic Review Protocol

Vincenza Gianfredi [1,*], Alessandro Berti [1], Marilena D'Amico [1], Viola De Lorenzo [1] and Silvana Castaldi [1,2]

1 Department of Biomedical Sciences for Health, University of Milan, Via Pascal, 36, 20133 Milan, Italy
2 Fondazione IRCCS Ca' Granda Ospedale Maggiore Policlinico, Via Francesco Sforza, 35, 20122 Milan, Italy
* Correspondence: vincenza.gianfredi@unimi.it

Abstract: A new coronavirus, SARS-CoV-2, was identified at the end of 2019. It swiftly spread all over the world, affecting more than 600 million people and causing over 6 million deaths worldwide. Different COVID-19 vaccines became available by the end of 2020. Healthcare workers and more vulnerable people (such as the elderly and those with comorbidities) were initially prioritized, followed by the entire population, including pregnant and breastfeeding women. Despite the safety and efficacy of COVID-19 vaccines, a certain level of skepticism was expressed, including among pregnant and breastfeeding women. There were several reasons for this reluctance, among them, fear of side-effects for both women and fetuses. Nevertheless, acceptance, as well as hesitancy, were time, country and vaccine specific. This review will collect available evidence assessing knowledge, attitudes, behaviour, practice and acceptance/hesitancy of pregnant/breastfeeding women in relation to the COVID-19 vaccination. The PubMed/MEDLINE, Scopus and EMBASE databases will be consulted. A predefined search strategy that combines both free text and MESH terms will be used. The systematic review will adhere to the PRISMA guidelines and the results will be reported in both narrative and summary tables. A meta-analysis will be conducted if data are available.

Keywords: pregnant women; lactating; breastfeeding; COVID-19 vaccine; acceptance

Citation: Gianfredi, V.; Berti, A.; D'Amico, M.; De Lorenzo, V.; Castaldi, S. Knowledge, Attitudes, Behavior, Acceptance, and Hesitancy in Relation to the COVID-19 Vaccine among Pregnant and Breastfeeding Women: A Systematic Review Protocol. *Women* **2023**, *3*, 73–81. https://doi.org/10.3390/women3010006

Academic Editors: Claudio Costantino and Maiorana Antonio

Received: 28 December 2022
Revised: 16 January 2023
Accepted: 16 January 2023
Published: 20 January 2023

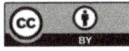

Copyright: © 2023 by the authors. Licensee MDPI, Basel, Switzerland. This article is an open access article distributed under the terms and conditions of the Creative Commons Attribution (CC BY) license (https://creativecommons.org/licenses/by/4.0/).

1. Introduction

Vaccine hesitancy is a complex phenomenon that is listed as one of the ten threats to global health by the World Health Organization (WHO) due to the consequent decrease in vaccination coverage [1]. Several definitions of vaccine hesitancy have been proposed. The WHO defines vaccine hesitancy as a delay in the acceptance or refusal of vaccines despite their availability. Dubè et al. considered vaccine hesitancy to comprise a spectrum, with active demand for vaccines or their complete refusal at the two ends and vaccine-hesitant individuals in between [2]. However, heterogeneities in attitudes/practices/knowledge exist, with some people refusing some vaccines but agreeing to take others, or some others delaying or accepting vaccines but being unsure to do so. In addition, Peretti-Watel et al. defined vaccine hesitancy as a complex decision-making process influenced by several contextual factors [3]. On this basis, in 2015, the Strategic Advisory Group of Experts on Immunization (SAGE) Working Group on vaccine hesitancy developed a theoretical model named the 3Cs to explain the complexity of vaccine hesitancy and its determinants [4]. The 3Cs refers to the three main factors: *complacency*, *convenience* and *confidence*. From 2015 to the present, the 3Cs model was revised based on the outcome of literature reviews and theoretical considerations [5]. The new 5Cs model is based on five psychological antecedents of vaccination: (1) *confidence* in the safety and efficacy of vaccines and trust in the system and providers that deliver them, (2) *complacency*, reflecting a low-perception of the risks linked to the vaccine-preventable disease and the consequent belief that the vaccination is not necessary; (3) *constraints*, physical and psychological barriers that cause vaccination to be perceived as inconvenient, threatening the conversion of vaccination intention into actual behavior; (4) *calculation*, the active effort in searching for information about risks and benefits of vaccination, though this commitment is not always associated with the ability to understand studies and data; and (5) *collective* responsibility, defined as "the willingness to protect others by one's own vaccination by means of herd immunity. The flipside is the willingness to have a free ride when a sufficient number of other people are vaccinated".

The 3C or 5C models provide a framework within which vaccine hesitancy/acceptance can be analyzed. In this respect, many studies have been conducted to date to better understand factors associated with vaccine hesitancy/acceptance. These factors include sociodemographic factors, such as ethnicity, age, sex, education, and employment; factors that depend on geographic or social context, such as accessibility and cost; the safety and efficacy of a new vaccine, lack of information or vaccine misinformation; and more personal factors, such as individual responsibility and risk perceptions and trust in health authorities and vaccines [6].

Among sociodemographic factors, pregnancy or breastfeeding represents a crucial period in which women seek information that will guide health decisions in relation to themselves and the unborn child. The safety of the unborn infant has been suggested to be the primary driver of decision-making during pregnancy [7]. In this context, exploring the knowledge, behavior and practice of vaccine acceptance/hesitancy among pregnant/breastfeeding women is important to plan counseling/education actions. This is particularly apposite considering the COVID-19 pandemic and the ensuing availability of new vaccines. A growing body of evidence suggests that COVID-19-related morbidity and mortality has been higher among pregnant women compared with age-matched non-pregnant individuals [8]. However, the novelty of the type of vaccines used, as well as the paucity of data about long-term effects (safety and efficacy) of the COVID-19 vaccine among the general population and pregnant/breastfeeding women, might impact on vaccination acceptance [9]. Emerging data from the Center for Disease Control and Prevention suggests that there has been no increase in side-effects or complications among pregnant women vaccinated against COVID-19 [10]. Considering data on the safety and efficacy of COVID-19 vaccines, public health programs have prioritized pregnant women as a high-risk group for COVID-19 infection and its complications. However, a certain level of vaccine hesitancy is commonly observed among pregnant women [11]. Moreover, pregnancy represents a time during which women, and the related family, are looking for information that can guide their own health choices and those of the unborn child [12]. Considering the above, the novelty of the COVID-19 vaccines, and recognising that vaccine hesitancy is vaccine-specific and depends on the socio-cultural background, we designed a systematic review and meta-analysis protocol with the purpose of better understanding the mechanisms underlying COVID-19 vaccine hesitancy among pregnant/breastfeeding women. Specifically, we aimed to assess the knowledge, beliefs, attitudes, barriers and facilitators relating to acceptance/refusal of the COVID-19 vaccine. Understanding the mechanisms underlying vaccination hesitancy is key to the design, testing and implementation of interventions that can improve vaccine acceptance and coverage in routine and outbreak settings.

2. Experimental Design

This systematic review protocol was developed based on The Preferred Reporting Items for Systematic Reviews and Meta-Analyses 2015 guidelines, as extended for systematic review protocols (PRISMA-P) [13]. The review protocol was developed, shared among the authors, and submitted to the journal in advance, prior to commencing the review. The review will be conducted in accordance with the Cochrane Collaboration [14] and the results will be reported based on the PRISMA 2020 guidelines [15]. Moreover, if the necessary data are available, we will proceed with statistical pooling and a meta-analysis will be performed. The latter will be carried out and documented in accordance with the Meta-analysis Of Observational Studies in Epidemiology (MOOSE) guidelines [16].

Research Question

The purpose of the systematic review (potentially with meta-analysis) is to answer the following questions: (1) What is the level of knowledge regarding COVID-19 vaccination among pregnant/breastfeeding women? (2) What are the facilitating/barrier factors associated with pregnant/breast-feeding women's acceptance/hesitancy to receive COVID-19 vaccine?

3. Materials and Equipment

3.1. Information Sources

A comprehensive, structured electronic search will be developed based on the research questions and conducted by checking three different scientific databases: PubMed/MEDLINE, Excerpta Medica Database (EMBASE) and Scopus. The electronic search will be conducted in the three databases during the same day by two different authors. If any discrepancy in records identification occurs between the two authors, it will be solved through discussion with a third (senior author) involved in retracing all the steps taken and checking for errors. The literature search will be supplemented by a review of the reference lists of included articles and, if available, by screening the reference lists of relevant similar reviews published previously in international scientific journals, consistent with previous research [17]. In addition, experts in the field will be contacted to potentially retrieve any additional relevant articles, as previously performed [18].

3.2. Search Strategy

A comprehensive and specific search strategy will be developed, combining medical subject headings (MeSH) and free text words. The search strategy will be defined according to the population, exposure, and outcome (PEO), as suggested by the Cochrane Collaboration [14]. We will first develop a search strategy for PubMed/MEDLINE. Then keywords and search terms will be adapted for use in the other two bibliographic databases. The Boolean operators AND and OR will be appropriately and logically combined in order to build the search strategy. The search strategy will be based on the following terms: (P) pregnant and breast-feeding women (and synonyms); (E) COVID-19 vaccination (and synonyms); and (O) knowledge, attitude, and practice (including factors associated with acceptance/hesitancy) regarding the COVID-19 vaccination (and synonyms). The specific search strategy will initially be created by a health specialist with extensive experience in conducting systematic reviews. Susequently, the search strategy will be adjusted based on input from the project team. The search strategy for PubMed/MEDLINE that will be adopted in the review is reported in Table 1.

Table 1. Search strategy developed in PubMed/MEDLINE.

Dataset	Search Strategy
PubMed/MEDLINE	"Breast Feeding"[Title/Abstract] OR "Pregnant Women"[Title/Abstract] OR "Maternal Behavior"[Title/Abstract] OR "Breast Feeding"[MeSH Terms] OR "Pregnant Women"[MeSH Terms] OR "Maternal Behavior"[MeSH Terms] OR "Postpartum Period"[MeSH Terms] OR "lactating"[Title/Abstract] AND ("attitude"[Title/Abstract] OR "knowledge"[Title/Abstract] OR OR "attitudes"[Title/Abstract] OR "behaviour"[Title/Abstract] OR "hesitancy"[Title/Abstract] OR "acceptance"[Title/Abstract] OR "barrier"[Title/Abstract] OR "barriers"[Title/Abstract] OR "behavior"[Title/Abstract] OR "behaviors"[Title/Abstract] OR "behaviour"[Title/Abstract] OR "behaviours"[Title/Abstract] OR "literacy"[Title/Abstract] OR "willingness"[Title/Abstract] OR "fear"[Title/Abstract] OR "facilitator"[Title/Abstract] OR "facilitators"[Title/Abstract] OR "determinant"[Title/Abstract] OR "determinants"[Title/Abstract]) AND ("COVID-19 Vaccines"[MeSH Terms] OR "2019-nCoV Vaccine mRNA-1273"[MeSH Terms] OR "BNT162 Vaccine"[MeSH Terms] OR "COVID-19 Vaccine"[Title/Abstract] OR "COVID-19 Vaccination"[Title/Abstract] OR "COVID-19 Vaccines"[Title/Abstract] OR "COVID-19 Vaccinations"[Title/Abstract] OR "Coronavirus Vaccine"[Title/Abstract] OR "Coronavirus Vaccines"[Title/Abstract])

4. Detailed Procedure

4.1. Inclusion/Exclusion Criteria

Studies will be selected based on the inclusion/exclusion criteria described below, defined according to the PEO strategy, along with additional information related to the study design, language, and time-span. Original population-based observational studies assessing the knowledge, attitudes and practice of pregnant or breastfeeding women in taking/refusing COVID-19 vaccination will be included in the review. By observational studies is implied all cross-sectional, case-control or cohort (prospective and retrospective) studies. Only English language, peer-reviewed articles published in international scientific journals will be considered. All articles published between 2019 and the date of the review's conclusion will be considered eligible for inclusion. The systematic review's exclusion criteria include the following: studies not performed among humans or that were conducted on a different population (for instance, the general public, women in general, parents or only mothers of children older than one year, and children's caregivers in general); studies combining data with different and multiple outcomes, or assessing different outcomes not listed in our inclusion criteria (for instance, articles assessing the efficacy, serology, immunology, safety, and development of the COVID-19 vaccine in pregnant or breastfeeding women); articles assessing acceptance/hesitancy/refusal against vaccines other than COVID-19; articles not written in the English language and those not published in peer-reviewed international journals; non-observational studies, e.g., trials (randomized or non-randomized controlled trials); and, lastly, non-original research papers, including reviews or meta-analyses, articles with no quantitative information or details, and non-full-text papers (e.g., letters to the editor, conference papers, commentary notes, expert opinions, abstracts). There will be no restrictions based on the type of setting, such as community-based or hospital-based populations.

4.2. Selection Process

All the retrieved studies will subsequently be downloaded to the EndNote software (EndNote® for Microsoft, Redmond, WA, USA, 2020). Duplicates will be removed using an automatic function in the EndNote software, followed by a manual check by one of the authors. The remaining articles will then be assessed for eligibility, firstly based on the title and abstract, followed by their full text. Two authors will independently undertake the two-step screening process by applying the inclusion/exclusion criteria detailed above. If any doubt or disagreement should arise during the two screening steps, this will be solved through a direct comparison between the views of the two authors. If divergences still persist, a final arbitrator will settle any disagreements over inclusion. Reviewer authors will be blind to the journal title, authors, and their institutions/affiliations. However, to increase agreement between the two reviewer authors, a pilot assessment will be conducted on 20 randomly selected retrieved articles [19]. Repeated articles and multiple publications from the same study will be excluded and all the reasons for exclusion will be reported. The results of the selection process will be detailed at each stage and reported using the PRISMA flow diagram.

4.3. Data Extraction

The data extraction process will be performed in duplicate by two reviewer authors. A standardized and pre-defined Excel (Microsoft Excel® for Microsoft 365 MSO, USA, 2019) spreadsheet will be used to extract data from the included studies [20]. The spreadsheet will initially be piloted on one-third (or no more than five, depending on the total number) of included articles to increase consistency between the two reviewer authors [21]. The following information will be extracted from each article included: author name, study period, country where the study was conducted, study settings, main characteristics and the study population's number, study completion rates (attrition), tool(s) used to assess the outcomes, number of items, whether the tool(s) was/were validated or not, manner in which the questionnaire was administered, recruitment methods, outcomes of interest, outcomes definition, main results, and funds and conflicts of interests, if any. Vaccine coverage will also be recorded, if available.

Nevertheless, recognising that outcomes of interest are composite measures, we will extract data directly as reported in the original articles even if unvalidated instruments are used to assess the outcomes. Furthermore, despite a general consensus on the definition of vaccine hesitancy/acceptance, no unequivocal tool or operationalization method is in place to evaluate it [22]. Rather, several instruments and statistical methods are commonly used. In light of this, we anticipate substantial variation in the methods used to report results. For this reason, when available, we will also extract methodological information, such as whether the tool was validated or not and the statistical analysis undertaken. Lastly, if studies report data using risk estimates, for instance, odds ratio (OR), risk ratio (RR) or hazard ratio (HR), we will collect the maximally adjusted data, along with the list of variables used for the adjustment [23].

The data collected will support the assessment of the study quality and will be used for data synthesis.

4.4. Quality Assessment

The risk of bias of the included studies will be independently assessed by two reviewers. Disagreements between the reviewers will be discussed and resolved by consensus. However, insights from a third reviewer will be sought if necessary. The Joanna Briggs Institute (JBI) quality assessment tools will be used to assess the potential risk of bias in each included article [24]. We opted to use the JBI tools due to the availability of separate checklists for each study design (e.g., cross-sectional, case-control, and cohort studies) [25]. The JBI tools are based on eight items that explore seven different domains: (i) participant selection, (ii) setting definition, (iii) ascertainment of the exposure; (iv) validity of condition measurement; (v) identification of confounders and dealing strategy, (vi) ascertainment of the outcome, and (vii) appropriateness of the statistical analysis [24].

Assessed papers will be categorized based on their methodological qualities by applying a scoring system available in [11]. Specifically, for each of the eight items, four options are allowed: Yes, No, Unclear and Not applicable. We will assign 2 points for yes, -2 points for no, -1 point for unclear and 0 points for not applicable. The total score could range between -16 and 16. Articles scoring from -16 to 4 will be classified as low quality, articles scoring from 5 to 9 as moderate, and articles scoring equal to or more than 10 (and up to 16) as high quality.

5. Expected Results

The quantitative and qualitative results of the literature will be presented using descriptive tables. As previously performed [26], a narrative description of the main characteristics of the study (for instance, the study design, study period, country where the study took place), the population characteristics (for instance, the age of the women and their status), the methodology (for instance, the manner in which the survey was administered, if the tools were validated), and the outcome, will be obtained from the included studies. This description will help to identify similarities and differences among the studies. The main results will be presented with reference to the 5C model and synthesized using a narrative approach [5].

A pilot exploration of how many results will result was conducted on PubMed/MEDLINE (13 January 2023). A total of 184 records were identified.

5.1. Quantitative Analysis

If at least two studies report data for the same outcome using OR, RR, or HR and their 95% confidence interval (CI), then we will proceed to pool data through meta-analysis. When two or more studies report estimated risks (OR, RR or HR) for a specific factor, both random and fixed effects models will be used to calculate the pooled effect size. The pooled effect size will be reported as the OR with a 95% CI. We will assess the heterogeneity of the studies using both the chi-square test and the I^2 statistic, as previously performed [27]. Heterogeneity will be classified into four categories based on the I^2 value (higher: $I^2 > 75\%$, moderate = I^2 ranging between 75% and 50%, low = I^2 ranging between 50% and 25%, and low = $I^2 < 25\%$). Publication bias will be assessed via visual inspection of the funnel plot and by means of the Egger regression asymmetry test, with statistical significance set at $p < 0.10$ [28]. If there is any publication bias, the trim and fill method will be performed [29]. All analyses will be conducted using Prometa3® software (Internovi, Cesena, Italy).

5.2. Subgroup and Sensitivity Analysis

If the necessary data are available, the analysis may be stratified according to the subjects' characteristics (e.g., pregnant or breastfeeding women), the country where the study took place and, lastly, the methodological quality of the studies (e.g., only including moderate/high methodological quality studies).

6. Ethical Considerations

This is a systematic literature review of the available literature using already published data. No interventions are planned, nor will there be any direct data collection from humans/animals. For these reasons, no ethical approval is required. The results of our review will be disseminated among academia, policymakers, healthcare professionals and the general public. For detailed information dissemination, scientific presentations at national and international congresses and conferences, peer-reviewed scientific publications, and posts on both academic and generalist social network platforms will be used.

7. Discussion

The current review will offer a comprehensive overview of the existing literature on the knowledge, attitudes, behaviour, acceptance, and hesitancy regarding the COVID-19 vaccine among pregnant and breastfeeding women. Although previous reviews have focused on knowledge, attitudes or behaviour in accepting/refusing vaccines, in general, the current review will focus on specific vaccines for COVID-19, which largely differ from other type of vaccines [30]. The differences include, first and foremost, the availability of several vaccines developed by numerous pharmaceutical companies (for instance, seven different vaccines were approved and authorised to be marketed in Europe) [31] that may increase uncertainty among individuals. Despite the fact that all these vaccines showed satisfactory levels of safety and efficacy in clinical trials [31–34], they were all administered to the general public, albeit with different indications [31]. This could cause people to be uncertain about vaccine preferences, which may raise doubts regarding vaccination [35]. Some vaccines share the same technology, while others were developed using different approaches. The first COVID-19 vaccines approved were those using viral mRNA (for example, those from Pfizer and Moderna). Subsequently, recombinant, adjuvanted vaccines (for example, those from Novavax), inactivated, adjuvanted vaccines (for example, from Valneva), and, finally, those using recombinant DNA technology (for example, from Janssen) were developed and approved [31]. Secondly, COVID-19 vaccines were the first mRNA vaccine administered to humans, which may have contributed to fear of long-term side-effects [36]. Thirdly, due to the novelty of the virus and its rapid global spread, there was an urgent need for safe and effective vaccines. For this reason, many efforts were made to expedite the testing and licensing of the vaccines. Consequently, the public could also have been affected by fear of poorly executed experimental trials and possible unknown side-effects [37]. Additionally, during the COVID-19 pandemic, the general public and pregnant/breastfeeding women directly experienced fear of the disease itself, fear not commonly perceived for other "old" vaccine-preventable diseases for which the vaccination programmes are known to have prevented millions of cases, dispelling the fear of the disease itself and leaving, instead, room for fear of possible, albeit rare and mostly non-serious, vaccine adverse effects [38]. Last, but not least, the great volume of information (and even disinformation) readily available, especially on the internet and social networks, the so-called infodemic, has a substantial impact on vaccination acceptance [38–40].

The ultimate aim of the current review is to shed light on this still evolving area of research on the assumption that the results could help in understanding the barriers and facilitators of COVID-19 vaccine acceptance among a specific vulnerable sub-population. Pregnant women have a higher risk of severe complications from COVID-19 compared to non-pregnant women of reproductive age [41]. According to a large study conducted by the Centers for Disease Control and Prevention, pregnant women affected by COVID-19 have a higher risk of intensive care unit admission, invasive ventilation, extracorporeal membrane oxygenation, and death than non-pregnant women of reproductive age [8]. In light of this, and the associated high burden, it is of utmost importance to understand the reasons for hesitancy towards or acceptance of COVID-19 vaccines with the ultimate purpose of raising the vaccination rate among pregnant/breastfeeding women.

Some potential limitations of our work should be acknowledged. First, we will only be including articles written in English. This may exclude potentially relevant articles written in other languages, for instance, Chinese, the language of the country where the virus originally appeared. Moreover, we recognize the heterogeneity of outcomes, although this is a methodological weakness directly attributable to the content of the original studies published in the literature. However, the approach taken will enable us to assess a large number of studies, offering a broad overview of the phenomenon.

Despite the above-mentioned limitations, we conclude that our findings may be useful for both healthcare professionals and policy makers, as they can assist healthcare professionals in guiding pregnant and breastfeeding women through the decision-making process associated with receiving the COVID-19 vaccine [42–45]. Similarly, our findings could inform public health policies with respect to future vaccine communication strategies.

Author Contributions: Conceptualization, V.G.; methodology, V.G.; writing—original draft preparation, V.G., A.B., M.D. and V.D.L.; writing—review and editing, V.G. and S.C.; supervision, V.G. All authors have read and agreed to the published version of the manuscript.

Funding: This research received no external funding.

Institutional Review Board Statement: Not applicable.

Informed Consent Statement: Not applicable.

Data Availability Statement: Not applicable.

Conflicts of Interest: The authors declare no conflict of interest.

References

1. World Health Organization. Top Ten Threats to Global Health in 2019. 2019. Available online: https://www.who.int/news-room/feature-stories/ten-threats-to-global-health-in-2019 (accessed on 3 December 2022).
2. Dube, E.; Laberge, C.; Guay, M.; Bramadat, P.; Roy, R.; Bettinger, J. Vaccine hesitancy: An overview. *Hum. Vaccin. Immunother.* **2013**, *9*, 1763–1773. [CrossRef] [PubMed]
3. Peretti-Watel, P.; Larson, H.J.; Ward, J.K.; Schulz, W.S.; Verger, P. Vaccine hesitancy: Clarifying a theoretical framework for an ambiguous notion. *PLoS Curr.* **2015**, *7*, 25. [CrossRef]
4. MacDonald, N.E.; Hesitancy, S.W.G.O.V. Vaccine hesitancy: Definition, scope and determinants. *Vaccine* **2015**, *33*, 4161–4164. [CrossRef] [PubMed]
5. Betsch, C.; Schmid, P.; Heinemeier, D.; Korn, L.; Holtmann, C.; Bohm, R. Beyond confidence: Development of a measure assessing the 5C psychological antecedents of vaccination. *PLoS ONE* **2018**, *13*, e0208601. [CrossRef] [PubMed]
6. Al-Sanafi, M.; Sallam, M. Psychological Determinants of COVID-19 Vaccine Acceptance among Healthcare Workers in Kuwait: A Cross-Sectional Study Using the 5C and Vaccine Conspiracy Beliefs Scales. *Vaccines* **2021**, *9*, 701. [CrossRef]
7. Kiefer, M.K.; Mehl, R.; Costantine, M.M.; Johnson, A.; Cohen, J.; Summerfield, T.L.; Landon, M.B.; Rood, K.M.; Venkatesh, K.K. Characteristics and perceptions associated with COVID-19 vaccination hesitancy among pregnant and postpartum individuals: A cross-sectional study. *BJOG* **2022**, *129*, 1342–1351. [CrossRef]

8. Zambrano, L.D.; Ellington, S.; Strid, P.; Galang, R.R.; Oduyebo, T.; Tong, V.T.; Woodworth, K.R.; Nahabedian, J.F., 3rd; Azziz-Baumgartner, E.; Gilboa, S.M.; et al. Update: Characteristics of Symptomatic Women of Reproductive Age with Laboratory-Confirmed SARS-CoV-2 Infection by Pregnancy Status-United States, January 22-October 3, 2020. *MMWR Morb. Mortal. Wkly. Rep.* **2020**, *69*, 1641–1647. [CrossRef]
9. Aw, J.; Seng, J.J.B.; Seah, S.S.Y.; Low, L.L. COVID-19 Vaccine Hesitancy-A Scoping Review of Literature in High-Income Countries. *Vaccines* **2021**, *9*, 900. [CrossRef]
10. Center for Disease Control and Prevention. New CDC Data: COVID-19 Vaccination Safe for Pregnant People. Available online: https://www.cdc.gov/media/releases/2021/s0811-vaccine-safe-pregnant.html (accessed on 3 December 2022).
11. Kilich, E.; Dada, S.; Francis, M.R.; Tazare, J.; Chico, R.M.; Paterson, P.; Larson, H.J. Factors that influence vaccination decision-making among pregnant women: A systematic review and meta-analysis. *PLoS ONE* **2020**, *15*, e0234827. [CrossRef]
12. Gencer, H.; Ozkan, S.; Vardar, O.; Serceskus, P. The effects of the COVID 19 pandemic on vaccine decisions in pregnant women. *Women Birth* **2022**, *35*, 317–323. [CrossRef]
13. Shamseer, L.; Moher, D.; Clarke, M.; Ghersi, D.; Liberati, A.; Petticrew, M.; Shekelle, P.; Stewart, L.A.; Group, P.-P. Preferred reporting items for systematic review and meta-analysis protocols (PRISMA-P) 2015: Elaboration and explanation. *BMJ* **2015**, *350*, g7647. [CrossRef] [PubMed]
14. Higgins, J.P.; Altman, D.G.; Gotzsche, P.C.; Juni, P.; Moher, D.; Oxman, A.D.; Savovic, J.; Schulz, K.F.; Weeks, L.; Sterne, J.A.; et al. The Cochrane Collaboration's tool for assessing risk of bias in randomised trials. *BMJ* **2011**, *343*, d5928. [CrossRef] [PubMed]
15. Page, M.J.; McKenzie, J.E.; Bossuyt, P.M.; Boutron, I.; Hoffmann, T.C.; Mulrow, C.D.; Shamseer, L.; Tetzlaff, J.M.; Akl, E.A.; Brennan, S.E.; et al. The PRISMA 2020 statement: An updated guideline for reporting systematic reviews. *BMJ* **2021**, *372*, n71. [CrossRef] [PubMed]
16. Stroup, D.F.; Berlin, J.A.; Morton, S.C.; Olkin, I.; Williamson, G.D.; Rennie, D.; Moher, D.; Becker, B.J.; Sipe, T.A.; Thacker, S.B. Meta-analysis of observational studies in epidemiology: A proposal for reporting. Meta-analysis of Observational Studies in Epidemiology (MOOSE) group. *JAMA* **2000**, *283*, 2008–2012. [CrossRef]
17. Nucci, D.; Marino, A.; Realdon, S.; Nardi, M.; Fatigoni, C.; Gianfredi, V. Lifestyle, WCRF/AICR Recommendations, and Esophageal Adenocarcinoma Risk: A Systematic Review of the Literature. *Nutrients* **2021**, *13*, 3525. [CrossRef]
18. Gianfredi, V.; Ferrara, P.; Dinu, M.; Nardi, M.; Nucci, D. Diets, Dietary Patterns, Single Foods and Pancreatic Cancer Risk: An Umbrella Review of Meta-Analyses. *Int. J. Environ. Res. Public Health* **2022**, *19*, 14787. [CrossRef]
19. Nucci, D.; Santangelo, O.E.; Provenzano, S.; Fatigoni, C.; Nardi, M.; Ferrara, P.; Gianfredi, V. Dietary Fiber Intake and Risk of Pancreatic Cancer: Systematic Review and Meta-Analysis of Observational Studies. *Int. J. Environ. Res. Public Health* **2021**, *18*, 11556. [CrossRef]
20. Nucci, D.; Fatigoni, C.; Amerio, A.; Odone, A.; Gianfredi, V. Red and Processed Meat Consumption and Risk of Depression: A Systematic Review and Meta-Analysis. *Int. J. Environ. Res. Public Health* **2020**, *17*, 6686. [CrossRef]
21. Gianfredi, V.; Albano, L.; Basnyat, B.; Ferrara, P. Does age have an impact on acute mountain sickness? A systematic review. *J. Travel Med.* **2020**, *27*, taz104. [CrossRef]
22. Cella, P.; Voglino, G.; Barberis, I.; Alagna, E.; Alessandroni, C.; Cuda, A.; D'Aloisio, F.; Dallagiacoma, G.; De Nitto, S.; Di Gaspare, F.; et al. Resources for assessing parents' vaccine hesitancy: A systematic review of the literature. *J. Prev. Med. Hyg.* **2020**, *61*, E340–E373. [CrossRef]
23. Gianfredi, V.; Bragazzi, N.L.; Nucci, D.; Villarini, M.; Moretti, M. Cardiovascular diseases and hard drinking waters: Implications from a systematic review with meta-analysis of case-control studies. *J. Water Health* **2017**, *15*, 31–40. [CrossRef] [PubMed]
24. Joanna Briggs Institute. Joanna Briggs Institute Critical Appraisal Tools. Available online: https://jbi.global/critical-appraisal-tools (accessed on 1 November 2022).
25. Santangelo, O.E.; Gianfredi, V.; Provenzano, S. Wikipedia searches and the epidemiology of infectious diseases: A systematic review. *Data Knowl. Eng.* **2022**, *142*, 102093. [CrossRef]
26. Ferrara, P.; Gianfredi, V.; Tomaselli, V.; Polosa, R. The Effect of Smoking on Humoral Response to COVID-19 Vaccines: A Systematic Review of Epidemiological Studies. *Vaccines* **2022**, *10*, 303. [CrossRef]
27. Perego, G.; Vigezzi, G.P.; Cocciolo, G.; Chiappa, F.; Salvati, S.; Balzarini, F.; Odone, A.; Signorelli, C.; Gianfredi, V. Safety and Efficacy of Spray Intranasal Live Attenuated Influenza Vaccine: Systematic Review and Meta-Analysis. *Vaccines* **2021**, *9*, 998. [CrossRef]
28. Egger, M.; Davey Smith, G.; Schneider, M.; Minder, C. Bias in meta-analysis detected by a simple, graphical test. *BMJ* **1997**, *315*, 629–634. [CrossRef]
29. Duval, S.; Tweedie, R. A nonparametric "Trim and Fill" method of accounting for Publication Bias in Meta-Analysis. *J. Am. Stat. Assoc.* **2000**, *95*, 89–98. [CrossRef]
30. Gianfredi, V.; Pennisi, F.; Lume, A.; Ricciardi, G.E.; Minerva, M.; Ricco, M.; Odone, A.; Signorelli, C. Challenges and Opportunities of Mass Vaccination Centers in COVID-19 Times: A Rapid Review of Literature. *Vaccines* **2021**, *9*, 574. [CrossRef]
31. European Medicines Agency (EMA). COVID-19 Vaccines: Authorised. Available online: https://www.ema.europa.eu/en/human-regulatory/overview/public-health-threats/coronavirus-disease-covid-19/treatments-vaccines/vaccines-covid-19/covid-19-vaccines-authorised#originally-authorised-covid-19-vaccines-section (accessed on 14 October 2022).

32. Gianfredi, V.; Minerva, M.; Casu, G.; Capraro, M.; Chiecca, G.; Gaetti, G.; Mantecca Mazzocchi, R.; Musaro, P.; Berardinelli, P.; Basteri, P.; et al. Immediate adverse events following COVID-19 immunization. A cross-sectional study of 314,664 Italian subjects. *Acta Biomed.* **2021**, *92*, e2021487. [CrossRef]
33. Vigezzi, G.P.; Lume, A.; Minerva, M.; Nizzero, P.; Biancardi, A.; Gianfredi, V.; Odone, A.; Signorelli, C.; Moro, M. Safety surveillance after BNT162b2 mRNA COVID-19 vaccination: Results from a cross-sectional survey among staff of a large Italian teaching hospital. *Acta Biomed.* **2021**, *92*, e2021450. [CrossRef]
34. Sultana, J.; Caci, G.; Hyeraci, G.; Albano, L.; Gianfredi, V. COVID-19 mRNA vaccine safety, immunogenicity, and effectiveness in a hospital setting: Confronting the challenge. *Intern. Emerg. Med.* **2022**, *17*, 325–327. [CrossRef]
35. Gorman, J.M.; Gorman, S.E.; Sandy, W.; Gregorian, N.; Scales, D.A. Implications of COVID-19 Vaccine Hesitancy: Results of Online Bulletin Board Interviews. *Front. Public Health* **2021**, *9*, 757283. [CrossRef] [PubMed]
36. Lazarus, J.V.; Wyka, K.; White, T.M.; Picchio, C.A.; Rabin, K.; Ratzan, S.C.; Parsons Leigh, J.; Hu, J.; El-Mohandes, A. Revisiting COVID-19 vaccine hesitancy around the world using data from 23 countries in 2021. *Nat. Commun.* **2022**, *13*, 3801. [CrossRef] [PubMed]
37. Jiang, S. Don't rush to deploy COVID-19 vaccines and drugs without sufficient safety guarantees. *Nature* **2020**, *579*, 321. [CrossRef] [PubMed]
38. Bendau, A.; Plag, J.; Petzold, M.B.; Strohle, A. COVID-19 vaccine hesitancy and related fears and anxiety. *Int. Immunopharmacol.* **2021**, *97*, 107724. [CrossRef] [PubMed]
39. Santangelo, O.E.; Provenzano, S.; Gianfredi, V. Infodemiology of flu: Google trends-based analysis of Italians' digital behavior and a focus on SARS-CoV-2, Italy. *J. Prev. Med. Hyg.* **2021**, *62*, E586–E591. [CrossRef]
40. Bragazzi, N.L.; Barberis, I.; Rosselli, R.; Gianfredi, V.; Nucci, D.; Moretti, M.; Salvatori, T.; Martucci, G.; Martini, M. How often people google for vaccination: Qualitative and quantitative insights from a systematic search of the web-based activities using Google Trends. *Hum. Vaccin. Immunother.* **2017**, *13*, 464–469. [CrossRef]
41. Rasmussen, S.A.; Jamieson, D.J. Pregnancy, Postpartum Care, and COVID-19 Vaccination in 2021. *JAMA* **2021**, *325*, 1099–1100. [CrossRef]
42. D'Ancona, F.; Gianfredi, V.; Riccardo, F.; Iannazzo, S. Immunisation Registries at regional level in Italy and the roadmap for a future Italian National Registry. *Ann. Ig.* **2018**, *30*, 77–85. [CrossRef]
43. Gianfredi, V.; Balzarini, F.; Gola, M.; Mangano, S.; Carpagnano, L.F.; Colucci, M.E.; Gentile, L.; Piscitelli, A.; Quattrone, F.; Scuri, S.; et al. Leadership in Public Health: Opportunities for Young Generations Within Scientific Associations and the Experience of the "Academy of Young Leaders". *Front. Public Health* **2019**, *7*, 378. [CrossRef]
44. Gianfredi, V.; Odone, A.; Fiacchini, D.; Rosselu, R.; Battista, T.; Signorelli, C. Trust and reputation management, branding, social media management nelle organizzazioni sanitarie: Sfide e opportunity per la comunita igienistica italiana. *J. Prev. Med. Hyg.* **2019**, *60*, E108–E109.
45. Gianfredi, V.; Grisci, C.; Nucci, D.; Parisi, V.; Moretti, M. [Communication in health.]. *Recenti. Prog. Med.* **2018**, *109*, 374–383. [CrossRef]

Disclaimer/Publisher's Note: The statements, opinions and data contained in all publications are solely those of the individual author(s) and contributor(s) and not of MDPI and/or the editor(s). MDPI and/or the editor(s) disclaim responsibility for any injury to people or property resulting from any ideas, methods, instructions or products referred to in the content.

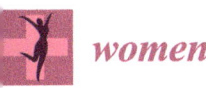

Article

Factors Influencing the Utilization of Antenatal Services among Women of Childbearing Age in South Africa

Putunywa Zandrina Nxiweni [1], Kelechi Elizabeth Oladimeji [1,2], Mirabel Nanjoh [3], Lucas Banda [1], Felix Emeka Anyiam [4], Francis Leonard Mpotte Hyera [1], Teke R. Apalata [2], Jabu A. Mbokazi [5] and Olanrewaju Oladimeji [1,4,*]

[1] Department of Public Health, Faculty of Health Sciences, Walter Sisulu University, Mthatha 5099, South Africa
[2] Department of Laboratory Medicine and Pathology, Faculty of Health Sciences, Walter Sisulu University, Mthatha 5099, South Africa
[3] Medical Education Unit, Faculty of Health Sciences, Walter Sisulu University, Mthatha 5099, South Africa
[4] Faculty of Health Sciences, Durban University of Technology, Durban 4003, South Africa
[5] Office of the Dean, Faculty of Health Sciences, Walter Sisulu University, Mthatha 5099, South Africa
* Correspondence: ooladimeji@wsu.ac.za

Abstract: Access to quality care before, during, and after childbirth remains an effective means of reducing maternal and neonatal mortality. Therefore, the study identified factors influencing the utilization of prenatal care services among women of childbearing age in South Africa. This is a retrospective study based on secondary data from the South African Demographic Health Survey (DHS) conducted from 1998 to 2016. In South Africa, 21.0% of mothers had used ANC services. Higher odds of seeking prenatal care were found in women aged 35 years and older (cOR = 1.26, 95% CI: 1.08–1.47, $p = 0.003$), married or cohabiting (cOR = 1.13, 95% CI: 1.004–1.27) observed, $p = 0.043$), higher level of education (tertiary education: cOR = 0.55, $p = 0.001$), female residents in urban areas (cOR = 1.35, 95% CI: 1.20–1.52, $p = 0.001$), higher wealth index (cOR = 1.32, 95% CI: 1.15–1.51, $p = 0.001$), employed (cOR = 1.48, 95% CI: 1.29–1.70, $p = 0.001$) and media exposure (cOR = 1.27, 95% CI: 1.12–1.44), $p = 0.001$). The findings of this study provide insight into the need to make maternal health services more accessible, more widely used, and of a higher quality. This requires effective strategic policies that promote patronage to reduce maternal mortality and improve newborn outcomes in South Africa.

Keywords: antenatal care utilization; antenatal care services; South Africa; maternal health

1. Introduction

Antenatal care (ANC) is an important factor in reducing maternal morbidity and mortality in pregnant women and in achieving a positive pregnancy experience [1–3]. The essence of this care pathway is to make sure that the health of both the unborn child and the pregnant mother is safe by monitoring the progress of the pregnancy vis-a-vis expected indicators for a normal pregnancy. Access to ANC gives a pregnant woman the opportunity to benefit from care services including health promotion, screening and diagnosis, and disease prevention, required to maintain normalcy and for timely identification of abnormalities that can pose a risk to the life of her unborn child and herself. Unfortunately, many women in developing countries do not have access to such services [1,4].

According to the South African Demographic Health Survey [5], there are approximately 536 prenatal deaths per 100,000 in South Africa. It shows that for every 1000 live births, five (5) women died during pregnancy. A higher proportion of women in South Africa receive prenatal care, also known as antenatal care (ANC) from healthcare professionals; doctors (18%), nurses or midwives (70%). Only a small fraction (2%) are cared for by traditional birth attendants, while 10% receive no prenatal care [5]. The benefits of ANC cannot be overstated, particularly when it comes to reducing maternal and prenatal

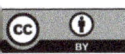

morbidity and mortality. Maternal morbidity refers to any health condition attributed to, or aggravated by, pregnancy and childbirth that negatively affects the woman's wellbeing [6,7].

WHO recommendations prior to 2016 call for at least four ANC visits [8] where a pregnant woman receives focused ANC, if eligible. Currently, a pregnant woman needs at least eight visits [9] to receive any significant evidence-based interventions. The South African Department of Health has classified the appropriate ANC based on the WHO criteria above. If a pregnant woman made at least four and eight visits between April 2006 and April 2017, she was considered booked or received an appropriate ANC. A 2.4% increase in the percentage of South African women who participated in at least four ANC visits from 1998 to 2016 was documented by Global Health data [10,11].

During this period, South Africa recorded 150 maternal deaths per 100,000 live births in 1998 [12] and 119 deaths in 2017 [13]. Despite the observed improvement, the country is far below the required 70 deaths per 100,000 live births to meet the Sustainable Development Goals (SDG) 3.1 [14]. Moreover, the rate of skilled delivery use, a predictor of Maternal Mortality Rate (MMR) in the country increased from 84% in 1998 to 97% in 2016 [15]; although, Bobo et al. [16] reported a higher rate of 96.7 percent. When it comes to pregnant women's health, adequate ANC services are essential.

It has been observed that increasing access to skilled attendants, which has a close link to ANC, emergency obstetric care, and family planning services can significantly reduce maternal mortality in low-income settings such as South Africa [17–19]. Despite the obvious importance of maternity care, including ANC, poor access to and utilization of such services remains an important determinant of maternal mortality and morbidity worldwide [11,17].

Previous research has shown a link between ANC utilization and accessibility, sociodemographic factors, knowledge, and the quality of care provided [20–22], but the extent to which these factors influence ANC utilization has not been adequately documented in the region of South Africa. Consequently, this study investigated the critical factors that influence the utilization of ANC and other maternal health services between the years 1998 and 2016 among women of reproductive age in South Africa. The insights provided by this study will further help to shape the strategic policy that South Africa will use to reduce the number of maternal deaths and improve neonatal outcomes.

2. Results

2.1. Characteristics of Maternal Household Factors of Women within Reproductive Age in South Africa

As shown in Table 1, of the 67,645 women included in the analysis, 77.5% were para 1–2, 12% were equally nulliparous, and para ≥3. Timing of ANC (in months) was more among those that have attended between 3–6 months (72.2%), followed by <3 months (17.4%). Almost three-quarters (72.2%) had their first ANC visit between 3–6 months of pregnancy, and slightly above one-sixth (17.4%) attended before three months. More participants resided in the urban area (56.6%), compared to rural (43.4%). The provinces with the most participants were Gauteng (23.5%), Kwazulu-Natal (19.7%), Limpopo (12.6%), and Eastern Cape (12.5%).

Table 1. Characteristics of women within reproductive age in South Africa and factors influencing the use of antenatal care among them (*n* = 67,645).

Variables	Weighted Frequency	Weighted %
Socio-demographics		
Age (years)		
15–24	20,933	30.9
25–34	31,531	46.6

Table 1. *Cont.*

Variables	Weighted Frequency	Weighted %
35+	15,181	22.4
Marital Status		
Married/Co-habiting	33,683	49.8
Single	33,962	50.2
Educational Level		
No Education	3542	5.2
Primary	12,505	18.5
Secondary	45,612	67.4
Tertiary	5986	8.8
Race		
Black/African	58,172	86.3
White	2256	3.3
Colored	5692	8.4
Indian/Asian	1261	1.9
Obstetric and Household Factor Parity		
Nulliparity	7833	11.6
Para 1–2	52,397	77.5
Para ≥3	7415	11.5
Timing of ANC (months) (n = 64,463) $^\gamma$		
<3	11,217	17.4
3–6	46,549	72.2
6+	6697	10.4
Place of Residence		
Urban	38,295	56.6
Rural	29,350	43.4
Province		
Gauteng	15,928	23.5
Kwazulu-Natal	13,344	19.7
Limpopo	8540	12.6
Eastern Cape	8429	12.5
Mpumalanga	5811	8.6
Western Cape	5624	8.3
North West	52,928	7.7
Free State	3471	5.1
Northern Cape	1286	1.9
Economic Status Wealth Index		
Poorest	12,177	18.0
Poorer	15,762	23.3
Middle	15,430	22.8

Table 1. Cont.

Variables	Weighted Frequency	Weighted %
Richer	13,007	19.2
Richest	11,269	16.7
Employment Status (n = 65,646) $^\gamma$		
Employed	20,095	30.6
Not employed	45,551	69.4
Own a Car/Truck (n = 66,442) $^\gamma$		
Yes	15,226	22.9
No	51,216	77.1
Own a Motorcycle/Scooter (n = 66,381) $^\gamma$		
Yes	1094	1.6
No	65,287	98.4
Own a Bicycle (n = 66,442) $^\gamma$		
Yes	9420	14.2
No	57,022	85.8
Own a refrigerator (n = 66,336) $^\gamma$		
Yes	39,090	58.93
No	27,246	41.07
Has Electricity (n = 66,417) $^\gamma$		
Yes	45,578	71.6
No	18,839	28.4
Media Exposure factor Own a Television (n = 66,371) $^\gamma$		
Yes	45,720	68.89
No	20,651	31.11
Own a Radio (n = 66,344) $^\gamma$		
Yes	43,316	65.29
No	23,028	34.71
Watches TV everyday/week (n = 67,220) $^\gamma$		
Yes	42,755	63.6
No	24,465	36.4
Listens to Radio everyday/week (n = 67,507) $^\gamma$		
Yes	41,424	61.4
No	26,083	38.6
Reads newspaper regularly (n = 67,491) $^\gamma$		
Yes	24,595	36.9
No	42,595	63.1
Health Institution factor Getting permission to go to the Health facility (n = 14,768) $^\gamma$		
Not a big Problem	12,828	86.9

Table 1. *Cont.*

Variables	Weighted Frequency	Weighted %
Big Problem	1940	13.1
Getting money to go to the Health facility for treatment (*n* = 14,768) $^\gamma$		
Not a big Problem	10,665	72.2
Big Problem	4103	27.8
Distance to Health facility (*n* = 14,768) $^\gamma$		
Not a big Problem	11,459	77.6
Big Problem	3309	22.4
Not wanting to go to the Health facility alone (*n* = 14,768) $^\gamma$		
Not a big Problem	12,989	88.0
Big Problem	1779	12.0

$^\gamma$ indicated variables with missing data.

2.2. Characteristics of Women within Reproductive Age in South Africa and Factors Influencing the Use of Antenatal Care among Them

The study analyzed the DHS data of 67,645 women, across South Africa. The majority of the participants (46.6%) were within the age 25–34; 30.9% were within 15–24 years; and 22.4% were 35 years and above. Almost half of the participants (49.8%) were married, and 50.2% were single. Those who have completed secondary education were more with 67.4%, followed by those who have completed primary education (18.5%). Black/African descent was the majority with 86.3%, followed by those of Colored descent (8.4%), White (3.3%), and Indian/Asian (1.9%). Among the women included in the analysis, 77.5% had 1 or 2 parities, 11.6% were nulliparous, and those with 3 or more parities were 11.5%. Almost three-quarters (72.2%) had their first ANC visit between 3 and 6 months of pregnancy while slightly above one-sixth (17.4%) attended before three months. More participants resided in the urban area (56.6%), compared to rural (43.4%) and the provinces with the most participants were Gauteng (23.5%), Kwazulu-Natal (19.7%), Limpopo (12.6%), and Eastern Cape (12.5%) as shown in Table 1.

As shown in Figure 1, the overall prevalence of Utilization of Antenatal care services among women of reproductive age in SA was 79%.

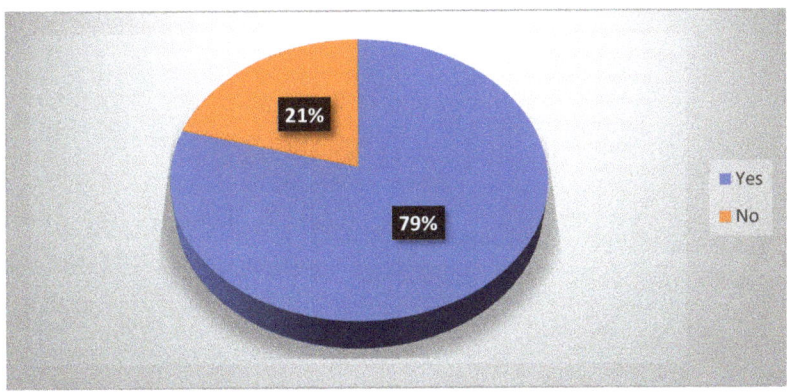

Figure 1. Utilization of Antenatal care services among women of reproductive age in South Africa.

As shown in Figure 2, the prevalence of Utilization of Antenatal care services among women of reproductive age in SA was statistically significantly highest in the province of Western Cape (88.6%), followed by Kwazulu-Natal (82.8%), Northern Cape (81.6%) and Northwest (80.5%) ($\chi^2 = 81.47$, $p = 0.001$).

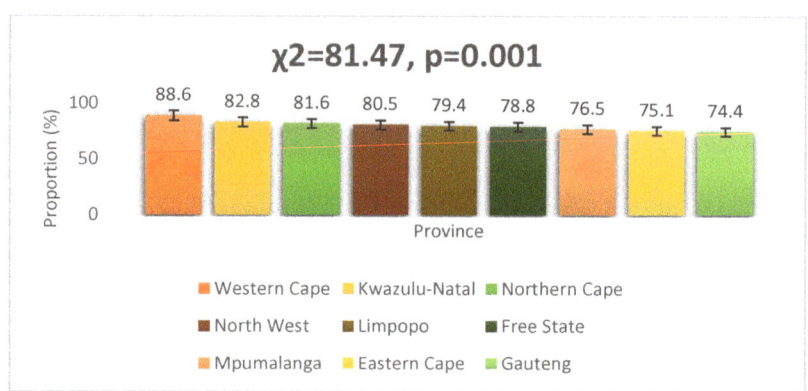

Figure 2. Utilization of Antenatal care by women of reproductive age in SA stratified by province.

Women in the poverty band of the wealth index were the majority (41.3%), those in the middle wealth index were 22.8% and barely one-third belonged to the rich band (35.9%). The majority were not employed (69.4%), and 77.1% neither owned a car, a motorcycle/scooter (98.4%), nor a bicycle (85.8%). A little over half owned a refrigerator (58.93%), and most had electricity (71.6%). Barely two-thirds owned a television (68.89%), a radio (65.29%), watched TV every day/week (63.6%), and listened to the radio every day/week (61.4%) and 36.9% read newspapers regularly. The overwhelming majority of the women had no problem getting permission (86.9%) and money (72.2%) to visit the health facility for treatment; had no problem with the distance to the health facility (77.6%); and had no problem going to the health facility alone (88.0%), as seen in Table 1.

As shown in Figure 1, the overall prevalence of the Utilization of Antenatal care services among women of reproductive age in SA was 79%.

As shown in Figure 2, the prevalence of the Utilization of Antenatal care services among women of reproductive age in SA was statistically significantly highest in the province of Western Cape (88.6%), followed by Kwazulu-Natal (82.8%), Northern Cape (81.6%) and North West (80.5%) ($\chi^2 = 81.47$, $p = 0.001$).

As shown in Table 2, the utilization of antenatal care varied across socio-demographic variables. Statistically significant higher prevalence of utilization of antenatal care was observed among those between 25 and 34 years in age ($p = 0.038$); married or cohabiting ($p = 0.001$); had a tertiary level of education ($p = 0.001$), and of the Indian/Asian race ($p = 0.001$). For obstetric and household factors, a significantly higher prevalence of utilization of antenatal care was observed among para 1–2 ($p = 0.001$), attended antenatal <3 months ($p = 0.001$), reside in the urban ($p = 0.004$), and the Western Cape Province ($p = 0.001$). Considering economic status, utilization of antenatal care has statistical significance for those in the richest wealth index ($p = 0.003$), are employed ($p = 0.001$), own a car ($p = 0.004$), own a motorcycle/scooter ($p = 0.001$), own a bicycle ($p = 0.032$), own a refrigerator ($p = 0.001$) and have electricity ($p = 0.001$). Moreover, there was statistically significant higher prevalence of utilization of antenatal care among those who own a television ($p = 0.001$), own a radio ($p = 0.001$), watches television every day/week ($p = 0.001$), listens to the radio every day/week ($p = 0.038$) and reads newspaper regularly ($p = 0.039$) under the media exposure factor. However, no statistically significant association was observed between health institutional factors and the utilization of antenatal care ($p > 0.05$).

Table 2. Associated factors for utilization of antenatal care services.

Variables	Utilization of Antenatal Care Services Weighted Freq (%)		Total	Chi-Square, p-Value
	Yes $n = 53{,}726$	No $n = 13{,}919$		
Socio-Demographics				
Age (Years)				$\chi^2 = 10.12$, $p = 0.038$
15–24	16,283 (77.8)	4650 (22.2)	20,933 (100.0)	
25–34	25,570 (81.1)	5961 (18.9)	31,531 (100.0)	
35+	11,873 (78.2)	3308 (21.8)	15,181 (100.0)	
Marital Status				$\chi^2 = 20.37$, $p = 0.001$
Married/Co-habiting	26,990 (80.1)	6693 (19.9)	33,683 (100.0)	
Single	26,736 (78.7)	7226 (21.3)	33,962 (100.0)	
Educational Level				$\chi^2 = 33.78$, $p = 0.001$
No Education	2611 (73.7)	931 (26.3)	3542 (100.0)	
Primary	9728 (77.8)	2777 (22.2)	12,505 (100.0)	
Secondary	36,140 (79.2)	9472 (20.8)	45,612 (100.0)	
Tertiary	5247 (87.7)	739 (12.3)	5986 (100.0)	
Race				$\chi^2 = 44.38$, $p = 0.001$
Black/African	45,504 (78.2)	12,668 (21.8)	58,172 (100.0)	
White	1952 (86.5)	304 (13.5)	2256 (100.0)	
Colored	4921 (86.5)	771 (13.5)	5692 (100.0)	
Indian/Asian	1179 (93.5)	82 (6.5)	1261 (100.0)	
Obstetric and Household factor				
Parity				$\chi^2 = 29.59$, $p = 0.001$
Nulliparity	5852 (74.7)	1981 (25.3)	7833 (100.0)	
Para 1–2	42,373 (80.9)	10,024 (19.1)	52,397 (100.0)	
Para ≥ 3	5501 (74.2)	1914 (25.8)	7415 (100.0)	
Timing of ANC (months)				$\chi^2 = 984.32$, $p = 0.001$
<3	10,881 (97.0)	336 (3.0)	11,217 (100.0)	
3–6	39,923 (85.8)	6626 (14.2)	46,549 (100.0)	
6+	2804 (41.9)	3893 (58.1)	6697 (100.0)	
Place of Residence				$\chi^2 = 8.21$, $p = 0.004$
Urban	30,565 (79.8)	7730 (20.2)	38,295 (100.0)	
Rural	23,161 (78.9)	6189 (21.1)	29,350 (100.0)	
Province				$\chi^2 = 81.47$, $p = 0.001$
Western Cape	4981 (88.6)	643 (11.4)	5624 (100.0)	
Eastern Cape	6334 (75.1)	2095 (24.9)	8429 (100.0)	

Table 2. Cont.

Variables	Utilization of Antenatal Care Services Weighted Freq (%)		Total	Chi-Square, p-Value
	Yes n = 53,726	No n = 13,919		
Northern Cape	1049 (81.6)	237 (18.4)	1286 (100.0)	
Free State	2734 (78.8)	737 (21.2)	3471 (100.0)	
Kwazulu-Natal	11,055 (82.8)	2289 (17.2)	13,344 (100.0)	
North West	4195 (80.5)	1017 (19.5)	5212 (100.0)	
Gauteng	11,856 (74.4)	4072 (25.6)	15,928 (100.0)	
Mpumalanga	4446 (76.5)	1365 (23.5)	5811 (100.0)	
Limpopo	7076 (82.9)	1464 (17.1)	8540 (100.0)	
Economic Status Wealth Index				$\chi^2 = 25.11$, $p = 0.003$
Poorest	9205 (75.6)	2922 (24.4)	12,177 (100.0)	
Poorer	12,185 (77.3)	3577 (22.7)	15,762 (100.0)	
Middle	12,563 (81.4)	2867 (18.6)	15,430 (100.0)	
Richer	10,554 (81.1)	2453 (18.9)	13,007 (100.0)	
Richest	9219 (81.8)	2050 (18.2)	11,269 (100.0)	
Employment Status				$\chi^2 = 27.07$, $p = 0.001$
Employed	16,706 (83.1)	3389 (16.9)	20,095 (100.0)	
Not employed	35,291 (77.5)	10,260 (22.5)	45,551 (100.0)	
Own a Car/Truck				$\chi^2 = 21.95$, $p = 0.004$
Yes	12,753 (83.8)	2473 (16.2)	15,226 (100.0)	
No	40,056 (78.2)	11,160 (21.8)	51,216 (100.0)	
Own a Motorcycle/Scooter				$\chi^2 = 36.18$, $p = 0.001$
Yes	950 (86.8)	144 (13.2)	1094 (100.0)	
No	51,831 (79.4)	13,456 (20.6)	65,287 (100.0)	
Own a Bicycle				$\chi^2 = 6.27$, $p = 0.032$
Yes	7776 (82.5)	1644 (17.5)	9420 (100.0)	
No	45,033 (79.0)	11,989 (21.0)	57,022 (100.0)	
Own a refrigerator				$\chi^2 = 27.92$, $p = 0.001$
Yes	31,917 (81.7)	7173 (18.3)	39,090 (100.0)	
No	20,788 (76.3)	6458 (23.7)	27,246 (100.0)	
Has Electricity				$\chi^2 = 29.54$, $p = 0.001$
Yes	38,627 (81.2)	8951 (18.8)	47,578 (100.0)	
No	14,164 (75.2)	4675 (24.8)	18,839 (100.0)	

Table 2. *Cont.*

Variables	Utilization of Antenatal Care Services Weighted Freq (%)		Total	Chi-Square, p-Value
	Yes n = 53,726	No n = 13,919		
Media Exposure factor Own a Television				$\chi^2 = 20.69$, $p = 0.001$
Yes	37,023 (81.0)	8697 (19.0)	45,720 (100.0)	
No	15,712 (76.1)	4939 (23.9)	20,651 (100.0)	
Own a Radio				$\chi^2 = 19.02$, $p = 0.001$
Yes	35,104 (81.0)	8212 (19.0)	43,316 (100.0)	
No	1766 (76.5)	5417 (23.5)	23,028 (100.0)	
Watches TV every day/week				$\chi^2 = 37.82$, $p = 0.001$
Yes	34,964 (81.8)	7791 (18.2)	42,755 (100.0)	
No	18,462 (75.5)	6003 (24.5)	24,465 (100.0)	
Listens to the Radio every day/week				$\chi^2 = 6.58$, $p = 0.038$
Yes	33,306 (80.4)	8118 (19.6)	41,424 (100.0)	
No	20,293 (77.8)	5790 (22.2)	26,083 (100.0)	
Reads newspaper regularly				$\chi^2 = 7.41$, $p = 0.039$
Yes	20,211 (81.2)	4685 (18.8)	24,896 (100.0)	
No	33,393 (78.4)	9202 (21.6)	42,595 (100.0)	
Health Institution factor α Getting permission to go to the Health facility				$\chi^2 = 0.253$, $p = 0.687$
Not a big Problem	10,013 (78.1)	2815 (21.9)	12,828 (100.0)	
Big Problem	1483 (76.4)	457 (23.6)	1940 (100.0)	
Getting money to go to the Health facility for treatment				$\chi^2 = 3.66$, $p = 0.167$
Not a big Problem	8439 (79.1)	2226 (20.9)	10,665 (100.0)	
Big Problem	3057 (74.5)	1046 (25.5)	4103 (100.0)	
Distance to Health facility				$\chi^2 = 1.75$, $p = 0.274$
Not a big Problem	8832 (77.1)	2627 (22.9)	11,459 (100.0)	
Big Problem	2664 (80.5)	645 (19.5)	3309 (100.0)	
Not wanting to go to the Health facility alone				$\chi^2 = 1.75$, $p = 0.274$
Not a big Problem	10,028 (77.2)	2961 (22.8)	12,989 (100.0)	
Big Problem	1468 (82.5)	311 (17.5)	1779 (100.0)	

Statistically significant ($p < 0.05$); α = A drop in sample population as institutional factor variables were not observed in the 1998 DHS data, rather only in the 2016 DHS data.

2.3. Multilevel Multivariate Logistic Regression Results

As shown in Table 3, statistically significant explanatory variables in the Chi-Square test of association were included for the multilevel multivariate logistic regression.

Table 3. Multilevel Multivariable Logistic Regression Results for Factors Associated with the Utilization of Antenatal Care Services among Women of Reproductive Age in South Africa (n = 67,645).

Variables	Model I cOR (95% CI)	Model II aOR (95% CI)	Model III aOR (95% CI)	Model IV aOR (95% CI)
Age (years)				
15–24 [R]				
25–34	0.98 (0.84–1.16)			
35+	1.26 (1.08–1.47) *			
Marital Status				
Single [R]				
Married/Co-habiting	1.13 (1.004–1.27) *			
Educational Level				
No Education [R]				
Primary	0.38 (0.26–0.53) ***			
Secondary	0.45 (0.34–0.60) ***			
Tertiary	0.55 (0.42–0.72) ***			
Race				
Black/African [R]				
White	0.25 (0.12–0.55) ***			
Colored	0.46 (0.19–1.09)			
Indian/Asian	0.35 (0.16–0.76) **			
Parity				
Nulliparity [R]				
Para 1–2	1.33 (1.06–1.68) **	0.95 (0.71–1.26)		
Para ≥3	1.63 (1.37–1.93) ***	1.29 (1.03–1.68) *		
Timing of ANC (months)				
<3 [R]				
3–6	41.91 (29.46–59.61) ***	0.029 (0.020–0.042) ***		
6+	9.73 (8.15–11.62) ***	0.29 (0.21–0.40) ***		
Place of Residence				
Rural [R]				
Urban	1.35 (1.20–1.52) ***	1.24 (1.04–1.49) *		
Province				
Western Cape [R]				
Eastern Cape	1.54 (1.09–2.18) *	0.54 (0.30–0.95) *		
Northern Cape	0.56 (0.45–0.69) ***	0.33 (0.19–0.58) ***		
Free State	0.94 (0.71–1.24)	0.23 (0.13–0.41) ***		
Kwazulu-Natal	0.84 (0.63–1.09)	0.31 (0.17–0.57) ***		
North West	0.98 (0.77–1.25)	0.38 (0.21–0.68) ***		
Gauteng	0.93 (0.49–0.81) ***	0.27 (0.15–0.50) ***		
Mpumalanga	0.63 (0.49–0.81) ***	0.34 (0.20–0.60) ***		
Limpopo	0.70 (0.55–0.89) ***	0.25 (0.15–0.43) ***		

Table 3. *Cont.*

Variables	Model I cOR (95% CI)	Model II aOR (95% CI)	Model III aOR (95% CI)	Model IV aOR (95% CI)
Wealth Index				
Poorest/Poorer [R]				
Middle	1.32 (1.15–1.51) ***	1.08 (0.93–1.25)	1.21 (1.0–1.47) *	
Richer/Richest	1.05 (0.89–1.25)	1.11 (0.94–1.31)	1.23 (1.007–1.51) *	
Employment Status				
Not employed [R]				
Employed	1.48 (1.29–1.70) ***	1.27 (1.102–1.49) ***	1.20 (1.004–1.44) *	
Own a Car/Truck				
No [R]				
Yes	1.44 (1.23–1.69) ***	1.01 (0.85–1.23)	1.15 (0.92–1.43)	
Own a Motorcycle/Scooter				
No [R]				
Yes	2.97 (1.37–6.44) **	2.11 (0.95–4.65)	2.69 (0.91–7.99)	
Own a Bicycle				
No [R]				
Yes	1.18 (0.99–1.41)	0.95 (0.79–1.15)	0.88 (0.71–1.12)	
Own a refrigerator				
No [R]				
Yes	1.58 (1.40–1.79) ***	1.20 (1.01–1.41) *	1.09 (0.89–1.33)	
Has Electricity				
No [R]				
Yes	1.62 (1.43–1.84) ***	1.27 (1.07–1.50) **	1.04 (0.85–1.28)	
Own a Television				
No [R]				
Yes	1.27 (1.12–1.44) ***	1.16 (1.0–1.35) *	1.33 (1.11–1.60)	1.18 (1.02–1.38) *
Own a Radio				
No [R]				
Yes	1.50 (1.33–1.69) ***	0.99 (0.84–1.19)	0.89 (0.72–1.11)	0.86 (0.70–1.04)
Watches TV every day/week				
No [R]				
Yes	1.68 (1.49–1.89) ***	1.44 (1.21–1.72) ***	1.39 (1.12–1.73) *	1.37 (1.15–1.65) ***
Listens to the Radio every day/week				
No [R]				
Yes	1.21 (1.07–1.36) **	0.95 (0.82–1.11)	0.90 (0.75–1.08)	0.95 (0.82–1.10)
Reads newspaper regularly				
No [R]				
Yes	1.47 (1.29–1.68) ***	1.12 (0.97–1.31)	1.18 (0.99–1.42)	1.18 (1.01–1.36) *

cOR = Crude OR, aOR = Adjusted OR, [R] = reference value, * significant at $p \leq 0.05$, ** significant at $p < 0.01$, *** significant at $p < 0.001$.

Model I: Non-adjusted (crude) aggregate model comprising all explanatory variable categories associated with the utilization of Antenatal care services

2.3.1. Socio-Demographic Factors

The study shows higher odds for the utilization of antenatal care among women aged 35 years and older than those 15–24 years (cOR = 1.26, 95% CI; 1.08–1.47, p = 0.003). Moreover, being married or cohabiting had higher odds for utilizing antenatal care than singles (cOR = 1.13, 95% CI; 1.004–1.27, p = 0.043). The odds for the utilization of antenatal care among women improved from primary to tertiary compared to those with no education (primary: cOR = 0.38, secondary: cOR = 0.45 and tertiary: cOR = 0.55, p = 0.001). White or Indian/Asian descent showed lower odds for the utilization of antenatal care compared to black/African (White: cOR = 0.25, Indian/Asian: cOR = 0.35, p = 0.001).

2.3.2. Obstetric and Household Factors

Women with Para 1–2 and Para $\geq$3 showed increased odds for the utilization of antenatal care compared to those that are nulliparous, with an increased odds in Para $\geq$3 compared to Para 1–2 (Para 1–2: cOR = 1.33, Para $\geq$3: OR = 1.63, p < 0.05). Women with the timing of ANC at 3 or more months of pregnancy showed increased odds for the utilization of antenatal care compared to those with the timing of ANC less than 3 months (3–6 months: cOR = 41.91, 6+ months: OR = 9.73, p = 0.001). Women residing in the urban area showed increased odds for the utilization of antenatal care compared to those in the rural area (cOR = 1.35, 95% CI; 1.20–1.52, p = 0.001). Only those residing in Eastern Cape showed increased odds for the utilization of antenatal care compared to Western Cape (cOR = 1.54, 95% CI; 1.09–2.18, p = 0.014). The other provinces, Northern Cape (cOR = 0.56, p = 0.001), Mpumalanga (cOR = 0.63, p = 0.001), Limpopo (cOR = 0.70, 0.001) and Gauteng (cOR = 0.93, p = 0.001) showed lower odds for the utilization of antenatal care compared to Western Cape.

2.3.3. Economic Status Factors

The study shows higher odds for the utilization of antenatal care among women in the middle wealth index compared to those in the poorest/poorer wealth index (cOR = 1.32, 95% CI; 1.15–1.51, p = 0.001). Higher odds for the utilization of antenatal care were observed among women who are employed (cOR = 1.48, 95% CI; 1.29–1.70, p = 0.001), own a car (cOR = 1.44, 95% CI; 1.23–1.69, p = 0.001), own a Motorcycle/Scooter (cOR = 2.97, 95% CI; 1.37–6.44, p = 0.006), own a refrigerator (cOR = 1.58, 95% CI; 1.40–1.79, p = 0.001), and have electricity (cOR = 1.62, 95% CI; 1.43–1.84, p = 0.001).

2.3.4. Media Exposure Factors

Higher odds for the utilization of antenatal care was observed among women who own a television (cOR = 1.27, 95% CI; 1.12–1.44, p = 0.001), own a radio (cOR = 1.50, 95% CI; 1.33–1.69, p = 0.001), watch television everyday/week (cOR = 1.68, 95% CI; 1.49–1.89, p = 0.001), listen to radio every day or week (cOR = 1.21, 95% CI; 1.07–1.36, p = 0.002), and read newspaper regularly (cOR = 1.47, 95% CI; 1.29–1.68, p = 0.001).

2.4. Model II: Household Factors, Economic Factors, and Media Exposure Factors Associated with Utilization of Antenatal Care Services, While Controlling for Their Socio-Emographic/Individual Factors

2.4.1. Obstetric and Household Factor

Women with Para $\geq$3 showed increased odds for the utilization of antenatal care compared to those who are nulliparous after adjusting for socio-demographic characteristics (aOR = 1.29, 95% CI; 1.03–1.68, p = 0.029). Women with the timing of ANC 3 or more months showed reduced odds for the utilization of antenatal care compared to those with the timing of ANC less than 3 months (3–6 months: aOR = 0.029, 6+ months: aOR = 0.29, p = 0.001). Women residing in the urban still showed increased odds for the utilization of antenatal care compared to those in rural areas after adjusting for confounding variables (aOR = 1.24, 95% CI; 1.04–1.49, p = 0.016).

All provinces showed lower odds for the utilization of antenatal care compared to Western Cape ($p < 0.05$).

2.4.2. Economic Status Factors

After controlling for socio-demographic characteristics, the study showed no statistically significant association between wealth index and the utilization of antenatal care ($p > 0.05$). Higher odds for the utilization of antenatal care were now observed among women for only those who were employed (aOR = 1.27, 95% CI; 1.10–1.49, $p = 0.001$), own a refrigerator (aOR = 1.20, 95% CI; 1.01–1.41, $p = 0.036$) and have electricity (aOR = 1.27, 95% CI; 1.07–1.50, $p = 0.006$). The variables own a car or own a Motorcycle/Scooter were no longer statistically significant.

2.4.3. Media Exposure Factors

After controlling for socio-demographic characteristics, higher odds for the utilization of antenatal care were still observed among women who own a television (aOR = 1.16, 95% CI; 1.0–1.35, $p = 0.049$) and watch TV every day/week (aOR = 1.44, 95% CI; 1.21–1.72, $p = 0.001$). The variables own a radio, listen to the radio every day or week, and read the newspaper regularly were no longer statistically significant ($p > 0.05$).

2.5. Model III: Economic Factors and Media Exposure Factors Associated with Utilization of Antenatal Care Services, While Controlling for Obstetric and Household Factors

2.5.1. Economic Status Factors

After controlling for obstetric and household factors, the study showed a statistically significant association between the wealth index and the utilization of antenatal care. Higher odds for the utilization of antenatal care among women were observed in those in the middle wealth index (aOR = 1.21, 95% CI; 1.0–1.47, $p = 0.047$) and richer/richest wealth index (aOR = 1.23, 95% CI; 1.007–1.51, $p = 0.043$). Higher odds for the utilization of antenatal care were observed among employed women (aOR = 1.20, 95% CI; 1.004–1.44, $p = 0.046$), own a refrigerator (aOR = 1.20, 95% CI; 1.01–1.41, $p = 0.036$) and have electricity (aOR = 1.27, 95% CI; 1.07–1.50, $p = 0.006$). The variables own a car, own a Motorcycle/Scooter, own a refrigerator, and have electricity were no longer statistically significant ($p > 0.05$).

2.5.2. Media Exposure Factors

Only the variable, watches TV every day/week, was statistically significantly associated with the utilization of antenatal care. Those watching TV every day/week showed increased odds for the utilization of antenatal care services (aOR = 1.39, 95% CI; 1.12–1.73, $p = 0.02$).

2.6. Model IV: Media Exposure Factors Associated with Utilization of Antenatal Care Services, While Controlling for Economic Status Factors

Media Exposure Factors

After controlling for economic status factors, higher odds for the utilization of antenatal were was still observed among women who own a television (aOR = 1.18, 95% CI; 1.02–1.38, $p = 0.030$) and watch TV every day/week (aOR = 1.37, 95% CI; 1.15–1.62, $p = 0.001$). The variables, own a radio, listen to radio every day or week, and read the newspaper regularly, were no longer statistically significant ($p > 0.05$), similar to the findings when controlling for maternal household factors.

3. Discussion

Using nationally representative 1998 to 2016 SADHS data, the goal of this study was to assess factors associated with the utilization of ANC services in South Africa. The cluster sampling methodology used ensured sample representativeness and the reliability of the study results. The study included 67,645 mothers of child-bearing age in nine provinces of South Africa whose complete information was available in the survey. In South Africa,

21.0% of mothers had utilized ANC services. There were variations in all the provinces. The highest provinces with the most prevalence were Western Cape and KwaZulu-Natal. The lowest are Eastern Cape and Gauteng, which could be as a result of the demographic and socioeconomic factors associated with both provinces. According to the findings of this study, women in South Africa's rural areas were less likely than women in the country's urban areas to use ANC services. This could be due to the disparities in the availability and accessibility of healthcare facilities, and women's awareness of ANC services in urban and rural areas. This finding was consistent with the findings of other studies conducted in Pakistan and Vietnam where ANC uptake was lower in rural areas [23,24]. This implies that more attention to health awareness, education, and promotion activities in rural areas is needed to improve ANC uptake. According to Rustagi et al. [25], the higher ANC coverage observed in the urban setting may likely be due to ANC accessibility at primary care facilities in these areas, highlighting the need for policy efforts to strengthen primary healthcare. ANC coverage has been found to be linked to primary healthcare availability in similar studies [26,27].

The present study observed a statistically significant relationship between a woman's age and adequate antenatal care utilization. The older the woman (35 years and older), the more likely she will use antenatal care appropriately. This suggests that young women have less experience with pregnancy care than older women. This is similar to findings to research by Adedokun and Yaya [21], who analyzed information obtained from the Demographic and Health Surveys (DHS) carried out in 31 different countries and involving 235,207 women aged 15–49 years old who had given birth to children within 5 years of the surveys. Similar findings were obtained by Joshi et al. [28] in Nepal, Dairo and Owoyokun [29] in Nigeria, Denny et al. [30] in Indonesia, and Ebonwu et al. [31] in South Africa. This may be due to older women placing more value on ANC, as a lack of knowledge about the benefits of ANC or the pregnancy being unwanted, which are common among adolescents, leads to seeking ANC care less frequently among younger women (including teenagers). Another study in Nigeria discovered that being 35 or older consistently increased the odds of using ANC by more than 200 percent [32]. Therefore, it is imperative for the South African Government to formulate policies that will protect adolescent pregnant women and provide for a tailored ANC to ensure utilization and a favorable pregnancy outcome for them. However, studies investigating the association between a woman's age and the use of ANC have not always reached consistent conclusions; as one study observed, the younger age utilization of ANC was found to be adequate because working women tend to postpone their first pregnancy and are more mature in terms of age during pregnancy than unemployed women [33].

The odds for the utilization of antenatal care among women improved from secondary to tertiary compared to those with no education. The findings indicated that women with higher levels of education have a greater likelihood of making appropriate use of antenatal care than women with lower levels of education. This suggests that a woman's likelihood of utilizing antenatal care increases in proportion to the level of education she possesses, which is similar to findings from previous studies [21,34,35]. A plausible explanation is that education fosters better enlightenment on issues, particularly health-related issues. This finding corroborated a study that alluded to increased utilization of maternal healthcare and women's empowerment through education, wealth, and decision making [36]. The girl child education policy needs to be strengthened, ensuring that no girl child is missed, thus improving their educational status and ANC utilization.

In addition, married or cohabiting had higher odds for utilizing antenatal care than singles. Rurangirwa et al. [33] in their study conducted in Rwanda, observed that the risk of poor utilization of ANC services was higher among single women. This may be due to the support that married and cohabiting women receive from their husbands or partners as a result of the ANC attendance sensitization campaign, which equally targets men and encourages them to follow their wife or partner to the clinic [37]. This is also consistent with the data from similar studies [38,39].

This study observed that women with a better economic status (wealth index) and who are employed had more antenatal care utilization than those with lower wealth indexes. Higher odds for the utilization of antenatal care among women were observed in those in the middle wealth index and richer/richest wealth index. When it comes to prenatal care, women from low-income families may not have the financial means to register at clinics or pay for their services. Studies conducted in Ethiopia and Gabon, and evidence from the Demographic Health Surveys data of 31 countries across sub-Saharan Africa corroborated this finding [21,40,41].

Women living in houses equipped with electricity were found to be utilizers of ANC services. It is possible that the presence of electricity in a household may be an indirect measure of accessibility to media services and may be a sign of a better or higher social class [23].

This study found that women exposed to mass media (own a television and watch TV every day/week, or listen to the radio) had a higher chance of ANC utilization than women who were not, as seen in some similar studies, with the propensity to enjoy essential obstetric care from skilled birth attendants [22,42,43]. This may be due to the fact that mass media can reach a large number of people at once, thereby increasing awareness of the benefits of maternal health services and influencing family behavior.

Limitations and Strengths of the Study

A limitation of this study is that the use of secondary data. One of the strengths of the study is that the DHIS survey is national data with geographical representation; hence, the study results are a true representation of the national data.

4. Materials and Methods

4.1. Research Design

This is a retrospective study based on secondary data obtained from the South African Demographic Health Survey (DHS), which was carried out between the years 1998 and 2016.

4.2. Population

Administratively, South Africa is divided into nine provinces. In 2020, the middle-year population estimated by Statistics South Africa was 59.62 million, of which approximately 51.1% are females. The infant mortality rate for 2020 was estimated at 23.6 per 1000 live births.

4.3. Sample Size and Sampling Frame

A curated and concatenated dataset on ANC utilization was obtained from demographic and health surveys conducted in South Africa from 1998 to 2016 The targeted study population was women of reproductive age (15–49 years).

The survey involved a two-stage cluster stratified sampling method. In the first stage, the country was divided into clusters, using the enumeration areas (EA); clusters for the study were selected using simple random sampling and the households within each cluster were line listed. Women between 15 and 49 years of age who were citizens or permanent residents were randomly selected from the listed households and enrolled in the study in the second stage [44].

4.4. Instruments

Data for the DHS were collected through interviewer-administered semi-structured validated questionnaires. Information obtained with this questionnaire includes socioeconomic characteristics, reproductive history, antenatal, delivery, post-natal care, and breastfeeding.

4.5. Validity and Reliability of the Data Collection Instrument

DHS questionnaire is a validated tool that has been used for many decades. The DHS survey data collection tool's reliability has been tested and established through repeated use by DHS and other experienced research investigators [44].

4.6. Variables of Interest

The independent variables: These include, sociodemographic characteristics such as age, marital status, education, and race; household factors such as parity (zero, one and two, three or more), the timing of ANC, place of residence, and region; economic status factors such as wealth index, employment, own a car/truck, own a motorcycle/scooter, own a bicycle, own a refrigerator, and electricity; media exposure factors such as own a television, own a radio, watch television regularly, listen to the radio regularly and read newspapers regularly; institutional factors such as access to a health facility and distance to a health facility.

The dependent (outcome) variable: ANC utilization during the women's pregnancy period was the outcome variable. This was categorized as 'not utilized—women who did not attend ANC', and 'utilized'—women who utilized. ANC not utilized was defined by <4 clinic visits and ANC utilized by ≥4 clinic visits across the study years.

4.7. Data Analysis

The data were analyzed using the SPSS package for data analysis. Descriptive analyses such as count, frequencies, and percentages are presented using a frequency table and bar/pie charts where appropriate. Pearson chi-square test was used to establish relationships between the independent and outcome variables, using a statistical significance of p-value less than or equal to 0.05 ($p \leq 0.05$).

Bivariate and multivariate logistic regression analyses were used to measure the associations between the independent and outcome variables.

The study further used a regression model expression to simulate a nested approach in which a non-adjusted aggregate model comprising all explanatory variable categories and utilization of Antenatal care services would be iterated to generate Model 1. Model 2 was simulated using obstetric and household factors; economic factors; and media exposure factors while controlling for their socio-demographic/individual factors. Simulation using economic factors and media exposure factors while controlling for household factors was for Model 3 and lastly, Model 4 was simulated using only media exposure factors and controlling for economic status factors. The primary benefit of the model selected is avoiding confounding effects by analyzing the association between all variables simultaneously. Confounding effects were tested in the four models among different factors. After defining the technique, the fundamental interpretation of the results was emphasized. A p-value set at 0.05 was considered statistically significant.

5. Conclusions

The study uncovered factors that influence women's use of antenatal care in South Africa. Age, marital status, having a tertiary education, living in an urban area, and socioeconomic factors, such as being in the richest wealth index and employed, having electricity, and media exposure, all influenced antenatal care utilization. Antenatal care enables the early detection and treatment of diseases that may affect both the mother and the child. It also allows a pregnant woman to be cared for during prenatal, antenatal, childbirth, and post-natal periods, reducing the chances of complications leading to maternal and neonatal death. Introducing targeted health promotion and education programs in communities would empower young and illiterate rural women to use available ANC services more often during pregnancy. Strengthening antenatal care visits becomes critical to the government in promoting and improving the health of the mother and child. This will lead to improved maternal and neonatal outcomes and minimize rural–urban reproductive health indices in South Africa. Maternal health services need to be accessible, used more frequently, and of higher quality. In addition, strengthening girl child education is paramount, not only to improve women's empowerment, but also to improve ANC utilization among those who are pregnant. Further, health promotion in the primary and secondary levels of education needs to be intensified to change the narrative of poor ANC utilization among these categories of people.

Author Contributions: Conceptualization, O.O. and P.Z.N.; methodology, O.O.; validation, O.O., K.E.O. and L.B.; formal analysis, O.O. and F.E.A.; resources, O.O.; writing—original draft preparation, O.O.; writing—review and editing, O.O. and K.E.O.; visualization, M.N.; F.L.M.H., T.R.A. and J.A.M.; Supervision, O.O.; funding acquisition, O.O. All authors have read and agreed to the published version of the manuscript.

Funding: Financial support for OO from the Fogarty International Center and National Institute of Mental Health, National Institutes of Health Award (D43 TW010543), National Research Foundation Grant (132385) to Incentive Funding for Rated Researchers (IPRR), and The APC was funded by the Walter Sisulu Seed Funding. The content is solely the responsibility of the authors and does not necessarily reflect the opinion(s) of the sponsors and affiliated institutions.

Institutional Review Board Statement: The DHS team ensured that ethical approvals were obtained from the national department's health ethics committee before the surveys were conducted. Ethical approval was obtained from the WSU IRB (033/2021) before the secondary data were obtained from the DHS for retrospective analysis. Respondents in the DHS data were informed that participation in this study is voluntary and they were asked to sign a voluntary consent form prior to enrollment in the study. Confidentiality and privacy were respected.

Data Availability Statement: The datasets analyzed for this study are available at https://dhsprogram.com (accessed on 15 June 2021).

Conflicts of Interest: The authors declare no conflict of interest.

References and Note

1. Konje, E.T.; Magoma, M.T.N.; Hatfield, J.; Kuhn, S.; Sauve, R.S.; Dewey, D.M. Missed opportunities in antenatal care for improving the health of pregnant women and newborns in Geita district, Northwest Tanzania 11 Medical and Health Sciences 1117 Public Health and Health Services. *BMC Pregnancy Childbirth* **2018**, *18*, 394. [CrossRef]
2. Arunda, M.; Emmelin, A.; Asamoah, B.O. Effectiveness of antenatal care services in reducing neonatal mortality in Kenya: Analysis of national survey data. *Glob. Health Action* **2017**, *10*, 1328796. [CrossRef] [PubMed]
3. Bolarinwa, O.A.; Sakyi, B.; Ahinkorah, B.O.; Ajayi, K.V.; Seidu, A.A.; Hagan, J.E., Jr.; Tessema, Z.T. Spatial patterns and multilevel analysis of factors associated with antenatal care visits in nigeria: Insight from the 2018 nigeria demographic health survey. *Healthcare* **2021**, *9*, 1389. [CrossRef] [PubMed]
4. Mutowo, J.; Yazbek, M.; van der Wath, A.; Maree, C. Barriers to using antenatal care services in a rural district in Zimbabwe. *Int. J. Afr. Nurs. Sci.* **2021**, *15*, 100319. [CrossRef]
5. NDoH SS, SAMRC I. South Africa Demographic and Health Survey 2016. Pretoria, South Africa, and Rockville, Maryland, USA: National Department of Health (NDoH). Statistics South Africa (Stats SA), South African Medical Research Council (SAMRC), ICF. 2019
6. WHO. Maternal Health. World Health Organization. 2022, p. 1. Available online: https://www.who.int/health-topics/maternal-health#tab=tab_1 (accessed on 13 May 2022).
7. Lange, I.L.; Gherissi, A.; Chou, D.; Say, L.; Filippi, V. What maternal morbidities are and what they mean for women: A thematic analysis of twenty years of qualitative research in low and lower-middle income countries. *PLoS ONE* **2019**, *14*, e0214199. [CrossRef]
8. Fife, J.G. Antenatal Care. *Br. Med. J.* **1948**, *2*, 227. [CrossRef]
9. World Health Organization. WHO recommendations on antenatal Care for a Positive Pregnancy Experience. World Heal Organ 2018; pp. 1–172. Available online: https://apps.who.int/iris/bitstream/handle/10665/250796/9789241549912-eng.pdf?sequence=1 (accessed on 13 May 2022).
10. WHO. Global Health Observatory Data Repository: Antenatal Care Coverage Data by Country. *World Health Organization*. 2021, p. 1. Available online: https://apps.who.int/gho/data/view.main.ANTENATALCARECOVERAGE4v (accessed on 13 May 2022).
11. Olaitan, T.; Okafor, I.P.; Onajole, A.T.; Abosede, O.A. Ending preventable maternal and child deaths in western Nigeria: Do women utilize the life lines? *PLoS ONE* **2017**, *12*, e0176195. [CrossRef]
12. Odhiambo, A. "Stop Making Excuses": Accountability for Maternal Health Care in South Africa. *Human Rights Watch*, 8 August 2011.

13. World Health Organization. *Trends in Maternal Mortality: 2000 to 2017: Estimates by WHO, UNICEF, UNFPA, World Bank Group and the United Nations Population Division*; World Health Organization: Geneva, Switzerland, 2019.
14. Beitzel, M. Sustainable Development Goal# 3 Good Health and Well-Being: Maternal and Child Health. Available online: https://summit.plymouth.edu/handle/20.500.12774/168 (accessed on 25 August 2022).
15. SSA Statistics South Africa. *Maternal Health Indicators: Further Analysis of the 1998 and 2016 South Africa Demographic and Health Surveys*; Statistics South Africa: Pretoria, South Africa, 2020.
16. Bobo, F.T.; Asante, A.; Woldie, M.; Dawson, A.; Hayen, A. Spatial patterns and inequalities in skilled birth attendance and caesarean delivery in sub-Saharan Africa. *BMJ Glob. Health* **2021**, *6*, e007074. [CrossRef]
17. Nuamah, G.B.; Agyei-Baffour, P.; Mensah, K.A.; Boateng, D.; Quansah, D.Y.; Dobin, D.; Addai-Donkor, K. Access and utilization of maternal healthcare in a rural district in the forest belt of Ghana. *BMC Pregnancy Childbirth* **2019**, *19*, 6. [CrossRef]
18. Geleto, A.; Chojenta, C.; Musa, A.; Loxton, D. Barriers to access and utilization of emergency obstetric care at health facilities in sub-Saharan Africa: A systematic review of literature 11 Medical and Health Sciences 1117 Public Health and Health Services. *Syst. Rev.* **2018**, *7*, 183. [CrossRef] [PubMed]
19. Wabiri, N.; Chersich, M.; Shisana, O.; Blaauw, D.; Rees, H.; Dwane, N. Growing inequities in maternal health in South Africa: A comparison of serial national household surveys. *BMC Pregnancy Childbirth* **2016**, *16*, 256. [CrossRef] [PubMed]
20. Morón-Duarte, L.S.; Varela, A.R.; Bertoldi, A.D.; Domingues, M.R.; Wehrmeister, F.C.; Silveira, M.F. Quality of antenatal care and its sociodemographic determinants: Results of the 2015 Pelotas birth cohort, Brazil. *BMC Health Serv. Res.* **2021**, *21*, 1070. [CrossRef] [PubMed]
21. Adedokun, S.T.; Yaya, S. Correlates of antenatal care utilization among women of reproductive age in sub-Saharan Africa: Evidence from multinomial analysis of demographic and health surveys (2010–2018) from 31 countries. *Arch. Public Health* **2020**, *78*, 134. [CrossRef]
22. Okedo-Alex, I.N.; Akamike, I.C.; Ezeanosike, O.B.; Uneke, C.J. Determinants of antenatal care utilisation in sub-Saharan Africa: A systematic review. *BMJ Open* **2019**, *9*, e031890. [CrossRef]
23. Aziz Ali, S.; Aziz Ali, S.; Feroz, A.; Saleem, S.; Fatmai, Z.; Kadir, M.M. Factors affecting the utilization of antenatal care among married women of reproductive age in the rural Thatta, Pakistan: Findings from a community-based case-control study. *BMC Pregnancy Childbirth* **2020**, *20*, 355. [CrossRef]
24. Tran, T.K.; Nguyen, C.T.; Nguyen, H.D.; Eriksson, B.; Bondjers, G.; Gottvall, K.; Ascher, H.; Petzold, M. Urban-Rural disparities in antenatal care utilization: A study of two cohorts of pregnant women in Vietnam. *BMC Health Serv. Res.* **2011**, *11*, 120. [CrossRef] [PubMed]
25. Rustagi, R.; Basu, S.; Garg, S.; Singh, M.M.; Mala, Y.M. Utilization of antenatal care services and its sociodemographic correlates in urban and rural areas in Delhi, India. *Eur. J. Midwifery* **2021**, *5*, 40. [CrossRef]
26. Venkateswaran, M.; Bogale, B.; Abu Khader, K.; Awwad, T.; Friberg, I.K.; Ghanem, B.; Hijaz, T.; Mørkrid, K.; Frøen, J.F. Effective coverage of essential antenatal care interventions: A cross-sectional study of public primary healthcare clinics in the West Bank. *PLoS ONE* **2019**, *14*, e0212635. [CrossRef]
27. Ogbo, F.A.; Dhami, M.V.; Ude, E.M.; Senanayake, P.; Osuagwu, U.L.; Awosemo, A.O.; Ogeleka, P.; Akombi, B.J.; Ezeh, O.K.; Agho, K.E. Enablers and barriers to the utilization of antenatal care services in India. *Int. J. Environ. Res. Public Health* **2019**, *16*, 3152. [CrossRef]
28. Joshi, C.; Torvaldsen, S.; Hodgson, R.; Hayen, A. Factors associated with the use and quality of antenatal care in Nepal: A population-based study using the demographic and health survey data. *BMC Pregnancy Childbirth* **2014**, *14*, 94. [CrossRef] [PubMed]
29. Dairo, M.D.; Owoyokun, K. Factors affecting the utilization of antenatal care services in Ibadan, Nigeria. *Benin J. Postgrad. Med.* **2011**, *12*, 1–11. [CrossRef]
30. Denny, H.M.; Laksono, A.D.; Matahari, R.; Kurniawan, B. The Determinants of Four or More Antenatal Care Visits Among Working Women in Indonesia. *Asia Pac. J. Public Health* **2022**, *34*, 51–56. [CrossRef] [PubMed]
31. Ebonwu, J.; Mumbauer, A.; Uys, M.; Wainberg, M.L.; Medina-Marino, A. Determinants of late antenatal care presentation in rural and peri-urban communities in South Africa: A cross-sectional study. *PLoS ONE* **2018**, *13*, e0191903. [CrossRef]
32. Dahiru, T.; Oche, O.M. Determinants of antenatal care, institutional delivery and postnatal care services utilization in Nigeria. *Pan Afr. Med. J.* **2015**, *21*, 1–17. [CrossRef]
33. Rurangirwa, A.A.; Mogren, I.; Nyirazinyoye, L.; Ntaganira, J.; Krantz, G. Determinants of poor utilization of antenatal care services among recently delivered women in Rwanda; a population based study. *BMC Pregnancy Childbirth* **2017**, *17*, 142. [CrossRef]
34. Basha, G.W. Factors Affecting the Utilization of a Minimum of Four Antenatal Care Services in Ethiopia. *Obstet. Gynecol. Int.* **2019**, *2019*, 5036783. [CrossRef]
35. Tessema, Z.T.; Teshale, A.B.; Tesema, G.A.; Tamirat, K.S. Determinants of completing recommended antenatal care utilization in sub-Saharan from 2006 to 2018: Evidence from 36 countries using Demographic and Health Surveys. *BMC Pregnancy Childbirth* **2021**, *21*, 192. [CrossRef]
36. Chopra, I.; Juneja, S.K.; Sharma, S. Effect of maternal education on antenatal care utilization, maternal and perinatal outcome in a tertiary care hospital. *Int. J. Reprod. Contracept. Obstet. Gynecol.* **2018**, *8*, 247. [CrossRef]

37. Teklesilasie, W.; Deressa, W. Husbands' involvement in antenatal care and its association with women's utilization of skilled birth attendants in Sidama zone, Ethiopia: A prospective cohort study. *BMC Pregnancy Childbirth* **2018**, *18*, 315. [CrossRef] [PubMed]
38. Alenoghena, I.O.; Isah, E.C.; Isara, A.R. Maternal health services uptake and its determinants in public primary health care facilities in edo state, Nigeria. *Niger. Postgrad. Med. J.* **2015**, *22*, 25–31. [PubMed]
39. Maduka, O.; Ogu, R. Non-Utilization of antenatal care services among women of reproductive age in the Niger delta region of Nigeria: Findings from 2595 women. *Clin. Obstet. Gynecol. Reprod. Med.* **2018**, *4*, 1–5. [CrossRef]
40. Yaya, S.; Bishwajit, G.; Ekholuenetale, M.; Shah, V.; Kadio, B.; Udenigwe, O. Timing and adequate attendance of antenatal care visits among women in Ethiopia. *PLoS ONE* **2017**, *12*, e0184934. [CrossRef] [PubMed]
41. Sanogo, N.A.; Yaya, S. Wealth Status, Health Insurance, and Maternal Health Care Utilization in Africa: Evidence from Gabon. *BioMed Res. Int.* **2020**, *2020*, 4036830. [CrossRef] [PubMed]
42. Acharya, D.; Khanal, V.; Singh, J.K.; Adhikari, M.; Gautam, S. Impact of mass media on the utilization of antenatal care services among women of rural community in Nepal. *BMC Res. Notes* **2015**, *8*, 345. [CrossRef]
43. Fatema, K.; Lariscy, J.T. Mass media exposure and maternal healthcare utilization in South Asia. *SSM-Popul. Health* **2020**, *11*, 100614. [CrossRef]
44. Login, S. The DHS Program. DHS 2016:1–2. Available online: https://dhsprogram.com/What-We-Do/Survey-Types/DHS-Questionnaires.cfm (accessed on 25 August 2022).

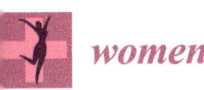

Article

Knowledge and Perception of Risk in Pregnancy and Childbirth among Women in Low-Income Communities in Accra

Patricia Anafi [1,*] and Wisdom Kwadwo Mprah [2]

[1] Department of Kinesiology and Health Sciences, College of Education and Health Professions, Columbus State University, Columbus, GA 31907, USA
[2] Centre for Disability and Rehabilitation Studies, Department of Health Promotion and Disability Studies, School of Public Health, Kwame Nkrumah University of Science and Technology, Kumasi PMB, Ghana
* Correspondence: anafi_patricia@columbusstate.edu; Tel.: +1-706-507-8506

Abstract: Perception and knowledge of risk factors for pregnancy influence health behaviors during pregnancy and childbirth. We used a descriptive qualitative study to examine the perception and knowledge of risk factors in pregnancy and childbirth in low-income urban women in Ghana. Over the course of three-months, 12 focus group discussions and six individual interviews were conducted with 90 participants selected from six communities in the study area. Data were analyzed using inductive-thematic content analysis. Findings revealed that participants had knowledge of some risk factors, although some had superstitious beliefs. Participants viewed pregnancy as an exciting and unique experience, but also challenging, with a host of medical and psychological risks. Pre-existing medical conditions (e.g., diabetes), lack of physical activity, poverty, poor nutrition, and lack of social support were identified as conditions that could lead to negative pregnancy outcomes. Superstitious beliefs such as exposure to "evil eye" during pregnancy, as well as curses and spells, were also identified as risk factors for pregnancy complications. This research has implications for policies and programs to improve pregnancy outcomes for low-income women in Ghana. Thus, we recommend social and economic support programs as well as health education to change misperceptions about pregnancy risk and to support other efforts being made to improve maternal health outcomes.

Keywords: perception; knowledge; risk in pregnancy; women; low-income communities

Citation: Anafi, P.; Mprah, W.K. Knowledge and Perception of Risk in Pregnancy and Childbirth among Women in Low-Income Communities in Accra. *Women* **2022**, *2*, 385–396. https://doi.org/10.3390/women2040035

Academic Editors: Claudio Costantino and Maiorana Antonio

Received: 17 October 2022
Accepted: 14 November 2022
Published: 22 November 2022

Publisher's Note: MDPI stays neutral with regard to jurisdictional claims in published maps and institutional affiliations.

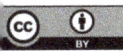

Copyright: © 2022 by the authors. Licensee MDPI, Basel, Switzerland. This article is an open access article distributed under the terms and conditions of the Creative Commons Attribution (CC BY) license (https://creativecommons.org/licenses/by/4.0/).

1. Introduction

Risk is defined as a factor that presents eminent danger or increases the probability of experiencing adverse outcomes [1,2]. Perception, on the other hand, refers to a mental image or subjective ideas about a potential occurrence of a phenomenon [3]. The concept of perception is important because it is a driver of health-seeking behavior and the management of health outcomes [4]. Risk perception, therefore, refers to risk interpretations or understanding, as well as subjective judgements about risk [2]. In the field of health, risk perception denotes subjective judgements about the likelihood of negative or adverse outcomes of conditions such as illnesses, injuries, diseases, or death. Perceptions and knowledge about risk are important determinants of health behaviors and risk-related decision-making, such as whether to adopt or not to adopt healthy behaviors and reject or accept a certain level of health risks [2,5].

Risk perception has two dimensions: the cognitive aspect, which relates to how much individuals know and understand risks; and the emotional aspect, which relates to how people feel about themselves and a potential risk [6]. Research on risk perception often begins with the presumption that how people feel about danger is determined by the level of knowledge and certainty they have regarding that risk. This idea is founded on the rational choice model of decision-making, which presents individuals as rational beings who evaluate the possibilities of health outcomes after first estimating the prospective costs and benefits. On the other hand, laypersons usually assess risk by using heuristics (for example, previous experiences) and other informal ways of thinking [2,7]. This means that, when people are aware of certain risks or potential risks, they tend to believe that those risks could happen more frequently than the risks actually occur, and vice versa. These risk misinterpretations, rooted in heuristics, can cause people to overestimate or underestimate the occurrence and severity of potential health threats [2].

According to Lennon [8], risk perception in pregnancy entails both the objective medical evaluation of risk as well as a subjective, socially constructed risk, guided by a complex web of personal, psychological, and cultural factors. It includes the assessment of the possibility of harm or negative health outcomes to either the mother or the newborn or both. However, sometimes this harm or risk is not related to a particular medical condition; instead, women may see pregnancy and childbirth as inherent risks rather than conditions that cause the risk. In recent years, risk perception and the way risks are construed in pregnancy have received a lot of scholarly attention [8]. This can be explained in part by the growing prevalence of a medicalized perspective on pregnancy and the social pressure placed on women to behave in a way that lessens the perceived risks [8]. Increasingly, medical interventions are seen as both necessary and desirable for successful pregnancies, as the state of pregnancy has become more and more medicalized. Thus, seeking preventive services such as antenatal screening, genetic screening, and testing, as well as health behavior modifications, are considered necessary to reduce any potential risk of pregnancy complications [8,9].

Furthermore, considerable evidence shows that perceptions and understanding (or knowledge) of risk are shaped by many factors, including socio-cultural background [10], levels of literacy [11], and religious or traditional beliefs [11,12]. An individual's knowledge and interpretation of risk is also dependent on their personal life philosophy and previous experience [9]. It has been documented that sometimes women perceive risk in relation to pregnancy from the social perspective, where risk is seen as being influenced by the social, cultural, and political milieu in which they reside [8,9]. Wheeler and colleagues [13], for example, reported women's employment experience during pregnancy as an important factor in determining their perception of risk in pregnancy. Furthermore, other scholars have reported that maternal age [14–16], personal and family history [17], knowledge about pregnancy and childbirth [18], as well as level of risk or complication in pregnancy [19] are important determinants of perception and understanding of risk in pregnancy. These factors can influence opinions, interpretations of and values put on the risks and even benefits associated with pregnancy [12]. In a qualitative study on pregnancy risk perception and preterm birth, Silva and colleagues [17] found that personal negative experiences in previous pregnancies, such as stillbirths, miscarriages, having a preterm birth or neonatal death, informed risk perceptions of the current pregnancy. Women's perception of risk in pregnancy has also been attributed to their knowledge-base of risk [20].

Perception and understanding of risk in pregnancy have the effect of influencing various critical pregnancy and childbirth decisions. They affect decisions such as when and where to seek antenatal care, where to give birth (or choice of maternity site), who supervises the birth and even the mode of delivery [8,21]. Silva and colleagues [17] also argued that a patient's risk perception of health guides his or her decisions on treatment and can further influence health-seeking behavior during serious conditions such as preterm births, one of the most critical potential risks faced during pregnancy. Janson [22], on childbirth decisions and traditional structures in Ghana, explained that women who viewed childbirth as a natural process, and without potential risks or ill health, may consider home delivery as the best option. Traditionally, in Ghanaian society, pregnancy and childbirth are viewed as a vulnerability and potentially dangerous experiences that do not only require biomedical care, but also spiritual intervention. Therefore, many women seek a combination of care: biomedical care, traditional care (which involves the use of herbal medicine) and spiritual support (faith healing and prayer) in the pregnancy period with the hope of averting any perceived or actual health risk to the pregnancy and during childbirth [23]. The focus of this paper, therefore, is to present findings from a study that investigated women's perception and knowledge of risk in pregnancy and childbirth, and how these affect their maternal healthcare seeking behavior in selected low-income communities in Accra. The implications of the findings for maternal and newborn health policies and programs are discussed.

2. Materials and Methods

2.1. Study Design

This was a descriptive qualitative study that targeted women in selected low-income communities in Accra, Ghana. The data were gathered over a three-month period through focus group discussions (FGDs) and interviews to examine women's perception and knowledge about risk in pregnancy and childbirth.

2.2. Study Area

The study was conducted in the Ashiedu-Keteke sub-metropolitan district in the city of Accra, Ghana's capital. Ashiedu-Keteke is one of the 3 sub-metropolitan districts of Accra Metropolitan City and has some of the poorest communities in the city. Using the Greater Accra region population growth of 3.1%, the sub-metropolis has an estimated population of about 143,990 in 2018 [24]. The sub-metropolis has the Central Business District (CBD), and it is the center of major commercial activities within the city of Accra, with an influx of approximately 2 million people from all parts of the country daily [24]. As the center of commerce, it houses the Markola and Agbogbloshie markets, which are two major markets within the Greater Accra region. The population of Ashiedu-Keteke is made up of the indigenous Ga people, who live in the coastal communities along the Gulf of Guinea (the Atlantic Ocean), and other migrant populations, who reside a bit further away from the coast. The main occupation of the indigenous Ga people is fishing; the men do the fishing, and the women smoke the fish for the market. The migrant population engages in small-scale commercial activities, mostly trading.

In terms of health care, the Ussher Polyclinic, the Prince Marie Louise Children's Hospital, and the James Town Maternity are among the major health facilities that provide care to residents in the sub-metropolitan district. Maternal health continues to be a health challenge as Ashiedu-Keteke has one of the poorest maternal health outcomes in Accra and has a persistently high teenage pregnancy rate in the city [25,26]. There is high prevalence of the use of informal maternal health care (traditional birth attendance, faith healing, and prayer) by pregnant women in the area, especially among the teenage and indigenous mothers. From available data, about 40% of pregnant women who reside in the sub metropolitan district do not seek antenatal care until the second and third trimesters, a situation quite a bit higher than the national average of 36% [27].

2.3. Sampling of Participants and Data Collection

Purposive sampling was utilized to select six communities within the study area for the FGDs and individual interviews. Altogether, 90 women between the ages of 17 and 45 years were recruited for 12 focus group discussions, and six individuals were involved in the interviews. For the FGDs, a snowball sampling approach was employed to recruit 84 women who had at least one child. We conducted two FGDs in each of the communities. We divided the women in the FGDs into two age cohorts: those aged 17 to 29 and those aged 30 to 45. Each FGD had an average of seven participants and lasted between 45–60 min. We conducted six FGDs with each age cohort. Additionally, six women with at least one child from each of the six communities (one mother from each community) were interviewed for about 30 min to elicit in-depth perspectives on the subject matter. Two community leaders assisted with the recruitment of the study participants.

The FGDs and individual interviews both used comparable questions, which were framed around our research objectives. We asked participants about their knowledge and risk perceptions with regard to pregnancy and childbirth and how these factors influenced their healthcare seeking decisions and behaviors during pregnancy and childbirth. Both

FGDs and interviews were carried out with the assistance of our two fieldworkers and in two local languages spoken in the study area. The two field assistants were native speakers of the two local languages (Ga and Twi). The FGDs and interviews were audio recorded with the participants' permission.

2.4. Ethical Consideration

The Human Subject Review Committee of the University of Massachusetts Amherst School of Public Health granted the ethical approval of the research. Additionally, we received authorization from the local health administration in the study area and verbal consent from all study participants prior to their enrollment in the study. Since most of our study participants had only a basic formal education, we only sought verbal consent from them prior to recruitment into the study and assured them that information obtained from the FGDs and interviews would be kept confidential, and only the lead researcher would have access to the raw data. Participation in the study was voluntary, and they had the option of withdrawing at any time.

2.5. Data Analysis

The data analysis began during the data collection phase and continued following FGDs and interview sessions. With the assistance of our two fieldworkers, audio recordings of both FGDs and interviews were transcribed from the local languages into English. Following transcription, we cross-checked the transcripts to confirm that the responses had been accurately transcribed and translated from the local languages to English. We reviewed the final transcripts in order to determine which words, phrases, and statements were pertinent to our primary research questions and objectives. We classified the data into nine themes using an inductive content analysis approach proposed by Corbin and Strauss [28] and Miles and colleagues [29].

We first identified and cataloged the major concepts and recurring ideas in each interview transcript. Second, we compared and classified the significant concepts and emerging themes from the interview transcripts. We did the same thing with the transcript data from the FGDs; we compared significant concepts and developing themes within and across FGDs. The raw text section containing the essential concepts and ideas were coded manually and classified according to the emergent themes. To ensure the findings' internal validity, we compared and contrasted data segments from the FGDs with the individual interviews [28,29]. In this article, we present data on nine themes that emerged from our analysis.

3. Results

The nine themes were identified as the following factors: first trimester experience; medical conditions; lack of physical activity; antenatal care; lack of social support; poverty and poor nutrition; sleeping posture and hot showers; exposure to certain conditions; and spells and curses.

3.1. First Trimester Experience

According to most of the participants, pregnancy during the first trimester period is associated with both joy and risk. The participants reported that the usual thought of being pregnant brings "joy" and "hope", but the experience during this period could be challenging for many women. Participants explained that during the first trimester, the pregnant woman is unable to eat, as she experiences general body weakness, morning sickness, fevers, severe headaches, dizziness, heart palpitations, and sleeplessness. Although these are normal, they could pose serious health risks to the woman during this period of the pregnancy. The women described psychological problems such as fears, anxiety, and stress that a woman could experience during early months of the pregnancy. Two participants explained it this way:

"When a woman is pregnant, she does not feel well as she used to be, the whole experience can make you feel sick and you know, this feeling of sickness can last during the whole pregnancy period for many women, the first three months can be hard on you, you become anxious and afraid ... " [FGD participant 1]

"In my case, I always felt like I was going to fall down in my early months. But this feeling happens to many pregnant women, so its normal to feel that way because your body is adjusting, it begins to go away after the third months for most pregnant women." [Interview participant 1]

3.2. Medical Conditions

Both FGD and interview participants were of the view that complications could occur in pregnancy when a pregnant woman already has "a pre-existing disease". They explained that pre-existing diseases or infections such as "malaria", "diabetes", candidiasis ("odeepu") or "HIV" can increase the vulnerability of a pregnant woman. This is because "it is not easy to carry a pregnancy when you are already sick or have a disease." [Interview participant 2] Having a chronic condition " ... like AIDS or sugar disease [diabetes] and becoming pregnant could be challenging as you don't sit at home. You will need to go to the clinic for regular and proper care." [FGD participant 2] These medical conditions could expose the woman to the risk of experiencing a difficult pregnancy, labor, and delivery, and could affect the baby's health as well.

According to the participants in the FGDs, other medical conditions indicating that the pregnant woman is at risk of complications are high blood pressure, swelling in the hands and feet, anemia, and delay in the delivery of the afterbirth or the placenta. Participants also mentioned bleeding during pregnancy and childbirth as a major health risk for the mother and the baby. These views were also expressed by the women in the individual interviews, as exemplified by a personal experience of an interview participant who said:

"I don't have an easy pregnancy. My second pregnancy was the worst of all. I had swollen feet and hands, and they [nurses] said my blood pressure was going up at some point, and I thought those were not good signs for my pregnancy, especially when they told me my pressure was going high and I had to come in for regular review." [Interview participant 3]

3.3. Lack of Physical Activity

Another risk factor identified was being physically inactive during pregnancy. According to some of the participants, a pregnant woman who is physically inactive or does not exercise could likewise be at risk for a difficult and prolonged labor, as explained in the following statement by an FGD participant.

"You see, there are pregnant women who don't do any work, they don't walk, they just sit at one place, and they stop coming to the market. But there are others who work with their pregnancy. They go to the farm and do everything. When you are not active, the baby will not be active. The baby cannot turn or move in the womb, and you will have problem during delivery ... " [FGD participant 3]

3.4. Antenatal Care

Most of the participants said women who do not seek medical care or attend antenatal clinics could be at risk of pregnancy complications. During the FGDs, participants recounted that a pregnant woman should seek regular health care to prevent potential complications that could affect the pregnancy and to ensure a successful birth. A participant in the FGDs noted, "a situation where the mother failed to seek antenatal screening for early risk detection and treatment, it leads to conditions such as fetal malpresentation or malposition, a critical condition for prolonged labor." [FGD participant 4]

Similar views were also shared by participants in the interviews, who identified prolonged labor as a risk a pregnant woman could be exposed to during childbirth if she fails to attend an antenatal clinic.

3.5. Lack of Social Support

According to the participants, pregnant women who do not have adequate spousal or family support could experience difficult pregnancy and childbirth because pregnancy could be stressful and emotionally demanding. As a result, if the pregnant woman is not adequately supported, it could negatively affect her health and that of the unborn baby. Two FGD participants explained the effect of a lack of social support on pregnancy outcomes in the quotation below.

> "I know a young woman that the man who made her pregnant refused to accept the pregnancy. Her parents are not living here [referring to her community] and she does not have any other family member in Accra here. The baby she delivered was very small. You know ... she didn't have any support; she was always by herself and only got a little help from neighbors and that affected the baby." [FGD participant 5]

> "Sometimes, these young mothers work long hours. The kayaye [teen girls head porters] who are pregnant ... they carry heavy loads in the market for people who come to shop or do groceries. They don't have their families or anybody here to help them ... It is stressful to do this kind of job when you are pregnant ... " [FGD participants 6]

These findings were corroborated by the interview participants who reported a lack of social support for young migrant pregnant women in the study area as a major risk factor for negative pregnancy outcomes. The following remark was made by a participant in support of this assertion, "when you go to the market right now, you see them [young female migrant porters] carrying big bowls full of load for people with their pregnancy. Some of them don't even know the fathers of their babies, and their parents are not here to help them, and this is not good for the pregnancy." [Interview participant 4]

3.6. Poverty and Poor Nutrition

Poverty emerged as an important risk factor for pregnancy and childbirth complications. Both FGDs and interview participants agreed that poverty could lead to poor nutrition among pregnant women, leading to poor pregnancy outcomes because "a pregnant woman should ensure she eats well, on time, and the right portions", which is a major problem for some women. According to the participants, some pregnant women "don't have the money to buy enough food" and that could affect their health and the pregnancy as well. A pregnant participant in one of the FGDs confirmed this and said, "the poor mothers who don't have families here, their general health begins to become worse after delivery. This is because when they go home, there is nothing there to eat and their babies cannot grow because they don't feed them well since they themselves don't eat well". [FGD Participant 7] According to some participants, the young pregnant migrant mothers who lived in the study area relied on neighbors for meals when they became pregnant. One FGD participant also put it this way:

> " ... if they don't get this assistance, they don't eat. Some pregnant mothers eat small portions of meal in the morning, and they don't eat until evening because they don't have families here [Accra] and the men who made them pregnant didn't accept the pregnancy." [FGD participant 8]

These findings were supported by some of the interview participants who said that the young pregnant migrant mothers usually worked for long hours, carrying heavy loads to make a living, and to save towards delivery, which exposes them to pregnancy-related risks. The quotation below highlights this issue.

"Oh, when you go there (markets) right now you will see them working in the market, they carry loads in the market. Some sell under the hot sun [and], this is not too good for the pregnancy, but they need the money, so they and their babies can have food to eat the weeks following delivery." [Interview participant 5]

Furthermore, most of the participants thought that poverty made it difficult for pregnant mothers to attend antenatal clinics and delayed care during labor, exposing the pregnant woman and the baby to life-threatening complications.

3.7. Sleeping Posture and Hot Showers

Both the FGDs and interview participants agreed that when a pregnant mother sleeps on her back, it can affect the health of the mother and the unborn baby. They explained that when a pregnant mother sleeps on her back, it obstructs the flow of oxygen from the mother to the unborn baby, and this could be fatal for the unborn baby as well as the mother.

"This [sleeping on your back during pregnancy] is not good for your pregnancy ... when you are pregnant, you don't sleep on your back. You sleep by your side. People (pregnant women) who sleep on their back can hurt their baby, the baby cannot breath because air will not flow from you the mother to your baby ... so they tell us not to sleep on our back. They are not good practice for the baby, so you can kill your baby because the baby cannot get air from your when you sleep on your back ... " [FGD participants 9]

Some participants also reported that taking hot water showers and baths could negatively affect the pregnancy. Two participants explained:

" ... they say bathing with hot water is not good, warm water is okay ... hot water is not good for the baby too. It can make the baby temperature go up" [Interview participant 4]

"Bathing with hot water can make you the mother feel hot ... and you can pass heat on to the baby in your womb, so you don't take hot showers when you are pregnant." [FGD participants 10]

3.8. Exposure to Certain Conditions

One major perceived risk in pregnancy mentioned by the participants is the exposure of the unborn baby to conditions that can cause the child to acquire certain health defects such as cerebral palsy (called "asram" in the local language). This often happens if the pregnant woman does not take "very good care" of herself and her pregnancy. For example, if the pregnant woman does not dress well, she could expose herself and her pregnancy (unborn baby) to individuals with such conditions. This is based on the belief that cerebral palsy is transferrable spiritually from a person who has the condition to the mother, and then to the baby to be born. "Asram" is a spiritual disease that can be passed on through eye contact when a pregnant mother comes into contact with an individual who spreads the disease. One interview participant elaborated on this perception in the following quotation.

"For a disease like asram, when you are pregnant you don't have to eat everywhere. When some people see the pregnancy, they can transfer the disease to the unborn baby. You have to dress decently, so that you don't expose yourself and your pregnancy. Some people dress exposing their body when they are pregnant . . . . . . So when you dress like that and you come across someone with the disease, that individual can transfer the disease to the baby." [Interview participant 4]

Some participants also reported that cerebral palsy can kill, and that it can only be treated with traditional or herbal medicine. For example, during the FGDs, one mother recounted her experience with "asram", "it [asram] affected me and my baby, and I was taken to a certain woman for herbal treatment for almost a year before my baby was ok." [FGD participant 11].

3.9. Spells and Curses

Participants also narrated that a woman can be at risk of pregnancy complications and/or even death if she is cursed during pregnancy. According to most FGD participants, when a pregnant woman is disrespectful or often picks quarrels with neighbors, a curse could be cast on her, and this may lead to stillbirth and death during childbirth. This view was confirmed by a participant in the interviews in the following remarks:

> " . . . do you know that evil people can harm your pregnancy? They can cast a curse spell on you and your unborn baby, so the young pregnant women here who like quarreling and fighting, some ended up having a difficulty childbirth." [Interview participant 4]

This finding was supported by other participants who spoke of some young pregnant mothers visiting spiritual churches to seek protection for fear the effects of curses by people they might have wronged.

> "They [young pregnant mothers] go the spiritual churches to pray for successful pregnancy because they are afraid somebody that they have quarreled with or disrespected might have cursed them and the pregnancy." [FGD participants 12]

4. Discussion

Although the findings from this study do not represent the views of all Ghanaian women, they provide some insight into the general perception and knowledge of risk factors for negative pregnancy and childbirth outcomes among women in Ghana. The findings indicated that participants view pregnancy as an exciting and unique experience; however, they acknowledged the risks, both medical and spiritual, associated with it. This perception of risk could serve as a motivation for women to adopt positive health-seeking behaviors such as attending antenatal clinics, exercising, and eating good food during pregnancy. However, this perception of risk can also induce serious emotional experiences such as fear, anxiety, and stress that will require both informal and professional support. On the contrary, it seems that some women in the study area were not adequately receiving this support during pregnancy. This might be one of the reasons why maternal health outcomes in the study area are reported to be poor [26]. The findings of the study are consistent with previous studies where women were found to hold such perceptions of risks [30–32]. Anxiety and fear due to perceived risks in pregnancy and childbirth, such as prolonged and painful labor, lack of social support, as well as economic uncertainty, leading to stress, were identified among women in studies by Erickson et al. [33], Lyberg and Severinson [34], and Saisto and Halmesmaki [35]. Thus, pregnancy risk perceptions among pregnant women can affect their health and health care decisions and treatment options [17].

The findings that women perceived a lack of social support as a risk factor for pregnancy is relevant. As confirmed by previous studies, people with a high quality or quantity of social networks and economic stability have a decreased risk of mortality in comparison with those who have a low quality or quantity of social network engagement and are economically unstable [36–38]. In pregnancy, in particular, Hotelling and colleagues [39] found that women with continuous support, either emotionally or socially, were less likely to have complications in pregnancy that could lead to Caesarean deliveries than those without any support. Likewise, evidence from Ghana indicated that lack of support from friends and extended family, being abandoned by one's husband, and being compelled to live with unfriendly in-laws are risk factors that could expose pregnant women to psychological problems during pregnancy [12].

Several studies have illustrated that poor women are at higher risk of food insufficiency, insecurity, and poor feeding practices, leading to malnutrition and maternal morbidity [40–42]. Poverty hinders access to sufficient and nutritious food, and at the same time, acts as a barrier to accessing quality and timely maternal health care [43,44]. In Kenya, for example, Izugbara and Ngilangwa [45] found that poverty compelled pregnant women in slums to engage in tedious work for long hours in order to save enough money for delivery, risking their lives. Women in our study shared similar views regarding young migrant pregnant women who carry heavy loads and work longer hours for a living and in preparation for delivery.

The findings showed that participants had knowledge of some common medical risks associated with negative pregnancy outcomes in Ghana. In Ghana, like many other tropical countries, malaria is endemic, and it is known to be a major contributing factor to stillbirths [46,47]. Medical conditions such as diabetes, candidiasis, high blood pressure, HIV, anemia, and delayed placenta as well as lack of physical activity are also risk factors that were identified as dangers to pregnancy and childbirth. These findings are consistent with a study conducted in Kenya where participants identified similar conditions as threats to positive pregnancy outcomes [48].

Our participants had a strong belief in religious-spiritual factors such as curses as risk factors in pregnancy. These beliefs are rooted in the community and are not only widespread among Ghanaians, but also exist in many cultures in sub-Saharan Africa. This belief has an influence on health care choices and decisions during pregnancy and childbirth and motivates most women to resort to herbal medicine, spiritual care (faith healing and prayer), or a combination of medical and traditional treatments during pregnancy [12,49]. In rural Zimbabwe, for example, it has been discovered that women fear being bewitched because they are thought to be vulnerable to witchcraft in the early months of pregnancy. As such, they preferred to seek protection from faith healers who are believed to possess supernatural powers to protect them and their pregnancy [50]. Similar findings have also been observed in studies in Southern America [51] and indigenous Pilipino in Southeast Asia [52]. Interestingly, this notion, according to the authors, is parallel to the biomedical perspective, which describes the early months of pregnancy as the most critical period. Unlike in many western cultures, women in Ghana fully cover their pregnancy during the entire pregnancy period. This practice is believed to protect the pregnancy from a curse, spell, or witchcraft [53].

5. Implications

As governments are making efforts to address the challenges of poor maternal health outcomes, the need for research that has practical applications is essential. Our findings revealed many issues that are relevant for maternal and child healthcare policies and programs for low-income women in Ghana. First, the findings suggest that many pregnant women go through psychological issues during pregnancy due to the perceived risks associated with it. Although medical interventions such as antenatal care are important during pregnancy, psychological support is equally important. Pregnancy induces physical and emotional change and increases the risk of mental illness [54]. Psychological support for women during pregnancy is therefore very important for positive outcomes. The Ministry of Health, in consultation with other relevant stakeholders such as the department of Social Welfare, should consider the implementation of social and emotional support programs that can help to alleviate the emotional stress of pregnant women, especially for poor and single women. Counseling units, specifically focusing on pregnant women, could be set up at the maternal and childcare units of health care centers to support women who need help.

Second, the belief that pregnant women could be cursed has implications for safe motherhood policies and programs in Ghana. As the findings indicated, some pregnant women use traditional medical practitioners, including faith healers, due to the belief that they could be cursed. This does not promote safe motherhood practices and should be addressed. Public health education must focus on explaining to women and communities the risk and non-risk factors associated with pregnancy and childbirth, as well as correcting misperceptions that may have a negative impact on pregnancy outcomes.

Third, the impact of poverty was a major risk factor identified by the participants. Current socio-economic conditions in the country are having dire consequences on the poor, and this could seriously affect Ghana's quest to achieve its Sustainable Development Goal 1. Poverty among women needs serious attention through protective social interventions. The Ministry of Health and Ministry of Gender, Children and Social Protection could partner with community organizations, including churches and other religious groups, to augment government efforts to reduce poverty among deprived communities.

6. Conclusions

The findings of the study revealed that low-income urban women in Ghana have a wide range of knowledge and perceptions of risk factors for negative pregnancy and childbirth outcomes. The women viewed pregnancy as a unique experience, but they acknowledged that it could be affected by a host of medical and non-medical issues, which could lead to adverse pregnancy outcomes, including negatively affecting the health of the mother and the baby. Though the study focused on urban women, these risk perceptions and knowledge about pregnancy and childbirth are held by many Ghanaian women. The findings also suggest that despite efforts being made to reduce maternal morbidity and mortality in Ghana, many pregnant women are still at risk of pregnancy-related complications. This study therefore brings to the fore the need to employ multiple approaches to safe motherhood programs—social, economic, religious, and psychological—to help poor pregnant women. While these activities will reduce barriers to quality maternal healthcare, health education should be ramped up to address superstitious beliefs as well as cultural misperceptions about pregnancy risk factors.

Author Contributions: P.A. was the lead investigator; led the research design, data collection and analysis. P.A. and W.K.M. prepared the original manuscript, reviewed, and edited. All authors have read and agreed to the published version of the manuscript.

Funding: This research was funded by Compton Foundation International Dissertation Fellowship.

Institutional Review Board Statement: The study was conducted in accordance with the Declaration of Helsinki and approved by the Institutional Review Boards (or Ethics Committees) of University of Massachusetts-Amherst School of Public Health [SPHHS-HSRC file # 10:35].

Informed Consent Statement: Verbal informed consent was obtained from all subjects involved in the study. Additionally, authorization was granted from the sub metropolitan district health administration to conduct the research.

Data Availability Statement: The study data are available upon request from the corresponding author and with approval from the author's institution's Research Ethics Committee.

Acknowledgments: Authors profound gratitude goes to David R. Buchanan in the School of Public Health and Health Sciences at the University of Massachusetts-Amherst who supervised the original research. We also acknowledge our research participants and two field research assistants.

Conflicts of Interest: The authors declare that they have no conflict of interest.

References

1. Rajbanshi, S.; Norhayati, M.N.; Nik Hazlina, N.H. Risk perceptions among high-risk pregnant women in Nepal: A qualitative study. *BMC Pregnancy Childbirth* **2021**, *21*, 539. [CrossRef] [PubMed]
2. Paek, H.; Hove, T. Risk perceptions and risk characteristics. In *Oxford Research Encyclopedia of Communication*; Oxford University Press: Oxford, UK, 2017. [CrossRef]
3. Merriam-Webster Dictionary. Dictionary by Merriam-Webster: America's Most-Trusted Online Dictionary. Available online: https://www.merriam-webster.com/ (accessed on 2 March 2022).
4. McDonald, S.; Rishby, J.; Li, S.; de Sousa, A.; Dimoska, A.; James, C.; Tate, R.; Togher, L. The influence of attention and arousal on emotion perception in adults with severe traumatic brain injury. *Int. J. Psychophysiol.* **2011**, *82*, 124–131. [CrossRef] [PubMed]
5. Heaman, M.; Gupton, A.; Gregory, D. Factors influencing pregnant women's perceptions of risk. *Am. J. Matern. Child Nurs.* **2004**, *29*, 111–116. [CrossRef] [PubMed]
6. Slovic, P. (Ed.) *The Perception of Risk*; Earthscan: Sterling, VA, USA, 2000.
7. Kahneman, D.; Slovic, P.; Tversky, A. *Judgement under Uncertainty: Heuristics and Biases*; Cambridge University Press: Cambridge, UK, 1982.
8. Lennon, S.L. Risk perception in pregnancy: A concept analysis. *J. Adv. Nurs.* **2016**, *72*, 2016–2029. [CrossRef]

9. Carolan, M.C. Towards understanding the concept of risk for pregnant women: Some nursing and midwifery implications. *J. Clin. Nurs.* **2009**, *18*, 652–658. [CrossRef] [PubMed]
10. Kim, J.S.; Choi, J.S. Middle East respiratory syndrome-related knowledge, preventive behaviours and risk perception among nursing students during outbreak. *J. Clin. Nurs.* **2016**, *25*, 2542–2549. [CrossRef]
11. Agus, Y.; Horiuchi, S.; Porter, S.E. Rural Indonesia women' traditional belief about antenatal care. *BMC Res. Notes* **2012**, *5*, 589. [CrossRef]
12. Dako-Gyeke, P.; Aiken, M.; Aryeetey, R.; Mccough, L.; Adongo, P.B. The influence of socio-cultural interpretations of pregnancy threats on health-seeking behavior among pregnant women in urban Accra, Ghana. *BMC Pregnancy Childbirth* **2013**, *13*, 211. [CrossRef]
13. Wheeler, S.M.; Massengale, K.E.C.; Adewumi, K.; Fitzgerald, T.A.; Dombeck, C.B.; Swezey, T.; Swamy, G.T.; Corneli, A. Pregnancy vs. paycheck: A qualitative study of patient's experience with employment during pregnancy at high risk for preterm birth. *BMC Pregnancy Childbirth* **2020**, *20*, 565. [CrossRef]
14. Bayrampour, H.; Heaman, M.; Duncan, K.A.; Tough, S. Advanced maternal age and risk perception: A qualitative study. *BMC Pregnancy Childbirth* **2012**, *12*, 100. [CrossRef]
15. Radon-Pokracka, M.; Adrianowicz, B.; Plonka, M.; Danil, P.; Nowk, M.; Huras, H. Evaluation of pregnancy outcomes at advanced maternal age. *Maced. J. Med. Sci.* **2019**, *7*, 1951–1956. [CrossRef] [PubMed]
16. Sangrin, S.; Phonkusol, C. Perception of pregnancy risk and related obstetric factors among women of advanced maternal age. *Pac. Rim Int. J. Nurs. Res.* **2021**, *25*, 494–504.
17. Silva, T.V.; Bento, S.F.; Katz, L.; Pacagnella, R.C. "Preterm birth risk, me?" Women risk perception about premature delivery—A qualitative analysis. *BMC Pregnancy Childbirth* **2021**, *21*, 633. [CrossRef] [PubMed]
18. Londeree, J.; Nguyen, N.; Nguyen, L.H.; Tran, D.H.; Gall, M.F. Underestimation of pregnancy risk among women in Vietnam. *BMC Women's Health* **2020**, *20*, 159. [CrossRef]
19. Lee, S. Risk perception in women with high-risk pregnancies. *Br. J. Midwifery* **2014**, *22*, 8–13. [CrossRef]
20. Lee, S.; Holden, D.; Webb, R.; Ayers, S. Pregnancy related risk perception in pregnant women, midwives & doctors: A cross-sectional study. *BMC Pregnancy Childbirth* **2019**, *19*, 335.
21. Regan, M.; McElory, K. Women perceptions of childbirth risk and place of birth. *J. Clin. Ethics* **2013**, *24*, 239–252.
22. Janson, I. Decision making in childbirth: The influence of traditional structures in a Ghanaian village. *Int. Nurs. Rev.* **2006**, *53*, 41–46. [CrossRef]
23. Anafi, P.; Mprah, W.K.; Buchanan, D.R.; Gubrium, A.C.; Faulkingham, R.; Barton-Burke, M. Motivations for preference for non-formal maternal health care in low-income communities in urban Ghana. *Int. J. Health Sci.* **2016**, *4*, 1–10.
24. Accra Metropolitan Assembly. 2022. Available online: https://ama.gov.gh/ (accessed on 12 August 2022).
25. Brain, L.E.; Zweekhorst, M.B.M.; Amoako-Coleman, M.; Muftugil-Yalcin, S.; Abejirinde, I.O.; Becquet, R.; Buning, T. To keep or not to keep. Decision making in adolescent pregnancy in Jamestown, Ghana. *PLoS ONE* **2019**, *14*, e0221789. [CrossRef]
26. Greater Accra Regional Health Directorate, 2018 Annual Health Reviews. Unpublished Annual Report. Ghana Health Service.
27. Ghana Statistical Service (GSS); Ghana Health Service (GHS); ICF. *Ghana Maternal Health Survey Report 2017*; Ghana Statistical Service; Ghana Ministry of Health: Accra, Ghana; Demographic & Health Survey Program/ICF: Rockville, MD, USA, 2018.
28. Corbin, J.; Strauss, A. *Basics of Qualitative Research*, 3rd ed.; Sage Publications: Los Angeles, CA, USA, 2008.
29. Miles, M.B.; Huberman, A.M.; Saldana, J. *Qualitative Data Analysis. A Method Sourcebook*, 4th ed.; Sage Publications: Los Angeles, CA, USA, 2019.
30. Hadfield, K.; Akyirem, S.; Sartori, L.; Abdul-Latif, A.; Akaateba, D.; Bayrampour, H.; Daly, A.; Hadfield, K.; Abiiro, G.A. Measurement of pregnancy-related anxiety worldwide: A systematic review. *BMC Pregnancy Childbirth* **2022**, *22*, 331. [CrossRef] [PubMed]
31. Bright, K.S.; Premji, S.S. Cross-cultural perspectives of pregnancy-related anxiety. In *Pregnancy-Related Anxiety: Theory, Research and Practice*, 1st ed; Dryer, R., Brunton, R., Eds.; Routledge: London, UK, 2021; pp. 143–157.
32. Rubertsson, C.; Hellstrom, J.; Cross, M.; Sydsjo, G. Anxiety in early pregnancy: Prevalence and contributing factors. *Arch. Women's Ment. Health* **2014**, *17*, 221–228. [CrossRef] [PubMed]
33. Erickson, C.; Westman, G.; Hamberg, K. Experiential factors associated with child-birth related fear in Swedish women and men. A population-based study. *J. Psychosom. Obstet. Gynecol.* **2005**, *26*, 325–329.
34. Lyberg, A.; Severinson, E. Fear of childbirth: Mothers' experiences of team-midwifery care- a follow-up study. *J. Nurs. Manag.* **2010**, *18*, 383–390. [CrossRef]
35. Saisto, T.; Halmesmåki, E. Fear of Childbirth: A Neglected Dilemma. *Acta Obstet. Et Gynecol. Scand.* **2003**, *82*, 201–208. [CrossRef]
36. Ng, F.; Trauer, T.; Dodd, S.; Callaly, T.; Campbell, S.; Berk, M. The validity of the 21-Items version of the Depression Anxiety Stress Scales as a routine clinical outcome measure. *Acta Neuropsychiatr.* **2007**, *19*, 304–310. [CrossRef]
37. Richmond, A.M.; Ross, N.A.; Egeland, G.M. Social support and thriving health: A new approach to understanding the health of indigenous Canadians. *Am. J. Public Health* **2007**, *97*, 1827–1833. [CrossRef]
38. Surkan, P.J.; Rådestad, I.; Cnattingius, S.; Steineck, G.; Dickman, P.W. Social support after stillbirth for prevention of maternal depression. *Acta Obstet. Et Gynecol. Scand.* **2009**, *88*, 1358–1364. [CrossRef]
39. Hotelling, B.; Amis, D.; Green, J.; Sakala, C. Care practices that promote normal birth #3: Continuous labor support. *J. Perinat. Educ.* **2004**, *13*, 16–22.

40. Abdu, J.; Kahssay, M.; Gebremedhin, M. Household food insecurity, underweight status, and associated characteristics among women of reproductive age group in Assayita district, Afar regional state, Ethiopia. *J. Environ. Public Health* **2018**, *2018*, 7659204. [CrossRef]
41. Dupuis, S.; Hennink, M.; Wendt, A.S.; Waid, J.L.; Kalam, M.A.; Gabrysch, S.; Sinharoy, S.S. Women's empowerment through homestead food production in rural Bangladesh. *BMC Public Health* **2022**, *22*, 234. [CrossRef] [PubMed]
42. Horwood, C.; Haskins, L.; Hinton, R.; Connolly, C.; Luthuli, S.; Rollins, N. Addressing the interaction between food insecurity, depression risk and informal work: Findings of a cross-sectional survey among informal women workers with young children in South Africa. *BMC Women's Health* **2021**, *21*, 2.
43. Habibov, N.N. On the socio-economic determinants of antenatal care utilization in Azerbaijan: Evidence and policy implications for reforms. *Health Econ. Policy Law* **2010**, *10*, 1–29. [CrossRef]
44. Houweling, T.A.J.; Ronsmans, C.; Campbell, O.M.R.; Kunst, A.E. Huge poor–rich inequalities in maternity care: An international comparative study of maternity and child care in developing countries. *Bull. World Health Organ.* **2007**, *85*, 745–754. [CrossRef]
45. Izugbara, C.O.; Ngilangwe, D. Women, poverty and adverse maternal outcomes in Nairobi, Kenya. *BMC Women's Health* **2010**, *10*, 33. [CrossRef]
46. Chua, M.C.; Ben-Amor, K.; Lay, C.; Neo, A.G.E.; Chiang, W.C.; Rao, R.; Chew, C.; Chaithongwongwatthana, S.; Khemapech, N.; Knol, J.; et al. Effect of symbiotic on the gut microbiota of cesarean delivered infants: A randomized, double-blind, multicenter study. *J. Pediatr. Gastroenterol. Nutr.* **2017**, *65*, 102–106. [CrossRef]
47. Elphinstone, R.E.; Weckman, A.M.; McDonald, C.R.; Tran, V.; Zhong, K.; Mwayiwawo, M.; Kalilani-Phiri, L.; Khairallah, C.; Taylor, S.M.; Meshnick, S.R.; et al. Early malaria infection, dysregulation of angiogenesis, metabolism and inflammation across pregnancy, and risk of preterm birth in Malawi: A cohort study. *PLoS Med.* **2019**, *16*, e1002914. [CrossRef]
48. Magadi, M. Poor pregnancy outcomes among adolescents in South Nyanza region of Kenya. *Afr. J. Reprod. Health* **2006**, *10*, 26–38. [CrossRef]
49. Sackey, B. Faith healing and women's reproductive health. *Res. Rev.* **2002**, *18*, 5–12. [CrossRef]
50. Mathole, T.; Lindmark, G.; Majoko, F.; Ahlberg, B.M. A qualitative study of women's perspectives of antenatal care in a rural area of Zimbabwe. *Midwifery* **2004**, *20*, 122–132. [CrossRef]
51. Jesse, D.E.; Schoneboom, C.; Blanchard, A. The effect of faith or spirituality in pregnancy: A content analysis. *J. Holist. Nurs.* **2007**, *25*, 151–158. [CrossRef] [PubMed]
52. Abad, P.J.B.; Tan, M.L.; Baluyot, M.M.P.; Villa, A.Q.; Talapian, G.L.; Reyes, M.E.; Suarez, R.C.; Sur, A.L.D.; Aldemita, V.D.R.; Padilla, C.D.; et al. Cultural beliefs on diseases causation in the Philippines: Challenges and implications in genetic counseling. *J. Community Genet.* **2014**, *5*, 399–407. [CrossRef] [PubMed]
53. Anafi, P. Understanding Maternal Health Care Seeking Behavior in Low-Income Communities in Accra, Ghana. Ph.D. Thesis, Graduate School of the University of Massachusetts Amherst, Amherst, MA, USA, 2012. Available from Proquest. AAI3518207. Available online: https://scholarworks.umass.edu/dissertations/AAI3518207 (accessed on 3 August 2022).
54. Bedaso, A.; Adams, J.; Peng, W.; Sibbritt, D. The relationship between social support and mental health problems during pregnancy: A systematic review and meta-analysis. *BMC Reprod. Health* **2021**, *18*, 162. [CrossRef] [PubMed]

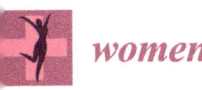

Article

Support Needs for Anxiety among Pregnant Women in Japan: A Qualitative Pilot Study

Ritsuko Shirabe [1,*], Tsuyoshi Okuhara [2], Hiroko Okada [2], Eiko Goto [2] and Takahiro Kiuchi [2]

1. Department of Health Communication, Graduate School of Medicine, The University of Tokyo, Tokyo 113-8655, Japan
2. Department of Health Communication, School of Public Health, Graduate School of Medicine, The University of Tokyo, Tokyo 113-8655, Japan
* Correspondence: rshirabe-tky@umin.ac.jp; Tel.: +81-3-5800-9754

Abstract: Support needs for pregnancy-related anxiety among low-risk pregnant women remain unclear. This study aimed to clarify the kinds of support for anxiety that women seek during pregnancy in Japan. Data were collected in a semi-structured focus group interview involving five pregnant women who were not in specific risk groups, recruited from three facilities in Tokyo. We generated themes using inductive thematic analysis. This paper adhered to the consolidated criteria for reporting qualitative research. From the data on support needs for anxiety during pregnancy, three themes were derived: (1) seeking tailored professional support; (2) seeking continuous support within informal relationships; and (3) seeking others' success stories in the same situation. These three types of support gave participants a sense of reassurance or raised concern, depending on the situation. We proposed a model comprising the three derived themes using social cognitive theory. We discussed how these three types of support influenced pregnant women's self-efficacy, which is the core concept of the social cognitive theory. Our findings may help to plan theory-based research and effective interventions to provide support for women's anxiety during pregnancy using a population approach. Our results also demonstrated the importance of collaboration with pregnant women in developing further research and interventions.

Keywords: pregnancy; pregnancy-related anxiety; needs assessment; social support; self-efficacy; social cognitive theory; qualitative study; health communication

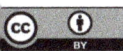

1. Introduction

Maternal mental health problems have become a major issue worldwide. Japan is no exception, as 10–20% of mothers become depressed after childbirth [1] and many more experience milder symptoms than depression. Support for maternal mental health should start from the antenatal period because more than one in five pregnant women experience anxiety or depression symptoms during pregnancy [2], which can predict the deterioration of their mental health in the following postpartum period [3]. Support during pregnancy may also be beneficial in terms of the feasibility of seamless care, because pregnant women in Japan can receive about fourteen antenatal checkups at public expense [4] and have opportunities to meet with specialists during pregnancy rather than postpartum.

To consider perinatal maternal mental health, numerous studies have explored psychosocial factors, such as parenting stress and social support. There is evidence that social support, which is considered an environmental factor in social cognitive theory [5], may be a major protective factor against perinatal anxiety and depression [6–11]. This theory has previously been used in the context of perinatal mental health problems [12–14]. In this theory, self-efficacy is the core concept for cognitive factors and interacting with environmental and behavioral factors [5], with one study indicating that self-efficacy for nurturing mediated the association between social support and postnatal depression [14]. However, we cannot ignore the negative aspects of social support, because support that did not meet needs was associated with an increased likelihood of postnatal depression [15]. Therefore, we should improve our understanding of the needs of pregnant women to ensure the provision of effective support in terms of mental health.

Multiple factors can lead to perinatal mental disorders, and it is difficult to identify high-risk individuals; therefore, a universal approach for preventing the deterioration of maternal mental health that extends beyond identified-risk groups is crucial. Previous qualitative studies have explored and clarified needs in medical situations among pregnant women, leading to one review which indicated that routine antenatal services might help only a small proportion of what matters to pregnant women without identified risks [16]. If routine antenatal services are not enough to help pregnancy-related anxiety, it is important to identify what kind of support pregnant women seek and what level of satisfaction and dissatisfaction they have in their daily lives in terms of their anxiety; however, at the present time, such details remain unclear.

We conducted this pilot study to explore pregnancy-related anxiety and support needs for anxieties among women residing in Japan, regardless of their specific risks. We believe these findings may be useful to conduct further quantitative studies and generate instruments or programs for a universal intervention to support pregnant women in Japan in the future.

2. Results

2.1. Participants' Characteristics

The participants' mean age was 31.8 years (range 27–36 years), and the mean gestational period was 28 weeks (range 23–33 weeks) at the time of the interview. Four of the five women were expecting their first baby. All participants were married and living with their husbands. All participants had completed university education and were working (Table 1).

Table 1. Participants' characteristics.

Participant	Age (Years)	GA (Weeks)	Facility	Number of Deliveries	Number of Abortions	IVF	Job	Education	Economic Comfort	Prenatal Class	Deliver at Same Facility	Risk
A	34	31	Hospital	0	0	Yes	Full-time worker	University	Some	Yes	Yes	NA
B	29	24	University hospital	0	0	No	Full-time worker	University	Not much	No	Yes	Been abused
C	33	33	Clinic	0	2	Yes	Contract worker	University	Not much	Yes	No	Fibroid
D	36	23	Hospital	1	3	No	Full-time worker	University	Not much	No	Yes	NA
E	27	31	Clinic	0	0	No	Full-time worker	University	Not much	Yes	No	NA

GA, gestational age; IVF, in vitro fertilization.

Participants expressed various anxieties based on their personal background and by hearing other participants' narratives. Table A1 shows the coded anxieties of this focus group.

2.2. Support Needs

We found three themes that described women's support needs for anxiety during pregnancy.
1. Seeking tailored professional support;
2. Seeking continuous support within informal relationships;
3. Seeking others' success stories in the same situation.

Table 2 shows the three derived themes with supporting quotes. The women's positive affects, derived from having received support that met their needs or was more than they expected, were coded as positive examples. Experiences where support for their needs was lacking (including negative affects caused by the support they received) were coded as negative examples.

Table 2. Themes and supporting quotes.

Themes	Affect	Supporting Quotes [1]
Seeking tailored professional support	Positive	Well ... the doctor at the clinic, and also the nurses and the receptionists, I like the way they behave towards myself, and I go to the checkups every time with a good feeling, well, I think I feel this way maybe because there is nothing wrong with my baby now, but I am very thankful that I can go to the checkups with a happy feeling. (Participant C)
	Negative	Well, as it turned out, it was okay, but should I search on Google? I didn't get much guidance on what and how much I should do in detail ... so I was a bit confused. (Participant B)
Seeking continuous support within informal relationships	Positive	Well, now that I'm on maternity leave, I have more time to spare, so I've been going to see my friends around me ... well, just going to see friends like who have children or who have recently born babies, well ... listening their opinions or ... I wonder ... just by talking with them, yes, I think I was able to relieve a lot of my worries. (Participant A)
	Negative	Well ... when I was pregnant with my first child, my husband always said something like that it would be fine if the baby was born healthy and without a physical defect, but that made me feel really anxious, and I thought "Please don't say things like that anymore." (Participant D)
Seeking others' success stories in the same situation	Positive	Let me see ... I did a lot of research on the Internet in English and so on, to find people who experienced bleeding, and when ... I read the stories of people who had done well, I was a little relieved ... (Participant B)
	Negative	There's a lot of information on the Internet that says [your partner] should quit smoking, but if I force him to do so, it might cause discord in my family, that's one of the things that happens ... so, in that respect, I recently would like to know positive feedback like what measures are taken by those who have husbands who smoke, or how their children grew up well even though they could only get this level of cooperation. (Participant E)

[1] Participants' narratives were translated into English for this publication.

2.2.1. Theme 1: Seeking Tailored Professional Support

In the professional sector, participants did not expect experts to only be involved with them in a manualized way. They wanted experts to see them not as "a pregnant woman" but as "myself". This did not have to involve difficult technology, as participants indicated that simple measures such as a friendly attitude toward "me", talking to "me", or listening to "my" minor physical problems and gaining a sense of the professionals' involvement was helpful.

In fact, it's like ... when I gave birth, the people around me were ... well ... only the midwives and the doctors, so I felt very reassured, and the doctors and midwives who were there and kept calling out to me were of course much more powerful than the stories I had heard. That's right. It was very reassuring. (Participant D)

Participants also expressed concerns about the professional sector, such as unclear explanations by medical professionals, uncertainty, and lack of options that allowed them to focus on their values, even if there was insufficient evidence. Beyond the manual or guideline, they needed guidance on how to bridge the gap between the scientific evidence of "correct answers" and their own real-world situations.

I tried to talk to a nurse or a doctor at the hospital about such things [partner's smoking], but all they said was that I should definitely stop him from smoking ... (Participant E)

2.2.2. Theme 2: Seeking Continuous Support within Informal Relationships

All participants agreed on the value of the existence of continued support within informal relationships. They especially valued support from people from the same generation who had previously experienced pregnancy or childbirth. Because of their high expectation of such support, one participant expressed concern about the lack of it.

> I don't have any friends who are pregnant or have children, so I don't really have anyone to talk to about something . . . like events during pregnancy, I guess I'm a little nervous about it. (Participant B)

Participants could get new information and felt reassured by just talking within such relationships without any specific purpose. Participants indicated they could talk easily and honestly within such relationships about what they hesitated to talk to experts about (e.g., weight gain during pregnancy and fear of childbirth).

> When I'm in the hospital, I feel a bit rushed and I don't feel like I can take my time to talk to the doctor, so I tend to ask [another] mother who is ahead of me such things about the pain of childbirth and daily life after childbirth. (Participant C)

Participants also reported encountering unexpected information or messages within informal relationships that they did not want.

> My number of gestational weeks is now 33, so I can't run any more tests of a definitive diagnosis at this week, well, like NIPT (noninvasive prenatal genetic testing). I'll tell you what . . . oh, I guess I should have taken it, although I can't take it anymore, when I've heard that my friend who is also pregnant got it, I was a little worried that maybe I should have taken the test, well, I made my own decision, but I think I [will] have anxiety about whether my decision was right all the way until my baby is born. (Participant C)

In particular, they valued support from their friends and relatives rather than cohabiting family, perhaps because they wanted "reasonable" nosiness. Some participants felt worried and anxious about the excessive involvement or indifferent attitudes of partners.

> My husband is a smoker, and we've talked about it, but the results haven't been to my satisfaction . . . (Participant E)

2.2.3. Theme 3: Seeking Others' Success Stories in the Same Situation

Most participants sought information about "success stories" of other people in the same situation, especially in their trouble. To seek this support, they often chose sources that did not have limitations in terms of time or access (i.e., the Internet, social networking services, and magazines), because information from people around them was not enough. They wanted to read or hear such stories at their convenience.

> Well, I'm not sure if I can really take care of my children properly . . . of course my niece and nephew are cute but . . . yes, this is my first baby so I guess I'm a little nervous about having to raise my baby day in and day out by myself, so . . . although I think the only way to solve it is to have a baby and raise it, I've been looking at pictures of cute babies on the Internet, or been reading blogs, by those things I can think babies are pretty cute, and it's kind of comforting. (Participant E)

Participants with concerns sought answers and solutions, even if they were not medically correct. Information biases, text-based one-way information, and inaccurate information in this type of support could damage participants physically and emotionally.

> (By reading information about non-evidence-based treatments on the Internet) Well, that's the emotional part, the bleeding may not be treatable, but if I receive some kind of treatment, and it might be good for my baby . . . that would make me feel like I'm doing my best, it's better than doing nothing . . . on the contrary,

I was doing nothing and just waiting to see what happens . . . oh, well, I think I was more worried. (Participant B)

2.3. Proposed Model

Based on our findings, we proposed a model of the needs of support for anxiety among pregnant women (Figure 1). Pregnant women in the focus group sought three types of support: tailored professional support; continuous support within informal relationships; available success stories.

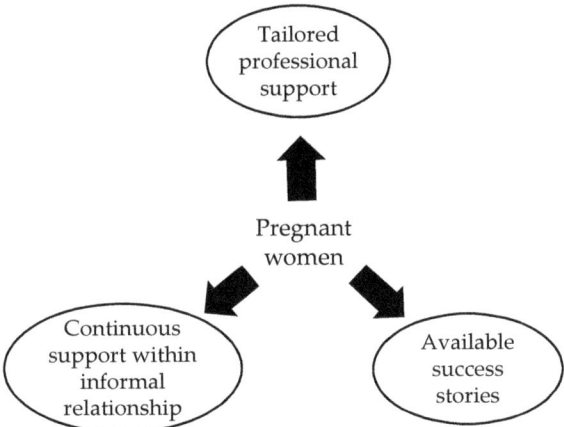

Figure 1. Needs of support for anxiety during pregnancy. White circles: type of support; Black arrows: needs.

In our study, participants sought these three types of support based on their individual preferences and environment. They used different types of support depending on their situation. To paraphrase using the Figure 1, black arrow thickness varies and fluctuates among individuals.

When it comes to normal checkups, I don't really have that much to talk about . . . In other words, I thought that it would be easier to ask someone closer to me. (Participant D)

Some participants relied on online information when they could not solve their own problems by talking to experts or to the people around them.

At first, I was very shocked, it is my first pregnancy, and no way, I was told that there was a possibility of a miscarriage. After that, I talked to the doctor about various things, let me see, like how likely it was, I asked a lot of questions about such things, but I was said the doctor didn't know . . . After I went home, I did a Google search and then it said that in my case, almost 100% my baby was going to be miscarried, so my shock got worse. (Participant B)

3. Materials and Methods

We used a narrative research design, whereby researchers study the lives of individuals and ask them to provide stories about their lives [17]. We conducted a semi-structured focus group discussion with pregnant women to explore a specific set of issues [18]. This is considered a useful method to elicit information on patient priorities and needs, with the aim of improving the quality of healthcare by collecting rich and detailed data in an interactional group structure [19,20]. One or two focus groups are said to be sufficient in exploratory studies [20], therefore we planned to conduct one focus group involving 4–12 women to analyze data over time [18]. This study adhered to the consolidated criteria for reporting qualitative research (COREQ) [21].

3.1. Participant Recruitment

This pilot study used convenience sampling to rapidly recruit participants for the following quantitative survey. To ensure that we recruited women from various backgrounds, this study was conducted across three facilities in Tokyo, Japan: a university hospital, a hospital, and a clinic. The university hospital is a regional perinatal center that manages normal and painless deliveries as well as high-risk pregnancies (e.g., maternal complications and fetal diseases). The hospital is also a regional perinatal center and manages various delivery types, including socially high-risk women, but does not deal with painless deliveries. The clinic only conducts pregnancy checkups and does not manage deliveries. Women who were pregnant, living in Japan, and fluent in Japanese were eligible for this study. In October 2020, the first author or research collaborators (obstetricians/midwives) approached eligible women who visited each facility face-to-face (e.g., "Would you like to talk about your anxieties during pregnancy?") and introduced this study using an information leaflet. The leaflet included a QR code that led to the first author's email address for further explanation, which was conducted face-to-face or in an online meeting. Of the 11 women who were approached and informed about this study (including the rationale) by the first author, eight women agreed to participate. Three women declined to participate; one did not want to show her home online; one believed that the research was useless and that policies (e.g., improving nursery schools) were the only support she needed; and the reason given by the third woman was unclear. After recruitment, three more women dropped out because of emergency hospitalization, schedule inconvenience, and inability to be contacted; therefore, we conducted a focus group with five women.

All participants provided written informed consent to participate in the study and to the publication of this paper. Each woman received a JPY 2000 (USD 20) gift certificate after the interview as a gesture of appreciation for their time. This study was approved by the Institutional Review Board of The University of Tokyo (approval code: 2020154NI).

3.2. Interview Procedure

Before the interview, we collected the participants' demographic information using an online questionnaire. This information included marital status, cohabiting family, job, education background, economic comfort (four-point Likert-scale; almost none to pretty much comfortable), and participation in any prenatal education class. Other information was collected from their medical records (age, expected delivery date, number of past deliveries and abortions, infertility treatment, planned delivery facility, and identified risk) by research collaborators at each facility.

The semi-structured focus group interview was held in an online meeting room (Zoom meetings: https://explore.zoom.us/ja/products/meetings/ (accessed on 2 February 2023)) to prevent infection during the current COVID-19 pandemic. The first author (female, MD, MPH) had conducted in-person medical interviews with pregnant women for seven years as an obstetrician. She felt challenged that the anxieties of pregnant women were unable to be fully addressed in their clinic visits. Therefore, this author facilitated the interview but concealed her occupation. Only the participants and the facilitator were present during the focus group. Following established focus group interview procedures [20], we created the goals of this pilot study: (1) to identify the needs of pregnant women without specific risks regarding the support that can be provided for their anxieties during pregnancy; (2) to get some idea and information from participants which lead to support and initiatives that pregnant women want to participate in. We designed guidelines and semi-structured questions for the interview based on these goals. The interview began with the general question, "Do you have any anxieties about this pregnancy or childbirth?" followed by us showing them a developing scale about pregnancy-related anxiety and discussing it. After clarifying and sharing each participant's anxieties during pregnancy, the facilitator gave semi-structured questions such as: "How are you dealing with your anxieties?"; "Do you want to share your anxieties with someone else?"; "How much are you satisfied with support during pregnancy?"; and "What are you satisfied or dissatisfied with?"

The facilitator took field notes throughout the interview with particular attention to the speaker's tone of voice and to the facial expressions and physical posture of speakers and listeners. The interview was audio- and video-recorded and lasted around one hour. Repeat interviews were not conducted because we intended to hear narratives of pregnant women in real time and all participants were no longer pregnant after data analysis.

3.3. Data Analysis

The unit of analysis was the individual who was pregnant. The first author transcribed the audio recording verbatim immediately after the interview. Participants' facial expressions and physical actions (e.g., nods, laughter, and raising their hands) were captured by the video recording and added to the transcript in words. The transcript was returned to participants for comment, with no corrections necessary. We applied inductive thematic analysis as proposed by Boyatzis [22]. The first author read the transcript carefully and repeatedly, and then coded it manually irrespective of the goals of the interview. The unit of coding was one sentence of the transcript. All derived codes were labeled with definitions and recorded in Microsoft® Excel® for Microsoft 365 MSO (version 2212 build 16.0.15928.20196) 64 bits as a code book. After coding, all similar codes were identified and grouped. Next, the first author and the second author (who had experience of qualitative studies) discussed the data in order to generate themes focused on the types of support participants wanted or perceived as helpful. Thematic codes were generated with consideration for the conditions proposed by Boyatzis, such as clear definitions, conditions for inclusion/exclusion, and specific positive and negative examples [22]. We classified codes as "positive" or "negative" focusing on the speaker's affects. Finally, the thematic codes were adapted to all derived codes. Codes that were judged to be irrelevant for the goals of the interview (e.g., anxiety about some specific risks) were then removed from the analysis. The first author wrote a report of the overall analysis and discussed the generated codes and themes among authors to reach a consensus. This report was returned to all participants, and no objections or changes were made. Two weeks after the final coding, the first author repeated the coding using non-marked transcripts. Minor inconsistencies were modified through discussion. All coding procedures were recorded in the code book.

4. Discussion

We extracted three types of support needs for anxiety during pregnancy based on the perceptions of the focus group participants: tailored professional support, mainly from the medical field; existence of informal relationships, especially with those in the same situation with adequate influence; and successful examples that could be easily accessed. With these three types of support, participants could have both positive and negative feelings depending on their situation. Even if there was an apparent supply of support, the support was not always appropriate for their needs.

To achieve positive pregnancy experience, the previous review questioned the tendency of routine antenatal care which focused on biomedical tests and treatment [16]. Pregnant women mostly sought healthcare support, such as access to healthcare services and experiences within medical/healthcare settings (i.e., positive interpersonal relationships with providers, skills and competencies of providers, and getting physiological, biomedical, and behavioral information) [16]. While our study also showed that the involvement of professionals can be both a positive and negative emotional experience for pregnant women, it also suggested that what they are looking for may differ depending on the place and person of support supplied. In other words, while they naturally sought biomedical tests and treatments from professionals, the degree to which they sought psychological support from professionals varied from person to person; some women were likely to turn to professional support, while others were more likely to turn to other sources, possibly due to the nature of their concern or because of a previous experience of seeking but not getting support. Our study covered both support in medical situations and their experiences in daily life to highlight their preferences and conflicts, details which have been difficult to ascertain in previous reviews and quantitative studies.

4.1. Theoretical Implications

Bandura outlined four factors that influenced self-efficacy: (i) previous experiences; (ii) vicarious experiences; (iii) verbal persuasion; and (iv) emotional arousal [23]. From this perspective, self-efficacy is developed by one's own experiences and by seeing successes and failures of other people (vicarious experiences). Verbal persuasion, which encompasses direct encouragement from a trustworthy person, is also effective in building self-efficacy. The three themes extracted in this study corresponded to two of Bandura's four factors (vicarious experiences and verbal persuasion). In other words, pregnant women in this study may have acted or sought support for building their self-efficacy. Therefore, the self-efficacy of pregnant women may be improved by creating a desirable support environment.

Our proposed model (Figure 1) suggests pregnant women can build their own self-efficacy if they can obtain the three types of support that meet their needs. However, the impact of support on self-efficacy may vary by the type of support, because each of Bandura's four factors has a different strength of impact on self-efficacy in various fields [23,24]. In addition, people appear to live in their own unique psychological world [23]. In other words, each person perceives, understands, and remembers events through their own unique "lens" [25]. The types of support to offer and focus on therefore depend on the unique lens of that individual. As seen in our study, pregnant women may choose (and change) the type of support they rely on based on their preferences and experiences. Therefore, to support every pregnant woman, interventions covering all three directions may be needed.

4.2. Practice Implications

The benefits and best methods of education or support programs during pregnancy remain unclear for a few reasons: it is difficult to conduct high quality research (e.g., randomized, controlled trials) in this population because of ethical considerations; and previous studies were conducted for various purposes using different methods [26]. Our findings also indicated that intervention with a single type of support may not be effective, which may explain the inconsistent results previously reported [26].

As in a previous review [16], the present study found examples in which pregnant women's needs were not met in the professional sector. Our results indicated that professional support has different functions from other types of support (e.g., friendship) because pregnant women may hesitate to talk about all of their concerns with experts. Consistent with the review that found that the provision of relevant, appropriate and timely information was a key factor in positive pregnancy experience [16], our study suggested that accurate descriptions, specific measures to resolve troubles, and reliable sources of information should be provided in the professional sector. Pregnant women may also need to share their values with professionals during treatment decisions and lifestyle transformations.

All participants in this study perceived the value of support from other experienced mothers, even if there were some disadvantages in encountering unexpected support. Although the lack of close relatives and friends with whom to talk and share similar problems was reported to predict the deterioration of mental health among pregnant women more than a decade ago [27], the present study revealed that not all pregnant women had such support. Previous interventions of lay-person-offered support only investigated the effect against adverse mental health outcomes (e.g., depression) among high-risk women [28]. However, our study suggested that such support may be theoretically effective for improving self-efficacy among pregnant women, regardless of specific risks. From the perspective of either vicarious experiences or verbal persuasion, further studies and interventions should be planned to connect anxious pregnant women with women who have had similar experiences to share real-life success or failure stories. In terms of informal relationships, it is worth noting that the present study found only negative statements about support from partners. Participants wanted support from their husbands. However, if their needs were not met, they may have remembered this as a negative experience that conflicted with the perception that they deserved support from their husbands. A systematic review found that marriage or cohabiting with the baby's father had no effect against maternal depressive symptoms after controlling for potential confounders [29], and support from partners that did not meet needs could raise the risk [15]. Education or support programs during pregnancy should therefore include pregnant women's partners.

As most women of reproductive age have smart phones and can easily access the Internet anytime and anywhere in Japan, online information has become a big source of support among pregnant women. Our study supported the previous finding that pregnant women often gained reassurance from other people's experiences online [30]. However, many pregnant women also felt scared by the information they read online [31]. We encountered similar cases in this study where participants were psychologically damaged by online information. Our study also indicated that pregnant women may be confused by information that may not be accurate. To offer effective support to any pregnant women in Japan, it may be valuable for professionals to create or recommend reliable websites from which women can find correct and unbiased information or read about other pregnant women's experiences.

Several limitations of this study should be acknowledged. First, although this study was conducted as a preliminary study to identify meaningful variables in the following large observational study, our findings were based on one focus group and additional focus groups may find other themes or key concepts. Although one or two focus groups are said to be sufficient in exploratory studies [20], we should use these results as a starting point to know what support needs may be needed during pregnancy in today's local Japanese context and should evaluate them in the next quantitative phase in a larger sample. Comparing this study with focus groups in different samples would also bring meaningful insights in the future. Second, by using convenience sampling, we might have failed to capture important perspectives from hard-to-reach women [32]. Although we tried to recruit a heterogeneous group, we found that some of the items we considered were homogeneous (such as parity, educational background, and marital status). A possible explanation for this was that this study was conducted in the urban area. Even though some items appeared to be homogeneous, all participants had different backgrounds that could not be measured. The results of this study would be helpful for considering better support in the urban areas in Japan or for populations with similar backgrounds, such as newly pregnant women. Further studies are needed to explore the other targeted groups that have different characteristics from our study. Third, the information leaflet used in recruiting the participants might have encouraged more anxious women to participate and therefore this study was not representative of the needs among pregnant women in Japan. However, gathering parties who have some opinions can stimulate discussion in focus groups and yield rich data. Despite these limitations, to our knowledge, this was the first report in the last decade of a focus group exploring support needs for anxiety during pregnancy among women without specific risks in an economically prosperous country.

5. Conclusions

Using a focus group among pregnant women without specific risks, we found three types of support needs for anxiety during pregnancy: (1) seeking tailored professional support; (2) seeking continuous support within informal relationships; and (3) seeking others' success stories in the same situation. We proposed a model of needs of support for pregnancy-related anxiety backed up by social cognitive theory. Because an individual's needs for each type of support may be influenced by their preferences and circumstances, professionals should be aware of all three types of support when considering effective universal support for pregnant women's mental health. Further research and interventions should also consider the narratives and collaborate with pregnant women, because a unilateral supply of support may cause negative feelings in pregnant women.

Author Contributions: Conceptualization, R.S.; methodology, R.S., H.O. and T.O.; validation, R.S.; formal analysis, R.S. and T.O.; investigation, R.S., T.O., H.O., E.G. and T.K.; resources, R.S.; data curation, R.S.; writing—original draft preparation, R.S. and T.O.; writing—review and editing, T.O., H.O., E.G. and T.K.; visualization, R.S. and T.O.; supervision, T.O. and T.K.; project administration, R.S. and T.O.; funding acquisition, R.S. All authors have read and agreed to the published version of the manuscript.

Funding: This research was funded by The Health Care Science Institute Research Grant.

Institutional Review Board Statement: This study was conducted according to the guidelines of the Declaration of Helsinki and approved by the Institutional Review Board of The University of Tokyo (approval code: 2020154NI, date of approval: 22 July 2020).

Informed Consent Statement: Informed consent was obtained from all participants involved in this study. Written informed consent was obtained from participants to publish this paper.

Data Availability Statement: The data presented in this study are available on request from the corresponding author. The data are not publicly available, for ethical reasons.

Acknowledgments: We thank all participants in the focus group as well as the women who could not participate even though they agreed. In addition, we thank Mie Yamada, Yuka Yamamoto, and Yo Takemoto as research collaborators, and the staff in each facility for their help in recruiting some of the participants in this study. We thank Audrey Holmes, MA, from Edanz (https://jp.edanz.com/ac (accessed on 2 February 2023)), for editing a draft of this manuscript.

Conflicts of Interest: The authors declare no conflict of interest.

Appendix A

Table A1. Coded anxieties and supporting quotes.

Anxiety Codes	Supporting Quotes [1]
Anxiety from Pregnancy Itself	
From confirmation of pregnancy to feeling fetal movement	Before I felt . . . the fetal movement, I was very anxious if my baby would be okay after I lost my morning sickness and entered the stable period, conversely. (Participant D)
Prenatal testing	I made my own decision (not to take prenatal testing), but I think I [will] have anxiety about whether my decision was right all the way until my baby is born. (Participant C)
Childbirth	As for my next concern, it is the first time I have given birth, so I am starting to feel a little scared about . . . childbirth. (Participant A)
Lack of preparation for childbirth and postpartum	The new anxiety that emerged was, as (Ms. G.) said, about what preparations I should make, whether there is anything I am missing or not, what and what timing I should prepare for the birth . . . I was starting to feel anxious about the birth? . . . little by little . . . (Participant C)
Postpartum attachment formation	Well, I'm not sure if I can really take care of my children properly . . . of course my niece and nephew are cute but . . . yes, this is my first baby so I guess I'm a little nervous about having to raise my baby day in and day out by myself . . . (Participant E)
Personal characteristics	
After miscarriage experience	My first child is four years old now, well, I'm four years away (before this pregnancy) and I had three miscarriages during that time . . . well . . . I was not anxious at all when I had my first child, but now that I experienced those miscarriages . . . I am always wondering . . . if my baby will be really okay. (Participant D)
Whether the pregnancy after infertility treatment can continue	(Like Ms. A,) I too had gone through infertility treatment, and since I had already gone through the full course of treatment, I was finally able to conceive on my third IVF cycle, so to be honest, I was more worried about whether this pregnancy would actually be successful than I was worried about the corona (COVID-19) disaster . . . (Participant C)
Complications during pregnancy	At first, well, I was in great shock . . . it was my first pregnancy, and I was told that I might have a miscarriage, which I didn't expect . . . (Participant B)

Table A1. *Cont.*

Anxiety Codes	Supporting Quotes [1]
Environment surrounding individuals	
Facilities and medical staffs	I was a little young when I had my first miscarriage, and I felt like a tragic heroine when I had a miscarriage ... the doctor's response was not very good, and I blamed it on the doctor and became displeased with the clinic ... I had such experience of being tossed around by the hospital ... so I am wondering what kind of criteria people use to choose a clinic, not just the proximity to their homes. (Participant C)
Home environment	If I impose it (the smoking cessation) [on my husband], it will make my family unhappy, and so on ... (Participant E)
Workplace	Well, I couldn't tell people at work (about my pregnancy) because of that (anxiety about miscarriage), and I finally reported it ... recently. (Participant D)
Outbreak of COVID-19	Of course, the world is getting so bad right now with corona (COVID-19) infections and things like that, so I was afraid of that ... (Participant B)

IVF, in vitro fertilization; COVID-19, coronavirus disease 2019. [1] Participants' narratives were translated into English for this publication.

References

1. Hahn-Holbrook, J.; Cornwell-Hinrichs, T.; Anaya, I. Economic and Health Predictors of National Postpartum Depression Prevalence: A Systematic Review, Meta-analysis, and Meta-Regression of 291 Studies from 56 Countries. *Front. Psychiatry* **2018**, *8*, 248. [CrossRef] [PubMed]
2. Dennis, C.-L.; Falah-Hassani, K.; Shiri, R. Prevalence of antenatal and postnatal anxiety: Systematic review and meta-analysis. *Br. J. Psychiatry* **2017**, *210*, 315–323. [CrossRef] [PubMed]
3. Grigoriadis, S.; Graves, L.; Peer, M.; Mamisashvili, L.; Tomlinson, G.; Vigod, S.N.; Dennis, C.-L.; Steiner, M.; Brown, C.; Cheung, A.; et al. A systematic review and meta-analysis of the effects of antenatal anxiety on postpartum outcomes. *Arch. Women's Ment. Health* **2019**, *22*, 543–556. [CrossRef] [PubMed]
4. *Pregnancy Health Examination*; No. 0227001; Notice by Director, Maternal and Child Health Division, Equal Employment and Child Family Bureau; Ministry of Health, Labor and Welfare: Tokyo, Japan, 27 February 2009.
5. Bandura, A. *Social Foundations of Thought and Action: A Social Cognitive Theory*; Prentice Hall: Hoboken, NJ, USA, 1986.
6. Chen, H.-H.; Hwang, F.-M.; Tai, C.-J.; Chien, L.-Y. The Interrelationships among Acculturation, Social Support, and Postpartum Depression Symptoms among Marriage-Based Immigrant Women in Taiwan: A Cohort Study. *J. Immigr. Minor. Health* **2013**, *15*, 17–23. [CrossRef] [PubMed]
7. Escribà-Agüir, V.; Royo-Marqués, M.; Artazcoz, L.; Romito, P.; Ruiz-Pérez, I. Longitudinal study of depression and health status in pregnant women: Incidence, course and predictive factors. *Eur. Arch. Psychiatry Clin. Neurosci.* **2013**, *263*, 143–151. [CrossRef]
8. Kritsotakis, G.; Vassilaki, M.; Melaki, V.; Georgiou, V.; Philalithis, A.E.; Bitsios, P.; Kogevinas, M.; Chatzi, L.; Koutis, A. Social capital in pregnancy and postpartum depressive symptoms: A prospective mother–child cohort study (the Rhea study). *Int. J. Nurs. Stud.* **2013**, *50*, 63–72. [CrossRef]
9. Leung, B.M.; Kaplan, B.J.; Field, C.J.; Tough, S.; Eliasziw, M.; Gomez, M.F.; McCargar, L.J.; Gagnon, L.; the APrON Study Team. Prenatal micronutrient supplementation and postpartum depressive symptoms in a pregnancy cohort. *BMC Pregnancy Childbirth* **2013**, *13*, 2. [CrossRef]
10. Bedaso, A.; Adams, J.; Peng, W.; Sibbritt, D. The relationship between social support and mental health problems during pregnancy: A systematic review and meta-analysis. *Reprod. Health* **2021**, *18*, 162. [CrossRef]
11. Biaggi, A.; Conroy, S.; Pawlby, S.; Pariante, C.M. Identifying the women at risk of antenatal anxiety and depression: A systematic review. *J. Affect. Disord.* **2016**, *191*, 62–77. [CrossRef]
12. Fathi, F.; Mohammad-Alizadeh-Charandabi, S.; Mirghafourvand, M. Maternal self-efficacy, postpartum depression, and their relationship with functional status in Iranian mothers. *Women Health* **2018**, *58*, 188–203. [CrossRef]
13. Mohammad, K.I.; Sabbah, H.; Aldalaykeh, M.; Albashtawy, M.; Abuobead, K.Z.; Creedy, D.; Gamble, J. Informative title: Effects of social support, parenting stress and self-efficacy on postpartum depression among adolescent mothers in Jordan. *J. Clin. Nurs.* **2021**, *30*, 3456–3465. [CrossRef] [PubMed]
14. Han, L.; Zhang, J.; Yang, J.; Yang, X.; Bai, H. Between Personality Traits and Postpartum Depression: The Mediated Role of Maternal Self-Efficacy. *Neuropsychiatr. Dis. Treat.* **2022**, *18*, 597–609. [CrossRef] [PubMed]
15. Gremigni, P.; Mariani, L.; Marracino, V.; Tranquilli, A.L.; Turi, A. Partner support and postpartum depressive symptoms. *J. Psychosom. Obstet. Gynecol.* **2011**, *32*, 135–140. [CrossRef]
16. Downe, S.; Finlayson, K.; Tunçalp, Ö.; Gülmezoglu, A.M. What matters to women: A systematic scoping review to identify the processes and outcomes of antenatal care provision that are important to healthy pregnant women. *BJOG Int. J. Obstet. Gynaecol.* **2016**, *123*, 529–539. [CrossRef]

17. Riessman, C.K. *Narrative Methods for the Human Sciences*; Sage Publications: Thousands Oaks, CA, USA, 2008.
18. Liamputtong, P. *Qualitative Research Methods*, 5th ed.; Oxford University Press: Oxford, UK, 2019.
19. Sofaer, S. Qualitative research methods. *Int. J. Qual. Health Care* **2002**, *14*, 329–336. [CrossRef] [PubMed]
20. Vaughn, S.; Schumm, J.S.; Sinagub, J.M. *Focus Group Interviews in Education and Psychology*; Sage Publications: Thousands Oaks, CA, USA, 1996.
21. Tong, A.; Sainsbury, P.; Craig, J. Consolidated criteria for reporting qualitative research (COREQ): A 32-item checklist for interviews and focus groups. *Int. J. Qual. Health Care* **2007**, *19*, 349–357. [CrossRef]
22. Boyatzis, R.E. *Transforming Qualitative Information: Thematic Analysis and Code Development*; Sage Publications: Thousands Oaks, CA, USA, 1998.
23. Bandura, A. *Self-Efficacy: The Exercise of Control*; W H Freeman & Co.: New York, NY, USA, 1999.
24. Ashford, S.; Edmunds, J.; French, D. What is the best way to change self-efficacy to promote lifestyle and recreational physical activity? A systematic review with meta-analysis. *Br. J. Health Psychol.* **2010**, *15*, 265–288. [CrossRef]
25. Kelder, S.H.; Hoelscher, D.; Perry, C.L. How Individuals, Environments, and Health Behaviors Interact. In *Health Behavior: Theory, Research, and Practice*, 5th ed.; Glanz, K., Rimer, B.K., Viswanath, K., Eds.; John Wiley & Sons: Hoboken, NJ, USA, 2015; pp. 159–182.
26. Gagnon, A.J.; Sandall, J. Individual or group antenatal education for childbirth or parenthood, or both. *Cochrane Database Syst. Rev.* **2007**, *2007*, CD002869. [CrossRef]
27. Brugha, T.S.; Sharp, H.M.; Cooper, S.-A.; Weisender, C.; Britto, D.; Shinkwin, R.; Sherrif, T.; Kirwan, P.H. The Leicester 500 Project. Social support and the development of postnatal depressive symptoms, a prospective cohort survey. *Psychol. Med.* **1998**, *28*, 63–79. [CrossRef]
28. Kenyon, S.; Jolly, K.; Hemming, K.; Hope, L.; Blissett, J.; Dann, S.-A.; Lilford, R.; MacArthur, C. Lay support for pregnant women with social risk: A randomised controlled trial. *BMJ Open* **2016**, *6*, e009203. [CrossRef]
29. Yim, I.S.; Stapleton, L.R.T.; Guardino, C.M.; Hahn-Holbrook, J.; Schetter, C.D. Biological and Psychosocial Predictors of Postpartum Depression: Systematic Review and Call for Integration. *Annu. Rev. Clin. Psychol.* **2015**, *11*, 99–137. [CrossRef] [PubMed]
30. Prescott, J.; Mackie, L. "You Sort of Go Down a Rabbit Hole . . . You're Just Going to Keep on Searching": A Qualitative Study of Searching Online for Pregnancy-Related Information During Pregnancy. *J. Med. Internet Res.* **2017**, *19*, e194. [CrossRef] [PubMed]
31. Bjelke, M.; Martinsson, A.-K.; Lendahls, L.; Oscarsson, M. Using the Internet as a source of information during pregnancy—A descriptive cross-sectional study in Sweden. *Midwifery* **2016**, *40*, 187–191. [CrossRef] [PubMed]
32. Elder, N.; Miller, W.L. Reading and evaluating qualitative research studies. *J. Fam. Pract.* **1995**, *41*, 279–285.

Disclaimer/Publisher's Note: The statements, opinions and data contained in all publications are solely those of the individual author(s) and contributor(s) and not of MDPI and/or the editor(s). MDPI and/or the editor(s) disclaim responsibility for any injury to people or property resulting from any ideas, methods, instructions or products referred to in the content.

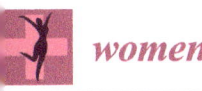

Article

Psychosocial Risk Factors and Psychopathological Outcomes: Preliminary Findings in Italian Pregnant Women

Maria Rita Infurna *, Eleonora Bevacqua, Giulia Costanzo, Giorgio Falgares and Francesca Giannone

Department of Psychology, Educational Sciences and Human Movement, University of Palermo, 90144 Palermo, Italy
* Correspondence: mariarita.infurna@unipa.it

Abstract: The perinatal period may represent a particularly challenging time for expecting parents. Previous studies have highlighted an association between several perinatal risk conditions (e.g., childhood maltreatment, poor social support, and stress levels) and the development of psychopathological symptoms in pregnant women, especially depression symptoms. The current study examined the effects of psychosocial risk factors (childhood maltreatment, poor social support, and stressful events) on anxiety, depression, perceived stress, irritability/anger, relationship problems, psychosomatic symptoms, specific physiological problems, and addiction/at-risk behaviors. Sixty-one pregnant women (age range = 24–45) participating in a larger study completed questionnaires about childhood maltreatment (CECA Q.), Maternity Social Support Scale (MSSS), questionnaire on stressful events, and the Perinatal Assessment of Maternal Affectivity (PAMA) during their pregnancy. Results from regression analysis indicated that the presence of childhood maltreatment predicted elevated depressive symptoms, elevated irritability and anger, and elevated relationship problems. Further, stressful events in the year prior to pregnancy predicted elevated psychosomatic symptoms during pregnancy. No other significant associations were found. In this study, traumatic childhood events were strongly associated with mental health symptoms during pregnancy. This is an important finding that suggests the importance of screening and targeting psychotherapeutic interventions for vulnerable women during pregnancy.

Keywords: childhood maltreatment; social support; stressful events; psychopathological outcomes; pregnancy

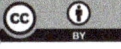

1. Introduction

The perinatal period, which is typically defined as from the beginning of pregnancy to one year after childbirth, is associated with major physiological and emotional changes related to pregnancy, childbirth, and the care of a newborn. Such intense changes can make the transition into parenthood a time of vulnerability for mothers and fathers. During gestation, caregivers are required to reorganize their internal experience and begin to change their identity to accommodate their new role as parents [1,2]. Pregnancy is usually defined as a generally positive and joyful time for most; nevertheless, there may also be severe stressors associated with the physical, emotional, and cognitive changes that affect women in the prenatal period [3]. These stressors may be exacerbated by recall of one's own childhood caregiving experiences [4,5].

As research has shown, experiences of childhood maltreatment can have long-term negative consequences on adult health [6–10]. Childhood adversities typically refer to a wide range of negative early experiences, including physical, sexual, and emotional abuse; physical and emotional neglect; exposure to domestic violence; the presence of a family member with mental illness and/or substance abuse problems; bullying; parental death or loss; serious accidents or injuries; and extreme poverty [10]. Among all experiences of childhood adversity, research has demonstrated a strong link between experiences of childhood maltreatment and several psychopathological conditions in the lifespan, such as post-traumatic stress disorder, suicidal and self-injurious behavior, depressive symptomatology, personality disorders, substance abuse, somatization, anxiety, and dissociation [6]. Considering the possible explanations of the association between childhood maltreatment experiences and psychopathological conditions, psychodynamic models highlight how experiences of childhood maltreatment can threaten fundamental human needs to belong and to create positive relationships, which are scaffolding for the development of self-worth and security feelings [11,12]. Given the importance of early nurturing bonds, traumatic experiences within the relationship between parents and their child can lead to the damaged development of all future relationships, including that of maltreated individuals with their offspring [13].

A growing body of research has shown interest in studying the relationship between childhood maltreatment and adverse psychological outcomes specifically during pregnancy [14,15]. The long-term consequences of early traumatic experiences are a serious public health concern. Therefore, identifying sensitive life periods when childhood maltreatment consequences are most salient may lead to successful intervention efforts. Research has shown that the perinatal period is one such sensitive time point [16].

In line with the attachment theory and psychodynamic models, the perinatal period is a time during which the negative effects of childhood maltreatment can manifest [13,14]. Indeed, early adverse experiences, particularly those of abuse and neglect, may be reactivated by the transition process to motherhood, potentially eliciting emotional and psychological responses associated with those experiences [17,18]. To confirm this theory, an interesting longitudinal study compared psychological distress in a group of pregnant and non-pregnant adolescents. Findings highlighted that early traumatic experiences can be considered predictors of psychopathological conditions among pregnant and parenting adolescents but not among nulliparous adolescents [19]. During pregnancy, emotional distress such as depression may be caused by recall of childhood maltreatment, which can elicit trauma-related thoughts and feelings [20,21].

Women who have experienced abuse in childhood may therefore be at particularly high risk for the development of psychopathological conditions such as post-traumatic stress disorder and post-partum depression during pregnancy and the postpartum period [22–25]. A recent systematic review of the empirical literature on the relationship between maternal histories of childhood maltreatment and perinatal mood and anxiety disorders revealed strong trends of association between adverse early experiences and perinatal depression, as well as post-traumatic stress disorder [20].

Research highlights that early traumatic experiences not only may affect mothers' psychological well-being during the perinatal period but also may have potential negative implications for their offspring's health and development. Indeed, strong associations were found between maternal psychological distress and increased risk for preterm birth, low birth weight, poor health, and other pregnancy and birth complications [26–28]. Moreover, evidence suggests that exposure to maternal psychopathology during the perinatal period also may have detrimental effects on the cognitive, behavioral, and emotional development of offspring, increasing the risk of psychiatric disorders in the adolescence and early adulthood of offspring [29,30].

The aforementioned studies show that pregnancy is a sensitive window during which to act promptly to avoid possible negative consequences for women and families. Among possible negative effects, previous studies have focused mainly on postpartum depression and have shown that it is associated with serious emotional distress, important social and occupational impairments, and increased healthcare utilization [31]. Postpartum depression may also affect women's parenting functioning and couples' relationships [32]. The potential link between a history of abuse and maternal depression during pregnancy has been less investigated [33] despite evidence suggesting that prenatal depression and postpartum depression may have similar negative effects and that pregnant women with a history of early traumatic experiences can manifest severe depression symptoms [34,35]. Further, as evidenced in some studies, almost 50% of women experience continued prenatal depression in the postnatal period [36,37].

For this reason, assessment during pregnancy is necessary to immediately detect, treat, and reduce depressive symptoms, as well as other forms of psychopathological distress [38,39].

Besides the serious negative consequences of childhood maltreatment, several risk factors associated with prenatal and postpartum psychopathological distress (anxiety, relationship, or psychosomatic problems), such as low social support and stressful life events, have been detected [40].

Knowing and understanding predictors of psychological negative conditions in pregnancy is crucial to avoid negative consequences for parents and children. One of the major obstacles to implementing effective prevention programs is inadequate programs for the early identification of women who are at risk of suffering from psychological problems during pregnancy and postpartum [41]. This situation has often left such disorders undetected and untreated or only detected at an advanced stage [42]. In this study, a wider range of potential risk factors (such as childhood abuse, lack of social support, and stressful events) for psychopathological outcomes was examined.

The current study aimed to present preliminary findings of larger ongoing research to garner a better understanding of the associations between potential risk factors and mental health outcomes in a sample of pregnant women. Targeting the risk factors of future mothers may help to reduce mental health problems for women, improve pregnancy outcomes, and offer a better family environment for children.

2. Materials and Methods

2.1. Procedure and Participants

Participants in this study (N = 61) comprised a convenience sample of Italian pregnant women. Eligibility requirements included the following: (a) being pregnant, (b) being at least 18 years of age, and (c) having the ability to understand and speak fluent Italian. Eligible participants provided informed consent after being provided with a thorough description of the purpose of the project. Following informed consent, participants completed a battery of self-report measures on their smartphone or computer/tablet. The project was conducted in accordance with the Declaration of Helsinki, and the protocol was approved by the Department of Psychology, Educational Science and Human Movement at the University of Palermo (V.8_22/05/2022).

Participants were recruited through the active involvement of birth centers and local health services and health workers (e.g., gynecologists, obstetricians, etc.); formal and informal birth support networks; and the posting of fliers in public healthcare service locations, hospitals, community prenatal clinics, and social service agencies serving pregnant women.

2.2. Measures

- Questionnaire on sociodemographic characteristics and pregnancy-related variables: an ad hoc questionnaire used to collect primary information such as date of birth, marital status, education level, gestational age (in weeks), primiparity (first pregnancy or not), other children, information on the current pregnancy (single/twin, high/low risk), and whether they were currently romantically involved with a partner. Further questions assess the presence of psychological distress (depression, anxiety, etc.) before the current pregnancy.
- *Stressful Events in the Previous Year*: a 15-item questionnaire assessing any stressful events that occurred in the previous year (economic problems, illness of a loved one, change or loss of work, etc.) through dichotomous questions. A final single item assesses the impact of reported stressful events (none, mild, medium, and strong levels).
- *Maternal Social Support Scale (MSSS)* [43]: The MSSS is a 6-item, 5-point Likert-type rating scale that measures perceived social support (i.e., friendship network, family support, help from spouse/partner, and conflict with spouse/partner). The total possible score is 30, with cutoff points suggested by Webster [43] as follows: 0–18 (low social support), 19–24 (medium support), and >24 (adequate support). The MSSI showed good psychometric properties.

- *Childhood Experience of Care and Abuse Questionnaire (CECA.Q)* [44]: a self-report measure designed to collect information concerning adverse events occurring before the age of 17 years. These experiences include physical abuse by the main mother and father figures, sexual abuse by any adult, parental antipathy (hostility, rejection, or coldness), and emotional or physical neglect (defined in terms of a parent's disinterest in material care, health, schoolwork, and friendships). It thus combines classic traumatic experiences with negative bonding experiences with each caregiver. This measure is considered the gold-standard measure for childhood experience assessment, and it has satisfactory levels of test–retest reliability and concurrent validity.
- *Perinatal Assessment of Maternal Affectivity* (PAMA) [45]: The PAMA is an 11-item screening instrument used to assess perinatal maternal affective disorders. The first eight items deal with the following dimensions: anxiety, depression, perceived stress, irritability/anger (irritability, hostility, arguments with others, and anger attacks), relationship problems (including couple, family, friends, and at work), abnormal illness behavior (somatization, functional medical syndromes, chronic pain syndromes, and hypochondriac complaints), physiological problems (with sleeping, eating, or sexual desire), addictions (smoking, drinking alcohol, taking drugs, gambling, and compulsive use of the Internet), and other risky behaviors (such as driving at high speed, dangerous sports, or taking unnecessary risks at work). The last three items are questions relating to motherhood and cultural factors. The questions are: "Do you think your answers to these questions are related to being, or becoming, a mother? If "YES" or "Possibly", in what way?"; "Do you feel happy or content with being, or becoming, a mother?", and "Are there other questions, or words, that would be better to describe how you have been feeling over the past two weeks? If "YES", please describe". A self-rating of 0–3 is elicited for nine scaled items, with a total maximum score of 27. A higher score indicates a greater risk for an affective disorder.

2.3. Data Analysis

All measures were scored according to published guidelines, and basic descriptive statistics were calculated. The associations between potential risk factors and specific types of psychopathological distress were examined using binary linear regressions. In each case, the independent variables were, the CECA Q. dichotomic score, MSSS total score, and the presence of stressful events in the last 12 months; dependent variables included the different PAMA subscales (e.g., anxiety, depression, relational problems, etc.). All analyses were carried out using SPSS version 28.0 (SPSS Inc., Chicago, IL, USA). The significance level was determined as 0.05.

3. Results

3.1. Sample Characteristics

The study population consisted of 61 Italian pregnant women, mainly from central (47.5%) and southern Italy (44.3%), aged between 24 and 45 years old. Most of the pregnant women were married or lived with their unmarried partner (91.8%), had a university degree (72.2%), and had paid work (85.2%). Only 18% of the sample reported a low economic state, whereas the rest of the sample reported an average (57.4%) or medium-high economic status (24.6%).

As regards current pregnancy, most participants had a planned pregnancy (86.9%), 72.1% of women were primipara, and 57.4% were in the third trimester.

From a clinical perspective, 82% of women reported a low-risk pregnancy, 81.3% reported no pharmacological treatment for psychological disorders, 83.6% had chosen a private gynecologist, and 54.1% attended childbirth preparation training.

A proportion of 65.3% of participants did not have a history of abortion, voluntary interruptions of pregnancy, perinatal death, or high-risk pregnancies. Table 1 indicates the main participant information.

Table 1. Characteristics of the study population (N = 61).

Variable	n	%
Age		
45–37 years old	18	29.5
36–30 years old	31	50.8
<29 years old	12	19.7
Country: Italy		
Northern	5	8.2
Central	29	47.5
Southern	27	44.3
Education		
Primary school	1	1.6
High school diploma	16	26.2
University degree	22	36.1
Postgraduate degree	22	36.1
Employment status		
Unemployed	4	6.6
Housewife	3	4.9
Student	2	3.3
Precarious employment	13	21.3
Stable employment	39	63.9
Marital status		
Unmarried	5	8.2
Married/cohabitant	56	91.8
Economic status		
Low	11	18
Middle class	35	57.4
Medium–high	15	24.6
Gestational age		
First trimester	7	11.5
Second trimester	19	31.1
Third trimester	35	57.4
Pregnancy		
Planned pregnancy	53	86.9
Unplanned pregnancy	8	13.1
First pregnancy		
Yes	44	72.1
No	17	27.9
Other children		
Yes	11	18
No	50	82
High-risk pregnancy		
Yes	11	18
No	50	82
Psychopharmacological treatment		
Yes	0	0
No	61	100

3.2. Risk Factors and Psychopathological Outcomes in Pregnancy

As regards child maltreatment, 59% of the total research sample (36 out of 61 women) reported at least one experience. Specifically, more than half (54.1%) reported emotional abuse (from mother and/or father), described as hostility or coldness toward the child; 8.2% experienced physical abuse, described as serious forms of physical violence toward the child (e.g., punching, hitting with an object, or threatening with a knife); and 6.6%

experienced sexual abuse, defined as any non-consensual sexual contact by any perpetrator (e.g., fondling, oral sex, or penetration) before the age of 16.

Over half of the sample (55.7%) reported the presence of stressful events in the last 12 months. The type of stressful events reported concerned serious illness or accidents involving oneself or loved ones, grief, being a victim of violence, change or loss of important lifestyle components (study, work, or home), marital separation, problems with justice, and problems with work or finances. Among those who reported the presence of stressful events in the last 12 months, more than half (18 out of 34) were in the third trimester of gestation; moreover, 38.2% and 35.3% reported medium and strong levels of discomfort, suffering, and stress caused by these events, respectively.

Results from the MSSS showed that the majority (88.5%) of pregnant women indicated a medium level of perceived social support (from partner, parents, and friends), while 6.6% indicated a low level, and only 4.9% indicated a high level. With the progress of the gestation trimester, this perception did not significantly change.

Detailed information on childhood maltreatment experiences, stressful events in the previous year, and perceived maternal social support are provided as Supplementary Materials.

3.3. Associations of Risk Factors and Psychopathology in Pregnancy

Subscales of the PAMA were related to different risk factors, such as childhood maltreatment, stressful events in the last year, and lack of social support.

Regression analysis (Table 2) showed that the presence of childhood maltreatment was significantly related to higher levels of depression symptoms ($R^2 = 0.07$, Adj $R^2 = 0.05$, $F(1,59) = 4.11$, $p = 0.047$), higher levels of irritability and anger ($R^2 = 0.07$, Adj $R^2 = 0.05$, $F(1,59) = 4.12$, $p = 0.047$), and higher levels of relational problems ($R^2 = 0.12$, Adj $R^2 = 0.10$, $F(1,59) = 7.68$, $p = 0.007$).

Table 2. Association between childhood maltreatment and PAMA subscales.

Dependent Variable	B	SE	Beta	p
Anxiety	0.12	0.21	0.08	0.555
Depression	0.35	0.17	0.26	0.047 *
Perceived stress	0.33	0.22	0.19	0.144
Irritability/anger	0.45	0.22	0.26	0.047 *
Relationship problems	0.54	0.19	0.34	0.007 **
Psychosomatic problems	0.10	0.21	0.06	0.643
Physiological problems	−0.14	0.22	−0.08	0.520
Addiction/at-risk behaviors	0.11	0.10	0.14	0.277

PAMA: Perinatal Assessment of Maternal Affectivity; B: unstandardized coefficient; SE: standard error; Beta: standardized coefficient. * $p < 0.05$. ** $p < 0.01$.

Regression analysis with stressful events in the last year as independent predictors indicated that the presence of stressful events predicted significantly more psychosomatic symptoms during pregnancy (Table 3; $R^2 = 0.10$, Adj $R^2 = 0.08$, $F(1,59) = 6.47$, $p = 0.014$), whereas no significant relations were found for other psychopathological subscales.

Table 3. Association between stressful events and PAMA subscales.

Dependent Variable	B	SE	Beta	p
Anxiety	−0.31	0.21	−0.19	0.138
Depression	−0.08	0.18	−0.06	0.660
Perceived stress	−0.19	0.22	−0.11	0.389
Irritability/anger	0.05	0.23	0.03	0.827
Relationship problems	−0.07	0.20	−0.04	0.734

Table 3. Cont.

Dependent Variable	B	SE	Beta	p
Psychosomatic problems	−0.51	0.20	−0.31	0.014 *
Physiological problems	−0.29	0.21	−0.17	0.184
Addiction/at-risk behaviors	<0.01	0.10	<.01	0.992

PAMA: Perinatal Assessment of Maternal Affectivity; B: unstandardized coefficient; SE: standard error; Beta: standardized coefficient. * $p < 0.05$.

Regression analysis with maternal social support as independent predictors indicated that higher levels of a lack of social support from partner, parents, or friends did not predict any psychopathological symptoms (Table 4).

Table 4. Association between perceived social support (MSSS) and PAMA subscales.

Dependent Variable	B	SE	Beta	p
Anxiety	−0.02	0.04	−0.05	0.697
Depression	−0.05	0.04	−0.17	0.199
Perceived stress	−0.02	0.05	−0.07	0.615
Irritability/anger	−0.01	0.05	−0.04	0.761
Relationship problems	−0.02	0.04	−0.07	0.592
Psychosomatic problems	−0.05	0.04	−0.15	0.247
Physiological problems	0.02	0.04	0.07	0.605
Addiction/at-risk behaviors	0.02	0.02	0.15	0.246

MSSS: Maternity Social Support Scale; PAMA: Perinatal Assessment of Maternal Affectivity; B: unstandardized coefficient; SE: standard error; Beta: standardized coefficient.

4. Discussion

This study reported preliminary findings from broader ongoing research that aims to establish links between several risk factors for psychopathological outcomes in pregnant women. Specifically, in the current study, the unique contribution of these risk factors to specific clinical manifestations (e.g., anxiety, depression) during pregnancy was examined. However, given the small sample size and the use of multiple tests, results from this study should be considered provisional.

The current study builds on the childhood maltreatment literature by linking childhood maltreatment to psychopathological problems specifically during the prenatal period, which is a phase of extensive psychological and physiological changes. The PAMA questionnaire is a tool for the screening of perinatal affective disorders that considers not only depressive symptoms but also anxiety; hostility; and somatic, relational, behavioral, and addiction problems.

It is well-recognized that childhood abuse is among the major risk factors for depression in adulthood [46]. Despite the detrimental effects of depression at any time during a woman's lifetime, the effects of depression during the prenatal and postpartum periods are of great importance due to their severe and protracted consequences for both women and their offspring [33,47]. Findings from this study indicate an association between childhood abuse and depressive symptoms during pregnancy. As suggested in previous research, pregnancy may be a particularly sensitive period due to the development of a new self-identity, as well as the substantial biological and emotional changes that occur during the transition to motherhood [25,33]. Therefore, identification of traumatic childhood experiences during pregnancy may allow pregnant women at risk for depression to be closely observed by healthcare professionals, enabling the implementation of important preventive strategies, as treatment of prenatal depression can ward off the onset of postpartum depression [37].

Furthermore, in our sample of pregnant women, childhood maltreatment was associated with higher levels of irritability and anger, as well as with relationship problems, including in couples, as well as with family and friends, and at work. These findings contribute important insights to current knowledge, highlighting the effect of childhood maltreatment not only on depressive symptoms but also on other areas of psychopathological distress. Significantly, dimensions such as irritability and anger (against others), and relationship problems appeared to be affected by traumatic childhood experiences. Indeed, from a psychodynamic point of view, an infant is shaped by his environment, interaction with his parents, and his own personal growth [48,49]. Psychologically, becoming a mother requires the activation of mental patterns that pregnant women and their own parents had reciprocally shaped. Unfortunately, this process may be problematic or impaired in women with traumatic childhood experiences, in whom traumatic memories can cause psychological distress, suggesting the need for greater attention to women's childhood histories during prenatal screening in order to achieve early detection of expectant mothers at risk of developing psychopathological conditions.

In line with previous research [4,50], this study considered not only childhood maltreatment but also the presence of several stressful events in the last year (economic problems, illness of a loved one, change or loss of work, etc.) and a lack of social support (from partner, parents, and friends) as potential risk factors for psychopathological symptoms during pregnancy.

Overall, the findings of regression analysis indicated that the presence of stressful events in the last 12 months predicted higher levels of psychosomatic symptoms but not other psychopathological problems. This result is in line with the literature considering recent stressful life events (including illness, accidents, domestic violence, etc.) among the main risk factors for the development of psychopathological outcomes in pregnancy and the perinatal period [51,52]. These data seem to underline the importance of clinicians and medical staff evaluating whether the presence of psychosomatic symptoms (such as somatization, headaches and migraines, skin rash, stomach ulcers, and hypochondriac complaints) may have a psychological rather than a physiological etiology during pregnancy in order to better identify the most accurate interventions.

Moreover, contrary to expectation, no associations between lack of social support from partners, parents, and friends and PAMA subscales were found. This result does not allow for validation of the research hypothesis suggested by the literature, according to which poor social support represents a strong risk factor for psychopathological outcomes during pregnancy and the perinatal period [53,54]. These unexpected findings may be attributable to the small sample size or factors unique to this sample and should be assessed further in future studies.

Limitations

In this preliminary study, several limitations can be noted. First, our sample was self-selected and not representative of pregnant women. It is expected that the psychopathological consequences would be more marked among women who have more psychosocial stress factors. Future studies are needed to ascertain whether or not these results can be generalized to the broader population of pregnant women.

Second, the sample was small since this study is part of a larger ongoing research project, which did not allow for more sophisticated statistical analysis. The use of multiple tests and the small sample size mean that findings from this study should be interpreted with caution.

Lastly, is important that future research broaden this study to a more representative sample of pregnant women, taking into account other risk factors that may contribute, and start to examine the mechanisms behind these associations. For example, a topic of particular interest but that is still neglected is fathers' experience of pregnancy and their influence on the well-being of women and children. For many years, the literature has mainly focused on expectant mothers, probably because women play a principal role during pregnancy and their experience is more physically and physiologically perceptible than that of fathers [55]. However, in the last few years, researchers have focused their attention on the paternal experience of pregnancy; however, to date, there is not enough evidence to propose appropriate gender-based screening for fathers [56–58]. This area of investigation, which remains understudied, may play a central role in the prevention and management of situations of vulnerability and psychopathological risk.

5. Conclusions

In conclusion, although results from this study should be considered provisional, they suggest that the experience of maternal maltreatment in childhood has an impact on a pregnant woman's mental health and well-being. The results of this study highlight the need to identify at-risk women during pregnancy so as to allow healthcare workers to offer them the necessary help. Women with early traumatic experiences and a state of psychological suffering can be considered at risk. Therefore, comprehensive prenatal screening should include the assessment of childhood maltreatment experiences and of the current psychopathological distress of all pregnant women. This assessment is essential for identifying pregnant women who would benefit from targeted intervention to help interrupt the intergenerational transmission of adversity before babies are born.

The risk of the intergenerational transmission of mental health problems to the next generation of children is well-recognized [59,60]; therefore, prevention and intervention efforts for this vulnerable population may be informed by a better understanding of processes by which traumatic experiences provoke the risk of psychopathological conditions among pregnant women.

Supplementary Materials: The following supporting information can be downloaded at: https://www.mdpi.com/article/10.3390/women3010010/s1, Table S1: Percentage (%) of Stressful events in the previous year, CECA Q., and Maternal Social Support Scale (n = 61); Table S2: Percentage (%) of PAMA subscale (n = 61).

Author Contributions: Conceptualization, M.R.I. and F.G.; data collection: E.B., G.C. and G.F.; writing—review and editing, M.R.I. and G.F. All authors have read and agreed to the published version of the manuscript.

Funding: This research received no external funding.

Institutional Review Board Statement: This study was conducted in accordance with the Declaration of Helsinki.

Informed Consent Statement: Informed consent was obtained from all subjects involved in the study.

Data Availability Statement: The data presented in this study are available upon reasonable request from the corresponding author.

Conflicts of Interest: The authors declare no conflict of interest.

References

1. Maas, A.J.B.M.; Vreeswijk, C.M.J.M.; de Cock, E.S.A.; Rijk, C.H.A.M.; van Bakel, H.J.A. 'Expectant Parents': Study protocol of a longitudinal study concerning prenatal (risk) factors and postnatal infant development, parenting, and parent-infant relationships. *BMC Pregnancy Childbirth* **2012**, *12*, 46. [CrossRef] [PubMed]
2. Stern, D.N. *The Motherhood Constellation: A Unified View of Parent–Infant Psychotherapy*; Routledge: Abington, UK, 1995.
3. Glynn, L.M.; Schetter, C.D.; Wadhwa, P.D.; Sandman, C.A. Pregnancy affects appraisal of negative life events. *J. Psychosom. Res.* **2004**, *56*, 47–52. [CrossRef] [PubMed]
4. Narayan, A.J.; Rivera, L.M.; Bernstein, R.E.; Harris, W.W.; Lieberman, A.F. Positive childhood experiences predict less psychopathology and stress in pregnant women with childhood adversity: A pilot study of the benevolent childhood experiences (BCEs) scale. *Child Abuse Negl.* **2018**, *78*, 19–30. [CrossRef] [PubMed]
5. Van der Kolk, B.A. Developmental trauma disorder: Towards a rational diagnosis for chronically traumatized children. *Prax. Kinderpsychol. Kinderpsychiatr.* **2009**, *58*, 572–586.
6. Cicchetti, D.; Toth, S.L. Child maltreatment. *Annu. Rev. Clin. Psychol.* **2005**, *1*, 409–438. [CrossRef]
7. Felitti, V.J.; Anda, R.F.; Nordenberg, D.; Williamson, D.F.; Spitz, A.M.; Edwards, V.; Koss, M.P.; Marks, J.S. Relationship of Childhood Abuse and Household Dysfunction to Many of the Leading Causes of Death in Adults: The Adverse Childhood Experiences (ACE) Study. *Am. J. Prev. Med.* **1998**, *14*, 245–258. [CrossRef]
8. Infurna, M.R.; Brunner, R.; Holz, B.; Parzer, P.; Giannone, F.; Reichl, C.; Fischer, G.; Resch, F.; Kaess, M. The Specific Role of Childhood Abuse, Parental Bonding, and Family Functioning in Female Adolescents with Borderline Personality Disorder. *J. Pers. Disord.* **2016**, *30*, 177–192. [CrossRef]
9. Infurna, M.R.; Giannone, F.; Guarnaccia, C.; Lo Cascio, M.; Parzer, P.; Kaess, M. Environmental Factors That Distinguish between Clinical and Healthy Samples with Childhood Experiences of Abuse and Neglect. *Psychopathology* **2015**, *48*, 256–263. [CrossRef]

10. Scott, K.M.; McLaughlin, K.A.; Smith, D.A.R.; Ellis, P.M. Childhood maltreatment and DSM-IV adult mental disorders: Comparison of prospective and retrospective findings. *Br. J. Psychiatry* **2012**, *200*, 469–475. [CrossRef]
11. Baumeister, R.F.; Leary, M.R. The need to belong: Desire for interpersonal attachments as a fundamental human motivation. *Psychol. Bull.* **1995**, *117*, 497–529. [CrossRef]
12. Charuvastra, A.; Cloitre, M. Social Bonds and Posttraumatic Stress Disorder. *Annu. Rev. Psychol.* **2008**, *59*, 301–328. [CrossRef]
13. McLaughlin, K.A.; Conron, K.J.; Koenen, K.C.; Gilman, S.E. Childhood adversity, adult stressful life events, and risk of past-year psychiatric disorder: A test of the stress sensitization hypothesis in a population-based sample of adults. *Psychol. Med.* **2009**, *40*, 1647–1658. [CrossRef]
14. Sanchez, S.E.; Pineda, O.; Chaves, D.Z.; Zhong, Q.-Y.; Gelaye, B.; Simon, G.E.; Rondon, M.B.; Williams, M.A. Childhood physical and sexual abuse experiences associated with post-traumatic stress disorder among pregnant women. *Ann. Epidemiol.* **2017**, *27*, 716–723.e1. [CrossRef]
15. Zhang, X.; Sun, J.; Wang, J.; Chen, Q.; Cao, D.; Wang, J.; Cao, F. Suicide ideation among pregnant women: The role of different experiences of childhood abuse. *J. Affect. Disord.* **2020**, *266*, 182–186. [CrossRef]
16. Souch, A.J.; Jones, I.R.; Shelton, K.H.M.; Waters, C.S. Maternal childhood maltreatment and perinatal outcomes: A systematic review. *J. Affect Disord.* **2022**, *302*, 139–159. [CrossRef]
17. Finy, M.S.; Christian, L.M. Pathways linking childhood abuse history and current socioeconomic status to inflammation during pregnancy. *Brain Behav. Immun.* **2018**, *74*, 231–240. [CrossRef]
18. Shapero, B.G.; Black, S.K.; Liu, R.T.; Klugman, J.; Bender, R.E.; Abramson, L.Y.; Alloy, L.B. Stressful life events and depression symptoms: The effect of childhood emotional abuse on stress re-activity. *J. Clin. Psychol.* **2014**, *70*, 209–223. [CrossRef]
19. Milan, S.; Ickovics, J.R.; Kershaw, T.; Lewis, J.; Meade, C.; Ethier, K. Prevalence, Course, and Predictors of Emotional Distress in Pregnant and Parenting Adolescents. *J. Consult. Clin. Psychol.* **2004**, *72*, 328–340. [CrossRef]
20. Choi, K.W.; Sikkema, K.J. Childhood maltreatment and perinatal mood and anxiety disorders: A systematic review. *Trauma Violence Abus.* **2016**, *17*, 427–453. [CrossRef]
21. Huth-Bocks, A.C.; Krause, K.; Ahlfs-Dunn, S.; Gallagher, E.; Scott, S. Relational Trauma and Posttraumatic Stress Symptoms among Pregnant Women. *Psychodyn. Psychiatry* **2013**, *41*, 277–301. [CrossRef]
22. Atzl, V.M.; Narayan, A.J.; Rivera, L.M.; Lieberman, A.F. Adverse childhood experiences and prenatal mental health: Type of ACEs and age of maltreatment onset. *J. Fam. Psychol.* **2019**, *33*, 304–314. [CrossRef] [PubMed]
23. Flach, C.; Leese, M.; Heron, J.; Evans, J.; Feder, G.; Sharp, D.; Howard, L. Antenatal domestic violence, maternal mental health and subsequent child behaviour: A cohort study. *BJOG Int. J. Obstet. Gynaecol.* **2011**, *118*, 1383–1391. [CrossRef] [PubMed]
24. Grekin, R.; O'Hara, M.W. Prevalence and risk factors of postpartum posttraumatic stress disorder: A meta-analysis. *Clin. Psychol. Rev.* **2014**, *34*, 389–401. [CrossRef] [PubMed]
25. Lev-Wiesel, R.; Chen, R.; Daphna-Tekoah, S.; Hod, M. Past Traumatic Events: Are They a Risk Factor for High-Risk Pregnancy, Delivery Complications, and Postpartum Posttraumatic Symptoms? *J. Women's Health* **2009**, *18*, 119–125. [CrossRef] [PubMed]
26. Brooker, R.J.; Kiel, E.J.; MacNamara, A.; Nyman, T.; John-Henderson, N.A.; Schmidt, L.A.; Van Lieshout, R.J. Maternal neural reactivity during pregnancy predicts infant temperament. *Infancy* **2019**, *25*, 46–66. [CrossRef]
27. Pare-Miron, V.; Czuzoj-Shulman, N.; Oddy, L.; Spence, A.R.; Abenhaim, H.A. Effect of Borderline Personality Disorder on Obstetrical and Neonatal Outcomes. *Women's Health Issues* **2015**, *26*, 190–195. [CrossRef]
28. Alderdice, F.; Lynn, F.; Lobel, M. A review and psychometric evaluation of pregnancy-specific stress measures. *J. Psychosom. Obstet. Gynecol.* **2012**, *33*, 62–77. [CrossRef]
29. Monk, C.; Lugo-Candelas, C.; Trumpff, C. Prenatal Developmental Origins of Future Psychopathology: Mechanisms and Pathways. *Annu. Rev. Clin. Psychol.* **2019**, *15*, 317–344. [CrossRef]
30. Stein, A.; Pearson, R.M.; Goodman, S.H.; Rapa, E.; Rahman, A.; McCallum, M.; Howard, L.M.; Pariante, C.M. Effects of perinatal mental disorders on the fetus and child. *Lancet* **2014**, *384*, 1800–1819. [CrossRef]
31. Webster, J.; Pritchard, M.; Linnane, J.W.; Roberts, J.A.; Hinson, J.; Starrenburg, S.E. Postnatal depression: Use of health services and satisfaction with health-care providers. *J. Qual. Clin. Pract.* **2001**, *21*, 144–148. [CrossRef]
32. Buist, A.E.; Janson, H. Childhood sexual abuse, parenting and postpartum depression—A 3-year follow-up study. *Child Abus. Negl.* **2001**, *25*, 909–921. [CrossRef]
33. Alvarez-Segura, M.; Garcia-Esteve, L.; Torres, A.; Plaza, A.; Imaz, M.L.; Hermida-Barros, L.; San, L.; Burtchen, N. Are women with a history of abuse more vulnerable to perinatal depressive symptoms? A systematic review. *Arch. Womens Ment. Health* **2014**, *17*, 343–357. [CrossRef]
34. Mezey, G.; Bacchus, L.; Bewley, S.; White, S. Domestic violence, lifetime trauma and psychological health of childbearing women. *BJOG Int. J. Obstet. Gynaecol.* **2005**, *112*, 197–204. [CrossRef]
35. Inanici, S.Y.; Inanici, M.A.; Yoldemir, A.T. The relationship between subjective experience of childhood abuse and neglect and depressive symptoms during pregnancy. *J. Forensic Leg. Med.* **2017**, *49*, 76–80. [CrossRef]
36. Martini, J.; Petzoldt, J.; Einsle, F.; Beesdo-Baum, K.; Höfler, M.; Wittchen, H.-U. Risk factors and course patterns of anxiety and depressive disorders during pregnancy and after delivery: A prospective-longitudinal study. *J. Affect. Disord.* **2015**, *175*, 385–395. [CrossRef]
37. Van Bussel, J.C.H.; Spitz, B.; Demyttenaere, K. Depressive symptomatology in pregnant and postpartum women. An exploratory study of the role of maternal antenatal orientations. *Arch. Womens Ment. Health* **2009**, *12*, 155–166. [CrossRef]

38. Gaillard, A.; Le Strat, Y.; Mandelbrot, L.; Keïta, H.; Dubertret, C. Predictors of postpartum depression: Prospective study of 264 women followed during pregnancy and postpartum. *Psychiatry Res.* **2014**, *215*, 341–346. [CrossRef]
39. Woody, C.A.; Ferrari, A.J.; Siskind, D.J.; Whiteford, H.A.; Harris, M.G. A systematic review and meta-regression of the prevalence and incidence of perinatal depression. *J. Affect. Disord.* **2017**, *219*, 86–92. [CrossRef]
40. Hutchens, B.F.; Kearney, J. Risk Factors for Postpartum Depression: An Umbrella Review. *J. Midwifery Women's Health* **2020**, *65*, 96–108. [CrossRef]
41. Austin, M.-P. Targeted group antenatal prevention of postnatal depression: A review. *Acta Psychiatr. Scand.* **2003**, *107*, 244–250. [CrossRef]
42. Buist, A.E.; Barnett, B.E.W.; Milgrom, J.; Pope, S.; Condon, J.T.; Ellwood, D.A.; Boyce, P.M.; Austin, M.-P.; Hayes, B.A. To screen or not to screen—That is the question in perinatal depression. *Med. J. Aust.* **2002**, *177*, S101–S105. [CrossRef] [PubMed]
43. Webster, J.; Linnane, J.W.; Dibley, L.M.; Hinson, J.K.; Starrenburg, S.E.; Roberts, J.A. Measuring social support in pregnancy: Can it be simple and meaningful? *Birth* **2000**, *27*, 97–101. [CrossRef] [PubMed]
44. Bifulco, A.; Bernazzani, O.; Moran, P.M.; Jacobs, C. The childhood experience of care and abuse questionnaire (CECA.Q): Validation in a community series. *Br. J. Clin. Psychol.* **2005**, *44*, 563–581. [CrossRef] [PubMed]
45. Baldoni, F.; Giannotti, M.; Casu, G.; Agostini, F.; Mandolesi, R.; Peverieri, S.; Ambrogetti, N.; Spelzini, F.; Caretti, V.; Terrone, G. The Perinatal Assessment of Paternal Affectivity (PAPA): Italian validation of a new tool for the screening of perinatal depression and affective disorders in fathers. *J. Affect. Disord.* **2022**, *317*, 123–130. [CrossRef] [PubMed]
46. Infurna, M.R.; Reichl, C.; Parzer, P.; Schimmenti, A.; Bifulco, A.; Kaess, M. Associations between depression and specific childhood experiences of abuse and neglect: A meta-analysis. *J. Affect. Disord.* **2016**, *190*, 47–55. [CrossRef]
47. McCoy, S.J.B.; Beal, J.M.; Shipman, S.B.M.; Payton, M.E.; Watson, G.H. Risk factors for postpartum depression: A retrospective investigation at 4-weeks postnatal and a review of the literature. *J. Am. Osteopath. Assoc.* **2006**, *106*, 193–198.
48. Bowlby, J. Attachment and loss: Retrospect and prospect. *Am. J. Orthopsychiatry* **1982**, *52*, 664–678. [CrossRef]
49. Marchetti, D.; Musso, P.; Verrocchio, M.C.; Manna, G.; Kopala-Sibley, D.C.; De Berardis, D.; De Santis, S.; Falgares, G. Childhood maltreatment, personality vulnerability profiles, and borderline personality disorder symptoms in adolescents. *Dev. Psychopathol.* **2022**, *34*, 1163–1176. [CrossRef]
50. Class, Q.A.B.; Lichtenstein, P.; Långström, N.; D'Onofrio, B.M. Timing of Prenatal Maternal Exposure to Severe Life Events and Adverse Pregnancy Outcomes: A Population Study of 2.6 Million Pregnancies. *Psychosom. Med.* **2011**, *73*, 234–241. [CrossRef]
51. Biaggi, A.; Conroy, S.; Pawlby, S.; Pariante, C.M. Identifying the women at risk of antenatal anxiety and depression: A systematic review. *J. Affect. Disord.* **2015**, *191*, 62–77. [CrossRef]
52. Byrnes, L. Perinatal mood and anxiety disorders: Findings from focus groups of at risk women. *Arch. Psychiatr. Nurs.* **2019**, *33*, 149–153. [CrossRef]
53. Aktan, N.M. Social support and anxiety in pregnant and postpartum women: A secondary analysis. *Clin. Nurs. Res.* **2012**, *21*, 183–194. [CrossRef]
54. Nakić Radoš, S.; Tadinac, M.; Herman, R. Anxiety during Pregnancy and Postpartum: Course, Predictors and Comorbidity with Postpartum Depression. *Acta Clin. Croat.* **2018**, *57*, 39–51. [CrossRef]
55. Cannella, B.L. Maternal-fetal attachment: An integrative review. *J. Adv. Nurs.* **2005**, *50*, 60–68. [CrossRef]
56. Baldoni, F.; Giannotti, M. Perinatal Distress in Fathers: Toward a Gender-Based Screening of Paternal Perinatal Depressive and Affective Disorders. *Front. Psychol.* **2020**, *11*, 1892. [CrossRef]
57. Berg, A.R.; Ahmed, A.H. Paternal perinatal depression: Making a case for routine screening. *Nurse Pract.* **2016**, *41*, 1–5. [CrossRef]
58. Hammarlund, K.; Andersson, E.; Tenenbaum, H.; Sundler, A.J. We are also interested in how fathers feel: A qualitative exploration of child health center nurses' recognition of postnatal depression in fathers. *BMC Pregnancy Childbirth* **2015**, *15*, 290. [CrossRef]
59. Leen-Feldner, E.W.; Feldner, M.T.; Knapp, A.; Bunaciu, L.; Blumenthal, H.; Amstadter, A.B. Offspring psychological and biological correlates of parental posttraumatic stress: Review of the literature and research agenda. *Clin. Psychol. Rev.* **2013**, *33*, 1106–1133. [CrossRef]
60. Goodman, S.H.; Rouse, M.H.; Connell, A.M.; Broth, M.R.; Hall, C.M. Maternal depression and child psychopathology: A meta-analytic review. *Clin. Child Fam. Psychol. Rev.* **2011**, *14*, 1–27. [CrossRef]

Disclaimer/Publisher's Note: The statements, opinions and data contained in all publications are solely those of the individual author(s) and contributor(s) and not of MDPI and/or the editor(s). MDPI and/or the editor(s) disclaim responsibility for any injury to people or property resulting from any ideas, methods, instructions or products referred to in the content.

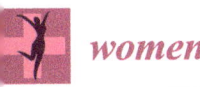

Article

Differentials in Maternal Mortality Pattern in Sub-Saharan Africa Countries: Evidence from Demographic and Health Survey Data

Osaretin Christabel Okonji [1,*], Chimezie Igwegbe Nzoputam [2,3], Michael Ekholuenetale [4,*], Emeka Francis Okonji [5], Anthony Ike Wegbom [6] and Clement Kevin Edet [7]

1. School of Pharmacy, University of the Western Cape, Cape Town 7530, South Africa
2. Department of Public Health, Center of Excellence in Reproductive Health Innovation (CERHI), College of Medical Sciences, University of Benin, Benin City 300001, Nigeria
3. Department of Medical Biochemistry, School of Basic Medical Sciences, University of Benin, Benin City 300001, Nigeria
4. Department of Epidemiology and Medical Statistics, Faculty of Public Health, College of Medicine, University of Ibadan, Ibadan 200284, Nigeria
5. School of Public Health, University of the Western Cape, Cape Town 7535, South Africa
6. Department of Public Health Sciences, College of Medical Sciences, Rivers State University, Port Harcourt 500101, Nigeria
7. Department of Community Medicine, College of Medical Sciences, Rivers State University, Port Harcourt 500101, Nigeria
* Correspondence: okonjichristabel@gmail.com (O.C.O.); mic42006@gmail.com (M.E.)

Abstract: Maternal mortality ratios in sub-Saharan Africa remain high and worrisome. Moreover, maternal health indicators have remained poor despite large efforts in the last two decades. This study assesses maternal mortality patterns by age and country. The demographic and health survey data were used for the study. Based on the results, countries with the lowest adult female mortality rate include Senegal, Comoros, Rwanda, Mauritania, Sao Tome and Principe, Gambia, and Ethiopia. In addition, Chad (44.7%), Niger (38.7%), the Congo Democratic Republic (34.8%), Nigeria (34.2%), Mauritania (32.0%), Senegal (29.2%), Liberia (28.8%), Benin (27.8%), and Guinea (27.5%), respectively, reported the highest female deaths that are pregnancy-related. Overall, Lesotho (1024; 95% CI: 731–1318), Liberia (913; 95% CI: 638–1189), Chad (860; 95% CI: 728–993), Congo Democratic Republic (846; 95% CI: 690–1003), Sierra Leone (796; 95% CI: 632–960) and Guinea (724; 95% CI: 531–916) had the leading pregnancy-related mortality ratio per 100,000 live births. The study found that the patterns of death vary across different countries. There is a need for concerted efforts to reduce pregnancy-related deaths in sub-Saharan countries.

Keywords: maternal mortality; trend; maternal health; prenatal care; sub-Saharan Africa

Citation: Okonji, O.C.; Nzoputam, C.I.; Ekholuenetale, M.; Okonji, E.F.; Wegbom, A.I.; Edet, C.K. Differentials in Maternal Mortality Pattern in Sub-Saharan Africa Countries: Evidence from Demographic and Health Survey Data. *Women* **2023**, *3*, 175–188. https://doi.org/10.3390/women3010014

Academic Editor: Mary V. Seeman

Received: 23 January 2023
Revised: 2 March 2023
Accepted: 6 March 2023
Published: 9 March 2023

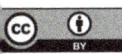

Copyright: © 2023 by the authors. Licensee MDPI, Basel, Switzerland. This article is an open access article distributed under the terms and conditions of the Creative Commons Attribution (CC BY) license (https://creativecommons.org/licenses/by/4.0/).

1. Background

Maternal mortality is a key public health concern, particularly in developing countries. In 2017, an estimated 810 women died from preventable causes associated with pregnancy and childbirth, with 94% of all maternal mortality occurring in resource-poor settings [1]. South Asia and sub-Saharan Africa (SSA) account for about 86% of maternal deaths worldwide [1]. SSA countries record the highest number of maternal deaths annually, with a maternal mortality ratio (MMR) of 553 deaths per 100,000 live births, which is over 50 times higher than the MMR for high-income countries with 11 deaths per 100,000 live births [2]. The burden of maternal deaths in the SSA region shows the inequities in access to maternal health services and the socioeconomic disparities between high-income and low-income countries.

The risk of maternal death remains high in low-income countries, as 1 in 45 women die from pregnancy-related causes, compared with 1 in 5400 in high-income countries. [1,2].

Women in the SSA region have the highest risk of maternal death at 1 in 38 [1,2]. Furthermore, women in low-income countries have a significantly higher fertility rate than women in high-income countries, making the risk of death due to pregnancy higher [1]. Additionally, the risk of complications from pregnancy and delivery is higher for adolescent and young mothers, respectively [1].

The number of maternal deaths has declined substantially worldwide in the past two decades, with SSA countries achieving about a 39% reduction between 2000 and 2017 [2]. Despite the substantial reduction in maternal deaths in the SSA region, the current burden remains worrisome. Research-based evidence from SSA countries shows that the highest number of deaths occur during the antepartum, intrapartum, and postpartum periods [3]. About 31% occurs during pregnancy, 36% during childbirth or the first week, and 33% happen between the first week and one year after termination of pregnancy [4].

Multiple studies conducted in the SSA countries have found obstetrical hemorrhage, eclampsia, and hypertensive conditions during pregnancy to be major causes of maternal deaths [5–7]. A recent systematic review found obstetrical hemorrhage, hypertensive conditions during pregnancy, non-obstetric complications, and infections related to pregnancy as the main causes of maternal deaths in SSA countries [5]. Similarly, another study reported haemorrhage and hypertensive conditions to account for about 40% of maternal deaths [8]. Among adolescents in low- and middle-income countries (LMICs), the main causes of maternal deaths were obstetrical hemorrhage, hypertensive conditions during pregnancy, and infections associated with pregnancy [9].

The Third Sustainable Development Goal (SDG 3.1) targets reduced maternal mortality and reduces the maternal mortality ratio (MMR) to 70 deaths for every 100,000 live births by 2030 [10]. To reduce maternal mortality in SSA countries, understanding the pattern and burden in various SSA countries is crucial. Therefore, we explore maternal mortality prevalence and patterns in SSA countries. The findings from this study would help policymakers implement health programs to reduce maternal mortality in SSA countries.

2. Methods

Data Source

We used 2006 to 2021, SSA countries' Demographic and Health Surveys (DHS) data [11–13]. A multistage cluster stratified sampling strategy is used by DHS to gather data. The respondents were divided into groups according to their geographic location, which was typically determined by their place of residence: urban versus rural, using the stratification method. The population was divided into first-level strata, second-level strata, etc. using a multi-level stratified approach. Geographic location and urban or rural status were used to determine the DHS's two levels of stratification. The following countries were examined in the study: Angola, Cameroon, Benin, Congo Democratic Republic Burkina Faso, Burundi, Egypt, Eritrea, Chad, Comoros, Nigeria, Congo, Cote d'Ivoire, Ethiopia, Gabon, Gambia, Liberia, Togo, Uganda, Guinea, Kenya, Lesotho, Madagascar, Morocco, Mozambique, Namibia, Malawi, Mali, Niger, Rwanda, Senegal, Sierra Leone, Sao Tome and Principe, South Africa, Tanzania, Zambia, Zimbabwe.

Since 1984, these surveys have been conducted every five years in more than 85 countries worldwide. One key advantage of DHS is the sampling approach to data collection, which is consistent across countries and enables results to be compared between countries. Even though the DHS was created to supplement the demographic, family planning, and fertility data collected by the World Fertility Surveys (WFSs) and Contraceptive Prevalence Surveys (CPSs), it has quickly evolved into the most significant base of population investigation for the monitoring of population health trends, particularly in areas with limited resources. The DHS collects data on immunizations, maternal and infant mortality, domestic violence, fertility, female genital mutilation, communicable and non-communicable diseases, nutrition, water and sanitation, lifestyle, family planning, and other health-related issues. The DHS is successful in gathering high-quality data by providing adequate interviewer training, nationwide coverage, uniform data collection tools, and methodological approaches to issues that are easy for legislators and decision-makers to understand. Using information from the

DHS, epidemiologic studies can be conducted to determine prevalence, movements, and disparities. Details about DHS have been reported previously [14].

3. Selection and Measurement of Variables

3.1. Outcome

- Adult female mortality rate: the adult female mortality rate over the seven-year period prior to the survey, expressed as a percentage of 1000 women-years of exposure.
- Female deaths that are pregnancy-related: the percentage of all female adult deaths that are pregnancy-related, including those from accidents or violence during pregnancy, delivery, and the two months following delivery.
- Pregnancy-related mortality rate: this is expressed as the number of deaths from pregnancy in the seven years prior to the survey, per 1000 woman-years of exposure.
- Pregnancy-related mortality ratio: the pregnancy-related mortality ratio is calculated as the age-adjusted pregnancy-related mortality rate multiplied by 100 divided by the age-adjusted general fertility rate, and it is expressed as the number of pregnancies lost during the seven years prior to the survey per 100,000 live births.
- Lifetime risk of pregnancy-related death: calculated as 1-(1-PRMR) TFR, where TFR is the total fertility rate for the seven years prior to the survey, is the lifetime risk of pregnancy-related death.

3.2. Explanatory Variable

The patterns of women's mortality were disaggregated by age (years): 15–19, 20–24, 25–29, 30–34, 35–39, 40–44, 45–49.

3.3. Analytical Approach

With the aid of the Stata survey module ('svy'), all sampling weights, clustering, and stratification were taken into account. The prevalence was evaluated using percentages. An analysis of forest plots was used to determine the variation in pregnancy-related mortality between the countries. The weighted effect size (w*es) for each country's prevalence in the forest plot was also calculated. To determine how heterogeneous a country is, we used the Q-test, which is comparable to the t-test. Using the same weights as those used in the pooling procedure, we also calculated this as the sum of squares of the variances between the effects in each individual study and the overall effect for all countries. With k-1 degrees of freedom, Q has a chi-square distribution (k being the total number of countries). Our null hypothesis is that all countries are equal. We reject the null hypothesis at the level of 5% significance. Stata 14.0 was used to conduct the analysis (StataCorp, College Station, TX, USA).

3.4. Ethical Approval and Informed Consent

Public domain datasets based on populations that had been anonymized were examined in this study. MEASURE DHS/ICF International granted the authors permission to use the data. The DHS Program adheres to all applicable standards for protecting respondents' personal information. ICF International ensures that the survey complies with the requirements of the Human Subjects Protection Act of the US Department of Health and Human Services. Before conducting the surveys, the DHS team received approval from the National Health Research Ethics Committees of several countries. For this investigation, no additional authorizations were required. Check out this link for more information on our data and ethical standards: http://goo.gl/ny8T6X (accessed on 5 January 2023).

4. Results

Table 1 shows that the adult female mortality rate was higher among older women aged 30 years and older across many countries. Countries with the lowest adult female mortality rate include Senegal (1.5 per 1000 women-years of exposure), the Comoros (1.58 per 1000 women-years of exposure), Rwanda (1.88 per 1000 women-years of exposure), Mauritania (2.4 per 1000 women-years of exposure), Sao Tome and Principe (2.52 per

1000 women-years of exposure), Gambia (2.72 per 1000 women-years of exposure), and Ethiopia (2.74 per 1000 women-years of exposure). See the details below in Table 1.

Table 1. Pattern of adult female mortality rate.

Country	Survey Year	Total Sample Size	Adult Female Mortality Rate							
			15–19	20–24	25–29	30–34	35–39	40–44	45–49	Total
Angola	2015–2016	14,379	1.99	2.48	2.86	3.87	4.13	5.63	2.41	3.04
Benin	2017–2018	15,928	2.45	2.23	2.32	4.02	3.82	3.9	4.71	3.06
Burkina Faso	2010	17,087	2.03	2.44	3.67	3.94	5.74	6.25	7.53	3.93
Burundi	2016–2017	17,269	1.92	1.77	2.46	3.27	4.25	6.54	7.4	3.24
Cameroon	2018	14,677	2.53	2.96	3.54	5.66	5.38	6.75	6.89	4.18
Chad	2014–2015	17,719	3.56	4.08	4.67	5.86	5.45	6.79	5.22	4.81
Comoros	2012	5329	0.53	1.09	1.43	2.08	2.08	3.72	2.68	1.58
Congo	2011–2012	10,819	2.22	3.07	4.44	7.05	6.6	11.36	10.2	5.36
Congo Democratic Republic	2013–2014	18,827	4.08	4.53	4.88	5.33	7.87	7.3	7.23	5.4
Cote d'Ivoire	2011–2012	10,060	2.86	3.75	4.13	8.62	8.87	11.87	11.46	6.15
Ethiopia	2016	15,683	2.22	2.23	2.32	3.68	2.2	3.85	4.57	2.74
Gabon	2012	8422	2.14	2.05	4.87	4.23	5.05	5.18	8.43	3.94
Gambia	2019–2020	11,865	0.93	1.55	2.24	3.27	3.57	6.27	6.25	2.72
Guinea	2012	9142	3.86	3.68	3.92	5.01	6.98	5.36	9.25	4.93
Kenya	2014	31,079	1.67	2.1	2.66	4.73	6.78	6.83	5	3.72
Lesotho	2014	6621	2.29	5.57	10.93	17.84	19.12	28.21	30.29	12.82
Liberia	2019–2020	8065	2.53	3.36	4.25	5.01	6	7.44	9.4	4.76
Madagascar	2008–2009	17,375	3.23	3.28	3.24	4.32	3.7	6.59	7.38	4.14
Malawi	2015–2016	24,562	1.7	3.29	4.38	5.62	6.56	9.41	9.66	4.77
Mali	2018	10,519	2.34	2.89	2.52	3.37	4.17	7.26	6.51	3.54
Mauritania	2019–2021	15,714	0.99	1.45	2.15	2.75	3.73	5.93	2.32	2.4
Mozambique	2011	13,745	2.38	4.78	6.4	7.07	7.45	5.44	10.71	5.71
Namibia	2013	10,018	1.56	2.29	4.71	6.74	7.71	6.47	6.44	4.53
Niger	2012	11,160	3.23	4.21	2.92	4.41	2.92	5.31	4.32	3.76
Nigeria	2018	41,821	1.59	2.39	2.52	3.25	4.01	5.35	5.86	3.18
Rwanda	2019–2020	14,634	0.82	1.21	1.32	2.09	2.51	2.36	5.06	1.88
Sao Tome and Principe	2008–2009	2615	1.18	2.1	1.51	2.65	3.21	4.32	6.45	2.59
Senegal	2017	16,787	0.79	0.89	1.06	2.12	1.98	2.85	2.45	1.5
Sierra Leone	2019	15,574	2.81	3.48	3.95	4.85	6.15	7.22	8.36	4.69
South Africa	2016	8514	1.02	3.65	4.48	9.82	9.13	11.39	8.32	6.34
Tanzania	2015–2016	13,266	1.27	2.32	2.78	4.67	6.35	9.67	10.82	4.37
Togo	2013–2014	9480	2.21	3.18	3.8	4.98	4.92	8.81	9.4	4.69
Uganda	2016	18,506	2.26	2.48	3.25	4.79	5	6.16	7.2	3.78
Zambia	2018	13,683	1.25	3.22	3.31	6.16	5.02	8.36	9.13	4.29
Zimbabwe	2015	9955	1.88	2.49	5.02	10.75	13.64	15.23	17.1	7.59

Figure 1 shows the total adult female mortality rate in SSA countries. Overall, Lesotho, Zimbabwe, South Africa, Mozambique, and Cote d'Ivoire reported the leading adult female mortality rate per 1000 women-years of exposure.

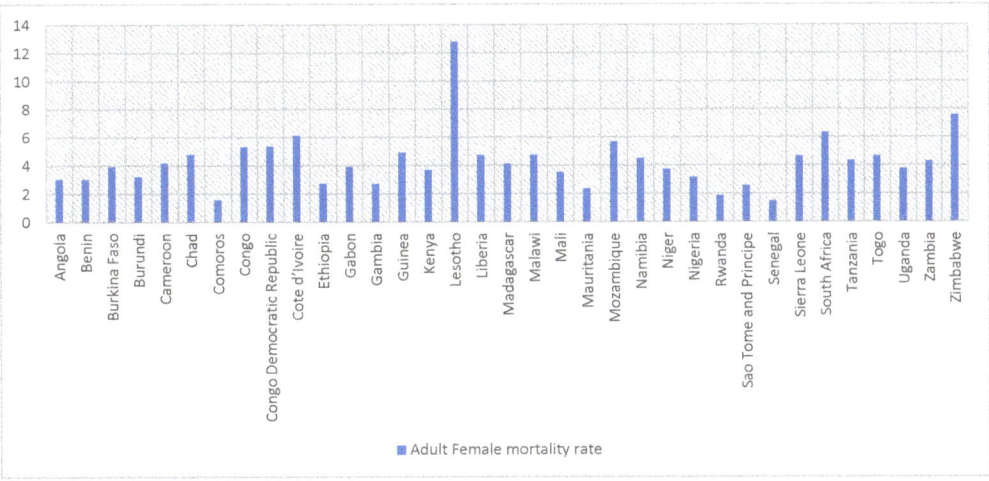

Figure 1. Adult female mortality rate.

Figure 2 shows the lifetime risk of pregnancy-related death across sub-Saharan countries. The Congo Democratic Republic (0.06), Chad (0.06), Guinea, Liberia, Niger, and Sierra Leone (0.04) reported the highest lifetime risk of pregnancy-related deaths, calculated as 1-(1-pregnancy-related mortality ratios (PRMR))^total fertility rate (TFR).

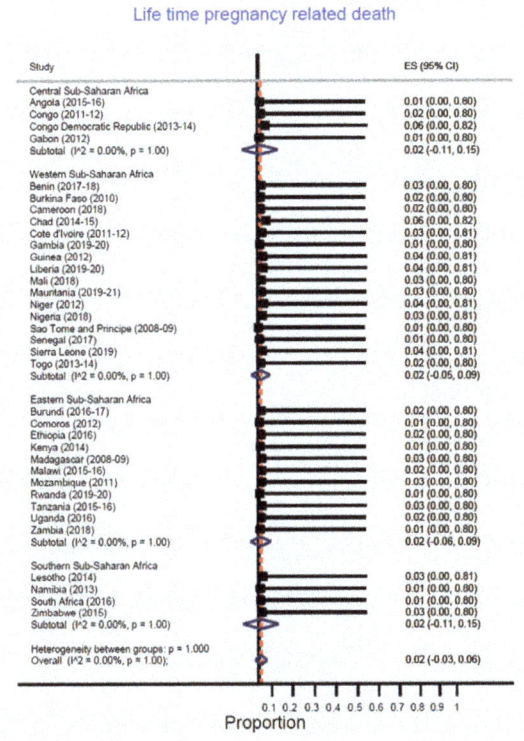

Figure 2. Lifetime risk of pregnancy-related death.

Table 2 shows female deaths that are pregnancy-related across sub-Saharan countries. The results show Chad (44.7%), Niger (38.7%), the Congo Democratic Republic (34.8%), Nigeria (34.2%), Mauritania (32.0%), Senegal (29.2%), Liberia (28.8%), Benin (27.8%), and Guinea (27.5%), respectively, reported the highest female deaths that are pregnancy-related.

Table 2. Female deaths that are pregnancy-related.

Country	Female Deaths That Are Pregnancy-Related							
	15–19	20–24	25–29	30–34	35–39	40–44	45–49	Total
Angola	16.5	21.2	13.8	12.7	23.5	10.3	14.1	16.3
Benin	18.1	35	32.9	35.2	24.7	20.9	14.1	27.8
Burkina Faso	14.3	29	19.3	21	18.2	11.4	9	18.6
Burundi	8	23.8	41.6	36.6	27.1	17.2	1.1	24.4
Cameroon	16	25.1	19.3	27	15.5	18.6	2.4	19.7
Chad	50.8	45.4	55.2	45.2	37.1	32	15.2	44.7
Comoros	0	0	45.6	26.6	18.7	1	0	16.9
Congo	19.6	17.5	11.8	15.7	19.6	2.6	7.6	13.2
Congo Democratic Republic	29.2	45.7	38.6	30.1	35.8	34.9	11.4	34.8
Cote d'Ivoire	14.8	21.9	22.7	13.1	22	10	11.8	16.9
Ethiopia	17.4	28.7	29.3	30	24.4	20.3	13.7	25.1
Gabon	33.8	10.2	9.3	4.1	11.9	7	1.9	10.6
Gambia	8.6	21	26.5	27.1	19.2	15.4	0	19.1
Guinea	30.1	35.3	31.3	30.4	25.4	15.4	7.5	27.5
Kenya	6.8	21.8	27.4	13.7	12.8	7.3	4.5	14.1
Lesotho	25	14.4	15.5	6.2	10.9	0.5	4.3	9.1
Liberia	27.1	58.8	23.6	27.6	31.6	20.5	7.8	28.8
Madagascar	25.8	22.3	27.4	21.3	25.8	11	6.6	20.6
Malawi	16.2	21.2	26.4	23.6	15.8	9.8	2.6	18.4
Mali	16.6	23.5	28	28.6	33.7	18.4	6	23.7
Mauritania	27	23.1	39.3	26	45.7	23.9	38.3	32
Mozambique	24.2	21.7	17.5	9	13.4	8.5	8.8	15.1
Namibia	11.9	11.9	8.8	9.6	13.8	0.8	5.5	9.4
Niger	34.4	41.7	45.4	42.9	46.5	23.4	15.1	38.7
Nigeria	40.8	42.7	43.5	41.2	33	14.8	11.8	34.2
Rwanda	5.5	6.7	16.2	22.7	22.7	29	15.2	18.2
Sao Tome and Principe	0	0	7.1	12.9	3.3	20.6	0	6.6
Senegal	16.4	34.4	35.2	35.6	32.3	22.7	11.5	29.2
Sierra Leone	22.6	28.2	28.5	30.8	31.2	17.6	7.7	25.6
South Africa	0	9.8	13	4.7	8.3	10.7	1.3	7.8
Tanzania	21.9	28.8	35.2	12.8	19.8	21.3	10.4	20.6
Togo	17.8	25.1	20.5	11.1	14.4	9.1	1.3	14.3
Uganda	18.3	28.2	23.4	20	15.1	19.2	2.3	19.2
Zambia	3.5	19.9	17.2	10.3	5.4	3.8	11.2	10.8
Zimbabwe	20.2	31	16.2	10.7	9.7	10.6	4.5	12.2

Figure 3 shows that Chad, Niger, Congo Democratic Republic, Nigeria, Mauritania, Senegal, Liberia, Benin, and Guinea reported the highest female deaths that are pregnancy-related.

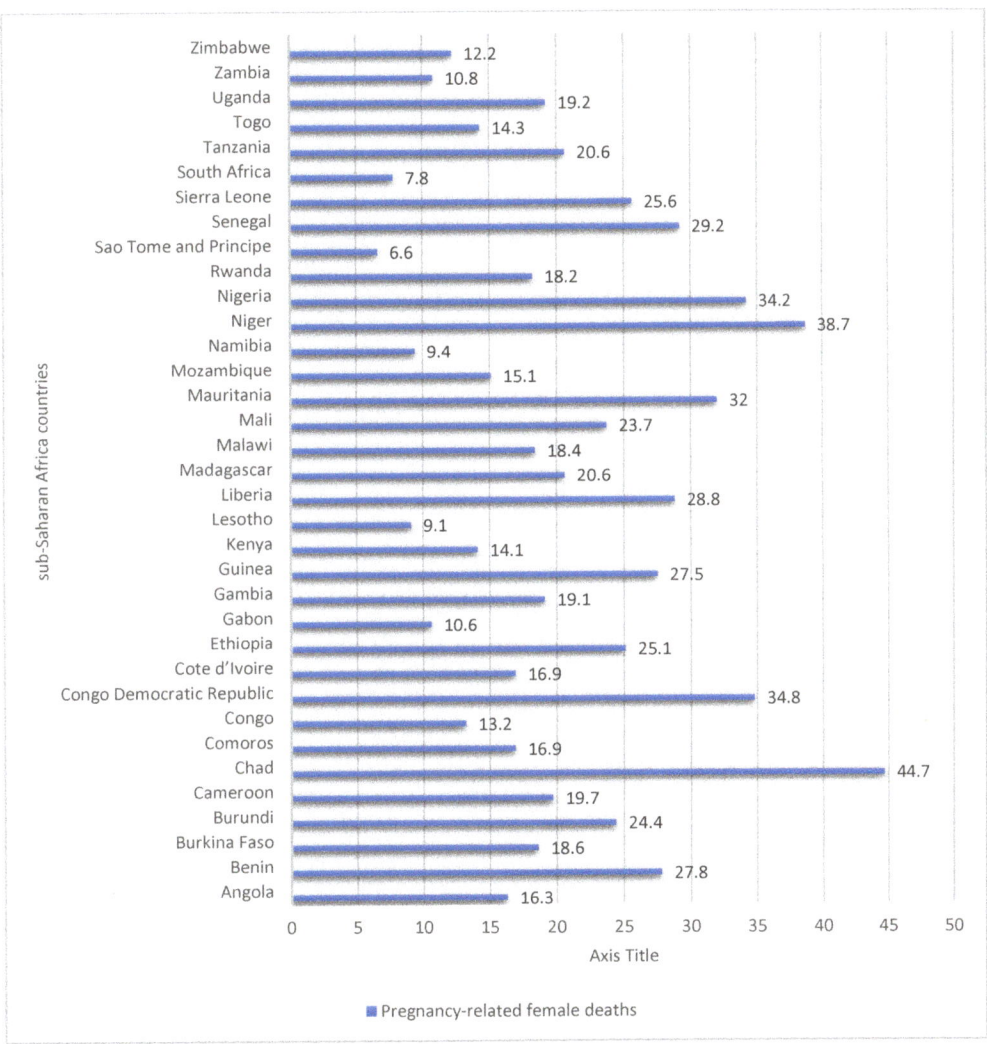

Figure 3. Pregnancy-related female deaths in sub-Saharan Africa 2006–2021.

Table 3 shows the pregnancy-related mortality rate and ratio. Overall, Lesotho (1024; 95% CI: 731–1318), Liberia (913; 95% CI: 638–1189), Chad (860; 95% CI: 728–993), the Congo Democratic Republic (846; 95% CI: 690–1003), Sierra Leone (796; 95% CI: 632–960), and Guinea (724; 95% CI: 531–916) reported the leading pregnancy-related mortality ratio per 100,000 live births.

Table 3. Pregnancy-related mortality rate and ratio.

	Pregnancy-Related Mortality Rate							Pregnancy-Related Mortality Ratio
	15–19	20–24	25–29	30–34	35–39	40–44	45–49	Total	
Angola	0.33	0.53	0.39	0.49	0.97	0.58	0.34	0.49	239 (CI: 164–313)
Benin	0.44	0.78	0.76	1.42	0.94	0.81	0.66	0.81	433 (CI: 339–527)
Burkina Faso	0.29	0.71	0.71	0.83	1.05	0.71	0.68	0.68	341 (CI: 275–406)
Burundi	0.15	0.42	1.02	1.2	1.15	1.13	0.08	0.7	392 (CI: 312–472)
Cameroon	0.4	0.74	0.68	1.53	0.83	1.25	0.16	0.78	467 (CI: 360–573)
Chad	1.81	1.85	2.58	2.65	2.02	2.17	0.8	2.06	860 (CI: 728–993)
Comoros	0	0	0.65	0.55	0.39	0.04	0	0.24	172 (CI: 60–284)
Congo	0.44	0.54	0.52	1.11	1.29	0.29	0.78	0.69	426 (CI: 274–579)
Congo Democratic Republic	1.19	2.07	1.88	1.61	2.82	2.55	0.82	1.83	846 (CI: 690–1003)
Cote d'Ivoire	0.42	0.82	0.94	1.13	1.95	1.19	1.36	1	614 (CI: 445–783)
Ethiopia	0.39	0.64	0.68	1.1	0.54	0.78	0.62	0.66	412 (CI: 273–551)
Gabon	0.72	0.21	0.45	0.17	0.6	0.36	0.16	0.41	316 (CI: 178–454)
Gambia	0.08	0.33	0.59	0.89	0.68	0.97	0	0.48	320 (CI: 231–409)
Guinea	1.16	1.3	1.23	1.52	1.77	0.82	0.69	1.25	724 (CI: 531–916)
Kenya	0.11	0.46	0.73	0.65	0.87	0.5	0.22	0.51	362 (CI: 254–471)
Lesotho	0.57	0.8	1.7	1.11	2.09	0.15	1.31	1.07	1024 (CI: 731–1318)
Liberia	0.69	1.98	1.01	1.38	1.89	1.52	0.74	1.31	913 (CI: 638–1189)
Madagascar	0.83	0.73	0.89	0.92	0.96	0.72	0.49	0.81	498 (CI: 402–594)
Malawi	0.28	0.7	1.16	1.33	1.03	0.92	0.25	0.8	497 (CI: 400–593)
Mali	0.39	0.68	0.71	0.97	1.41	1.34	0.39	0.8	373 (CI: 288–458)

Table 3. Cont.

	Pregnancy-Related Mortality Rate								Pregnancy-Related Mortality Ratio
	15–19	20–24	25–29	30–34	35–39	40–44	45–49	Total	
Mauritania	0.27	0.34	0.84	0.72	1.71	1.41	0.89	0.76	454 (CI: 333–575)
Mozambique	0.58	1.04	1.12	0.64	1	0.46	0.95	0.83	443 (CI: 328–559)
Namibia	0.19	0.27	0.41	0.65	1.06	0.05	0.35	0.41	358 (CI: 222–495)
Niger	1.11	1.76	1.33	1.89	1.36	1.24	0.65	1.41	535 (CI: 425–645)
Nigeria	0.65	1.02	1.1	1.34	1.33	0.79	0.69	1	556 (CI: 484–629)
Rwanda	0.05	0.08	0.21	0.47	0.57	0.68	0.77	0.34	274 (CI: 197–351)
Sao Tome and Principe	0	0	0.11	0.34	0.11	0.89	0	0.18	116 (CI: 25–207)
Senegal	0.13	0.31	0.37	0.76	0.64	0.65	0.28	0.42	273 (CI: 201–345)
Sierra Leone	0.63	0.98	1.12	1.49	1.92	1.27	0.65	1.12	796 (CI: 632–960)
South Africa	0	0.36	0.58	0.46	0.76	1.22	0.11	0.47	536 (CI: 270–802)
Tanzania	0.28	0.67	0.98	0.6	1.26	2.06	1.13	0.87	530 (CI: 405–655)
Togo	0.39	0.8	0.78	0.55	0.71	0.8	0.13	0.62	401 (CI: 290–512)
Uganda	0.41	0.7	0.76	0.95	0.75	1.19	0.16	0.69	368 (CI: 301–434)
Zambia	0.04	0.64	0.57	0.63	0.27	0.32	1.02	0.45	278 (CI: 182–375)
Zimbabwe	0.38	0.77	0.81	1.15	1.32	1.62	0.77	0.9	651 (CI: 473–829)

Figure 4 shows pregnancy-related mortality rate and ratio. Overall, Lesotho, Liberia, Chad, Congo Democratic Republic, Sierra Leone and Guinea reported the highest pregnancy-related mortality ratio per 100,000 live births.

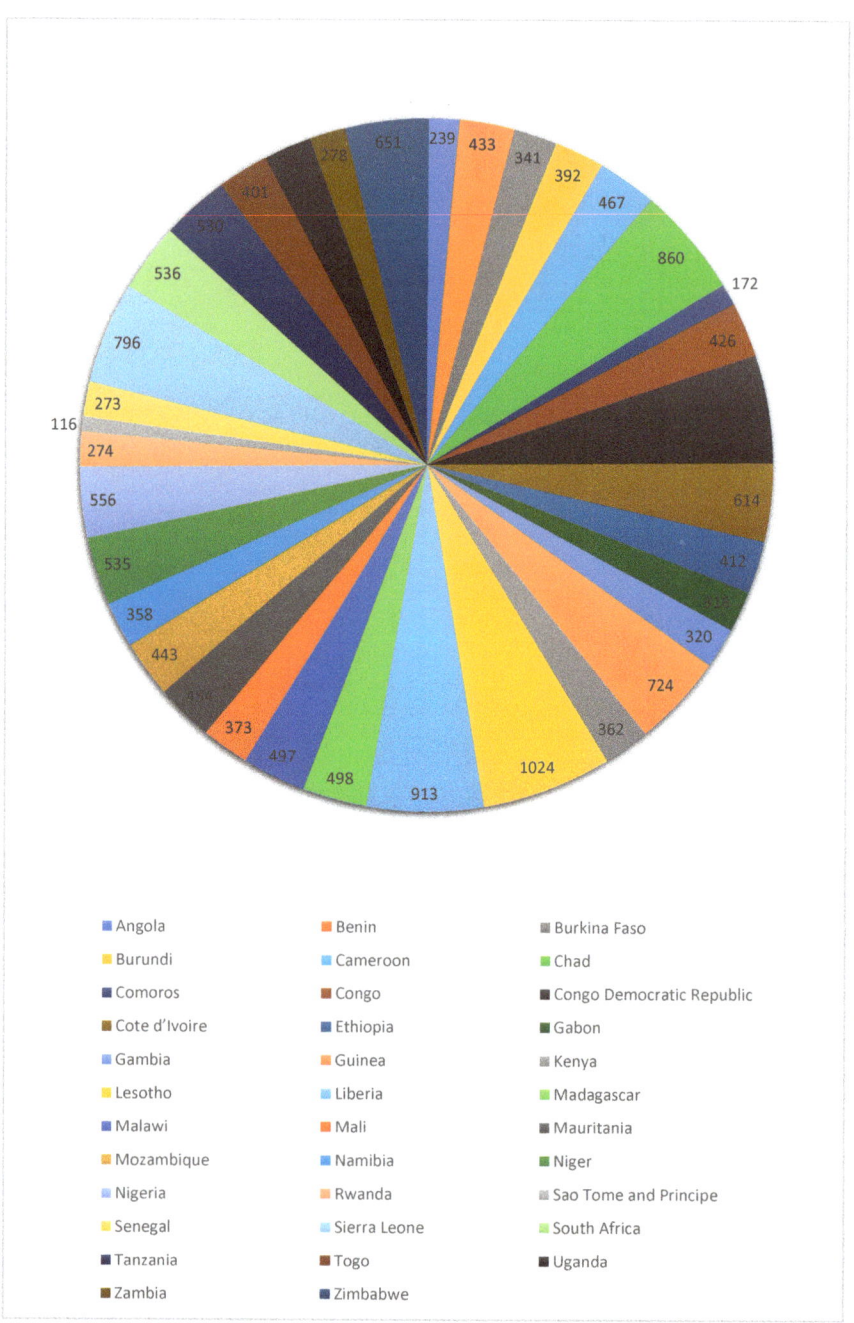

Figure 4. Pregnancy-related mortality ratio (maternal deaths per 100 000 live births).

5. Discussion

The study examined the differentials in maternal mortality in SSA countries. We observed a large variation in maternal deaths; the large variation in maternal deaths in this region is well known and documented [3,4]. Indicating that the various strategies implemented in health facilities across SSA countries to reduce maternal deaths and improve MMR have not produced the desired result as MMR remains high. Additionally, the contrast between SSA countries with the lowest and highest MMR is indicative of what remains to be done. Similarly, a study that looked at the trends in maternal mortality in SSA reported similar results in their estimation of maternal mortality ratios, where many countries have higher MMR than the national average despite comprehensive interventions to address this issue [4].

In developing countries, maternal deaths can cause long-term social and economic breakdown in a mother's immediate family and the wider community. The death of a mother can have a devastating impact on the livelihoods, quality of life, and survival chances of those she leaves behind. Households experiencing a maternal death spend roughly one-third of their income on pregnancy and child care, and funeral costs only add to the financial burden. Without the contribution of a mother, a family may be unable to meet basic needs such as food, shelter, and health care. In Africa, there are 985 people for every nurse-midwife and 3324 people for every medical doctor [15]. The African region has a shortage of maternity care providers, particularly midwives. Due to a lack of access to health care providers, pregnant women are unable to receive antenatal care, delivery care, or newborn care, increasing their risk of death from severe bleeding, infections, or other complications.

We examined the possibility of age-related death. The prevalence of death was higher among women who were 30 years and older than those aged 15 to 29 years. But a correlation with age in our study was only evident when comparing these two age groups. It has been hypothesized in other studies [16–18] that early (younger than 19) and late (above 35) pregnancy are risk factors for pregnancy-related maternal mortality, but we were not able to confirm this in our data. For women who are in their teens, their reproductive system may not be fully developed to withstand the physiological changes associated with pregnancy. Often, this age group is not psychologically, socially, or financially mature enough to make decisions concerning their health. On the other hand, women who are 35 years of age and older are at high risk of complications of pregnancy due to chronic health conditions; these health conditions expose women, particularly those aged 35 and older to a higher risk of an adverse outcome.

A notable finding from this study is the high prevalence of pregnancy-related maternal mortality among the study population. Women who were less than 30 years old in most of SSA countries had a higher prevalence of pregnancy-related death than women who were 30 years and older, though this pattern was not consistent across countries. It is well known that older women are at increased risk of maternal death. The low mortality rate among younger women less than 30 years old in some countries could be attributed to data limitations. The number of maternal deaths within each five-year age group on which these estimates are based was very small for some countries, making it difficult to reach clear conclusions and broaden uncertainty estimates. Another potential reason could be the under-reporting of maternal deaths in young women (<30 years); underreporting maternal deaths is well known in SSA [19,20] and is greater for young women than for other age groups [15]. Based on the country studied with low mortality rate in this study, maternal deaths among young women may be under-reported because of undisclosed pregnancies or fatalities linked to unsafe abortions. Further studies are needed to understand the factors that influence these different patterns.

Hemorrhage has been reported to be the leading cause of maternal death, accounting for more than one-quarter of all deaths. A similar proportion of maternal deaths were caused by pre-existing medical conditions that were exacerbated by pregnancy. A significant number of deaths are caused by hypertensive pregnancy disorders, particularly eclampsia, as well as sepsis, embolism, and complications from unsafe abortion [5,21]. The high maternal deaths observed in this study could be attributable to a lack of resources to provide quality maternal health care, as well as patient-related factors such as affordability and acceptability of maternal health services, which are common issues in SSA.

Despite established interventions to prevent and treat direct causes of maternal death, such as active management of the third stage of labor, the proportion of hemorrhage and hypertension deaths among pregnant women, especially in sub-Saharan countries, remains high. The proportion of maternal deaths caused by indirect causes has also continued to rise, and the perceived and technical quality of health care services provided is becoming increasingly important in the fight against maternal mortality, given the implications for both demand for and supply of services [22,23]. Our study observed that the pregnancy-related maternal mortality ratio was higher in western and southern sub-Saharan countries, with Lesotho, Liberia, Chad, Sierra Leone, Guinea, Zimbabwe, Cote d'Ivoire, Nigeria, South Africa, Niger, and Tanzania having the highest pregnancy-related maternal mortality ratios, in descending order. Sao Tome and Principe and Comoros have the lowest pregnancy-related maternal mortality ratios among the study countries. Differences in socioeconomic, demographic, and environmental characteristics across SSA may account for differences in maternal fatalities and MMR.

Although maternal mortality relating to pregnancy complications has not been drastically reduced in the sub-Saharan region. It is therefore necessary to affirm the submission by Batist, 2019, that maternal mortality is a human rights issue because the vast majority of maternal deaths in the sub-Saharan region are from pregnancy-related complications, which result from the region's inequitable and oppressive conditions. He further submitted that, through an examination of the intersecting social determinants of gender, economics, and education in the regional context, maternal mortality in sub-Saharan Africa is a violation of human rights [24]. Therefore, to effectively alleviate this systemic global health burden and promote human flourishing, maternal mortality should be structured and recognized as a fundamental human rights issue.

6. Strength and Limitation

We looked for plausible comparisons using large national datasets. The ability to combine multiple countries is a significant advantage. This research can be used as a scorecard for various countries to show how well their healthcare systems fare in terms of female reproductive health issues. A call to strengthen current programs relating to appropriate reproductive and sexual health care and practices may result from this, as well as more coordinated efforts, new policies, and programs. The findings of this study should prompt further research into pregnancy-related deaths in settings with scarce resources. Nevertheless, we gathered information from various countries at various times using a cross-sectional study. It might have potential influences on the socioeconomic state of each nation that are related to the variables of the study. Political climate, the expansion of medical facilities, and governmental health policies are just a few of the factors that could result in a different capture of socioeconomic conditions over time in each country. This may result in sampling bias. Additionally, other causes of maternal mortality in sub-Saharan Africa were not explored in this study. Future studies of maternal mortality should explore the contribution of socioeconomic factors influencing maternal deaths and identify specific causes of maternal deaths overall in the region.

7. Conclusions

Sub-Saharan African countries continue to experience unacceptably high risks of maternal deaths, indicating that a number of unaddressed challenges still exist, including sociodemographic and health care delivery. The persisting variation in maternal deaths in this region suggests a greater emphasis on improving the quality of care. These high rates of maternal deaths are a significant challenge for health systems, as they point to significant inequities in access to quality obstetric care. High-quality obstetric care is crucial to addressing the high levels of maternal deaths in this region. Universal health coverage services also need to be improved throughout SSA to reduce maternal mortality. At the same time, addressing the underlying social determinants of health, such as socio-economic status and disadvantaged communities and rural areas, is crucial to reducing maternal deaths since they are linked to health conditions that result in maternal morbidity and mortality. Additionally, policies and interventions that are aimed at reducing maternal morbidity and deaths need to be revised for better and more effective maternal health services in SSA. Women should be informed about the importance of maternal care and planned births at health facilities. The government and stakeholders in SSA countries should further enhance their policies in order to reduce maternal deaths and MMR by establishing and implementing strategies to improve maternal health.

Author Contributions: Conceptualization, O.C.O. and M.E.; Methodology, O.C.O. and M.E.; Software, M.E.; Validation, O.C.O., C.I.N., M.E. and E.F.O.; Formal analysis, O.C.O. and M.E.; Investigation, O.C.O., C.I.N., M.E., E.F.O., A.I.W. and C.K.E.; Resources, M.E.; Data curation, M.E.; Writing—original draft, O.C.O., C.I.N., M.E., E.F.O., A.I.W. and C.K.E.; Writing—review & editing, O.C.O., C.I.N., M.E., E.F.O., A.I.W. and C.K.E.; Visualization, O.C.O., C.I.N., M.E. and E.F.O.; Supervision, M.E.; Project administration, O.C.O., C.I.N., M.E., E.F.O., A.I.W. and C.K.E. All authors have read and agreed to the published version of the manuscript.

Funding: The Inner City Fund (ICF) provided technical assistance throughout the survey program with funds from the United States Agency for International Development (USAID). However, there was no funding or sponsorship for this study or the publication of this article.

Institutional Review Board Statement: Ethics approval was not required for this study because the authors used secondary data that was freely available in the public domain. As a result, IRB approval is not required for this study. More information about DHS data and ethical standards can be found at: http://dhsprogram.com/data/available-datasets.cfm (accessed on 5 January 2023).

Informed Consent Statement: The Demographic and Health Survey is an open-source dataset that has been de-identified. As a result, the consent for publication requirement is not applicable.

Data Availability Statement: Data for this study were obtained from the National Demographic and Health Surveys (DHS) of the studied African countries, which can be found at http://dhsprogram.com/data/available-datasets.cfm (accessed on 5 January 2023).

Acknowledgments: The authors are grateful to the MEASURE DHS project for granting permission to use and access to the original data.

Conflicts of Interest: The authors state that the research was carried out in the absence of any commercial or financial partnerships or connections that could be interpreted as potential conflicts of interest.

References

1. Maternal Mortality. Available online: https://www.who.int/news-room/fact-sheets/detail/maternal-mortality (accessed on 2 December 2022).
2. UNICEF DATA. Maternal Mortality Rates and Statistics. Available online: https://data.unicef.org/topic/maternal-health/maternal-mortality/ (accessed on 2 December 2022).
3. Merdad, L.; Ali, M.M. Timing of maternal death: Levels, trends, and ecological correlates using sibling data from 34 sub-Saharan African countries. *PLoS ONE* **2018**, *13*, e0189416. [CrossRef] [PubMed]
4. Onambele, L.; Ortega-Leon, W.; Guillen-Aguinaga, S.; Forjaz, M.J.; Yoseph, A.; Guillen-Aguinaga, L.; Alas-Brun, R.; Arnedo-Pena, A.; Aguinaga-Ontoso, I.; Guillen-Grima, F. Maternal Mortality in Africa: Regional Trends (2000–2017). *Int. J. Environ. Res. Public Health* **2022**, *19*, 13146. [CrossRef] [PubMed]
5. Musarandega, R.; Nyakura, M.; Machekano, R.; Pattinson, R.; Munjanja, S.P. Causes of maternal mortality in Sub-Saharan Africa: A systematic review of studies published from 2015 to 2020. *J. Glob. Health* **2021**, *11*, 04048. [CrossRef] [PubMed]
6. GBD 2015 Maternal Mortality Collaborators. Global, regional, and national levels of maternal mortality, 1990–2015: A systematic analysis for the Global Burden of Disease Study 2015. *Lancet Lond. Engl.* **2016**, *388*, 1775–1812. [CrossRef]
7. Say, L.; Chou, D.; Gemmill, A.; Tunçalp, Ö.; Moller, A.-B.; Daniels, J.; Gülmezoglu, A.M.; Temmerman, M.; Alkema, L. Global causes of maternal death: A WHO systematic analysis. *Lancet Glob. Health* **2014**, *2*, E323–E333. [CrossRef] [PubMed]
8. Institutional Maternal and Perinatal Deaths: A Review of 40 Low and Middle Income Countries—PubMed. Available online: https://pubmed.ncbi.nlm.nih.gov/28882128/ (accessed on 2 December 2022).

9. Neal, S.; Mahendra, S.; Bose, K.; Camacho, A.V.; Mathai, M.; Nove, A.; Santana, F.; Matthews, Z. The causes of maternal mortality in adolescents in low and middle income countries: A systematic review of the literature. *BMC Pregnancy Childbirth* **2016**, *16*, 352. [CrossRef]
10. Kumar, S.; Kumar, N.; Vivekadhish, S. Millennium development goals (MDGS) to sustainable development goals (SDGS): Addressing unfinished agenda and strengthening sustainable development and partnership. *Indian J. Community Med.* **2016**, *41*, 1. [CrossRef] [PubMed]
11. Demographic and Health Surveys (DHS) Data. Available online: http://api.dhsprogram.com/rest/dhs/indicators?f=html (accessed on 5 January 2023).
12. Owobi, O.U.; Okonji, O.C.; Nzoputam, C.I.; Ekholuenetale, M. Country-Level Variations in Overweight and Obesity among Reproductive-Aged Women in Sub-Saharan Countries. *Women* **2022**, *2*, 313–325. [CrossRef]
13. Ekholuenetale, M.; Nzoputam, C.I.; Okonji, O.C. Sub-Regional Variations in Sexually Transmitted Infections Manifesting as Vaginitis among Reproductive-Aged Women in Sub-Saharan Countries. *Venereology* **2022**, *1*, 245–261. [CrossRef]
14. Corsi, D.J.; Neuman, M.; Finlay, J.E.; Subramanian, S.V. Demographic and health surveys: A profile. *Int. J. Epidemiol.* **2012**, *41*, 1602–1613. [CrossRef]
15. Global Citizen. Why Maternal Mortality Is So High in Sub-Saharan Africa. In Global Citizen [Internet]. 2022. Available online: https://www.globalcitizen.org/en/content/maternal-mortality-sub-saharan-africa-causes/ (accessed on 5 January 2023).
16. Okonofua, F.E.; Abejide, A.; Makanjuola, R.A. Maternal mortality in Ile-Ife, Nigeria: A study of risk factors. *Stud. Fam. Plan.* **1992**, *23*, 319–324. [CrossRef]
17. Alkema, L.; Chou, D.; Hogan, D.; Zhang, S.; Moller, A.B.; Gemmill, A.; Fat, D.M.; Boerma, T.; Temmerman, M.; Mathers, C.; et al. Global, regional, and national levels and trends in maternal mortality between 1990 and 2015, with scenario-based projections to 2030: A systematic analysis by the UN Maternal Mortality Estimation Inter-Agency Group. *Lancet* **2016**, *387*, 462–474. [CrossRef] [PubMed]
18. Diguisto, C.; Saucedo, M.; Kallianidis, A.; Bloemenkamp, K.; Bødker, B.; Buoncristiano, M.; Donati, S.; Gissler, M.; Johansen, M.; Knight, M.; et al. Maternal mortality in eight European countries with enhanced surveillance systems: Descriptive population based study. *BMJ* **2022**, *379*, e070621. [CrossRef] [PubMed]
19. Abouchadi, S.; Zhang, W.-H.; De Brouwere, V. Underreporting of deaths in the maternal deaths surveillance system in one region of Morocco. *PLoS ONE* **2018**, *13*, e0188070. [CrossRef] [PubMed]
20. Said, A.; Malqvist, M.; Pembe, A.B.; Massawe, S.; Hanson, C. Causes of maternal deaths and delays in care: Comparison between routine maternal death surveillance and response system and an obstetrician expert panel in Tanzania. *BMC Health Serv. Res.* **2020**, *20*, 614. [CrossRef] [PubMed]
21. Horon, I.L. Underreporting of Maternal Deaths on Death Certificates and the Magnitude of the Problem of Maternal Mortality. *Am. J. Public Health* **2005**, *95*, 478–482. [CrossRef] [PubMed]
22. Alvarez, J.L.; Gil, R.; Hernández, V.; Gil, A. Factors associated with maternal mortality in Sub-Saharan Africa: An ecological study. *BMC Public Health* **2009**, *9*, 462. [CrossRef] [PubMed]
23. Filippi, V.; Chou, D.; Ronsmans, C.; Graham, W.; Say, L. Levels and Causes of Maternal Mortality and Morbidity. In *Disease Control Priorities*, 3rd ed.; Reproductive, Maternal, Newborn, and Child Health; The World Bank: Washington, DC, USA, 2016; Volume 2, pp. 51–70. [CrossRef]
24. Batist, J. An intersectional analysis of maternal mortality in Sub-Saharan Africa: A human rights issue. *J. Glob. Health* **2019**, *9*, 010320. [CrossRef] [PubMed]

Disclaimer/Publisher's Note: The statements, opinions and data contained in all publications are solely those of the individual author(s) and contributor(s) and not of MDPI and/or the editor(s). MDPI and/or the editor(s) disclaim responsibility for any injury to people or property resulting from any ideas, methods, instructions or products referred to in the content.

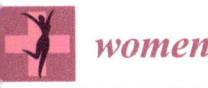

Article

Vaccine Hesitancy in Women of Childbearing Age and Occupational Physicians: Results from a Cross-Sectional Study (Italy, 2022)

Matteo Riccò [1,*], Antonio Baldassarre [2], Milena Pia Cerviere [3] and Federico Marchesi [4]

1. Occupational Health and Safety Service on the Workplace, Department of Public Health, AUSL–IRCCS di Reggio Emilia, 42122 Reggio Emilia, Italy
2. Department of Experimental and Clinical Medicine, University of Florence, 50134 Florence, Italy
3. Università Cattolica del Sacro Cuore, 00168 Rome, Italy
4. Department of Medicine and Surgery, University of Parma, 43126 Parma, Italy
* Correspondence: matteo.ricco@ausl.re.it or mricco2000@gmail.com; Tel.: +39-339-2994343 or +39-522-837587

Abstract: Italian occupational physicians (OPs) are instrumental in promoting vaccination practice in occupational settings, and this study aims to characterize their attitudes, knowledge, and practices (collectively, KAP) towards immunization practice in women of childbearing age. A convenience sample of 120 OPs (50.8% males, mean age of 48.2 ± 5.9 years old) completed a structured online questionnaire (potential recipients: 2034; response rate: 5.9%) assessing their understanding of official recommendations, their general knowledge of vaccine practice, their attitudes towards vaccines, and their risk perception about vaccine-preventable infectious diseases. The sampled OPs exhibited a good understanding of official recommendations, and they were largely favorable towards vaccination of pregnant women. Knowledge status was relatively good (potential range 0 to 100%, average score 22 74.5% ± 18.2), while risk perception towards sampled disorders was heterogenous: the greatest was the one for SARS-CoV-2 (52.7% ± 32.9), followed by seasonal influenza (45.3% ± 31.6), and pertussis (37.8% 24 ± 28.2). The main predictors for promoting vaccination were higher knowledge about seasonal influenza vaccine (SIV; adjusted Odds Ratio [aOR] 102.2, 95% Confidence Interval [95%CI] 9.68–1080.26), tetanus-diphtheria-acellular pertussis vaccine (Tdap; aOR 12.34, 95%CI 2.62; 58.22) 27 and SARS-CoV-2 vaccine (aOR 14.76, 95%CI 2.74–79.69). A better attitude towards SIV was positively associated with previous vaccination of the respondent (aOR 4.90, 95%CI 1.19–20.14), while higher risk perception towards SIV was characterized as a negative predictor (aOR 0.04, 95%CI 0.01–0.35), as was working as an OP in healthcare facilities (aOR 0.03, 95%CI 0.01–0.43). Tdap was positively associated with male gender of respondents (aOR 10.22, 95%CI 2.60 to 40.24) and higher risk perception about pertussis (aOR 10.38, 95%CI 1.47 to 73.47). Overall, our data suggest that improving the understanding of OPs about the health burden of frequently encountered pathogens could be instrumental in increasing their involvement in the promotion of vaccine practice. Because of the low rate of response to our survey, our conclusions remain tentative.

Keywords: pregnant women; vaccine-preventable diseases; knowledge; attitudes; practices; risk perception

Citation: Riccò, M.; Baldassarre, A.; Cerviere, M.P.; Marchesi, F. Vaccine Hesitancy in Women of Childbearing Age and Occupational Physicians: Results from a Cross-Sectional Study (Italy, 2022). Women **2023**, *3*, 237–262. https://doi.org/10.3390/women3020019

Academic Editors: Claudio Costantino, Maiorana Antonio, Mary V. Seeman and Maria Grazia Porpora

Received: 31 December 2022
Revised: 8 April 2023
Accepted: 4 May 2023
Published: 6 May 2023

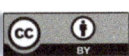

Copyright: © 2023 by the authors. Licensee MDPI, Basel, Switzerland. This article is an open access article distributed under the terms and conditions of the Creative Commons Attribution (CC BY) license (https://creativecommons.org/licenses/by/4.0/).

1. Introduction

Where implemented by the national legal framework, occupational physicians (OPs; please refer to Table A1 for a full summary of acronyms) are the medical professionals responsible for health surveillance and promotion across the workplaces [1,2]. Well before the inception of the SARS-CoV-2 pandemic, Italian OPs were actively involved in the implementation of specifically tailored preventive measures against biological risk factors [3–5], including prescription and/or delivery of appropriate vaccinations [2,6]. Not coincidentally, Italian OPs have been extensively involved in the implementation of SARS-CoV-2 vaccination campaigns [7].

Pregnant women may be exposed to various pathogens, including "conventional" ones such as seasonal and pandemic influenza, pertussis, measles, and rubella [8–10], and emerging ones such as Flaviviridae (e.g., Zika virus) [11–13], and most notably SARS-CoV-2 [14–20] not only as healthcare workers (HCWs) but also in settings such as forestry, zootechny, food, veterinary, biotechnology, treatment and waste disposal. Their exposure and contact with highly dangerous agents are associated with an increased risk of morbidity, mortality, and adverse pregnancy outcomes [21–24].

Consequently, the implementation of properly tailored immunization policies among female workers of childbearing age could represent a substantial duty for OPs [25–29]. Notably, since 2017, the Italian National Immunization Plan (NIP) recommends the vaccination of pregnant women with the pertussis vaccine, included in the trivalent formulation tetanus-diphtheria-acellular pertussis (Tdap) vaccine between the 27th and the 36th week of every pregnancy, regardless of prior Tdap history [30,31]. Similarly, Seasonal Influenza Vaccine (SIV) should be delivered at any stage of the gestational period as a preventive intervention targeting both the recipient and the offspring [30–33]. In both cases, the role of OPs in improving vaccination rates among female workers from high-risk settings (e.g., HCW) has been specifically stressed by official Italian guidelines [9,18,34–39]. Unfortunately, coverage rates for recommended vaccinations, including SIV and Tdap, among pregnant women remain very low [27,28,32,33,40–42].

Even SARS-CoV-2 vaccines have been recently addressed by official recommendations that support their delivery in pregnant women. While initially recommended for breastfeeding mothers and pregnant women at higher risk of exposure to the virus or at greater risk of developing a severe illness, since the second half of 2021, SARS-CoV-2 mRNA vaccines have been extended to all pregnant women in their second and third trimester who wish to be vaccinated [43–48]. More precisely, national vaccination guidelines prioritize women at greater risk of contracting SARS-CoV-2 infection because of their occupational exposures (e.g., HCWs) and/or at greater risk of developing severe COVID-19 disease (women with risk factors such as age >30 years, BMI >30, comorbidities, women from countries where the migration pressure is high) [43–45].

In such a setting, the role of OPs may be of particular interest, as they could contribute to the promotion of recommended vaccination in working age groups, which in women largely coincide with childbearing age. Unfortunately, previous studies have reported a high occurrence of false beliefs about vaccinations and a lack of knowledge about national vaccination policies among Italian OPs [2,6,46,47]. Interestingly, similar shortcomings have been reported also in other national settings [1,20,48].

As a consequence, the main endpoint of this study was to assess knowledge (how much the respondents understand a certain topic), attitudes (that is the feelings of sampled individuals towards the assessed subject, as well as any preconceived ideas they may have towards it), and practices (the ways in which they demonstrate their knowledge and attitude through their actions; collectively, KAP) of a sample of OPs about vaccinations and vaccination policies in women of childbearing age and pregnant women. The understanding of general and specific recommendations was specifically focused on, as well as how the KAP of sampled professionals related to these recommendations. Our results may contribute to identifying areas that may be potentially targeted by specific informative and educative campaigns dedicated to OPs.

2. Results

2.1. Descriptive Analysis

As reported in Figure 1, a total of 120 OPs (5.9% of the original population of 2034 OPs) participated in the inquiry.

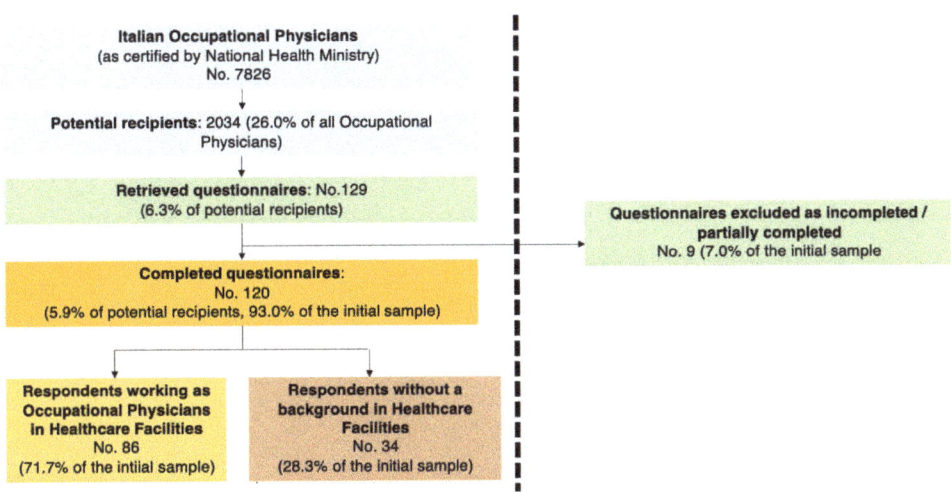

Figure 1. Flowchart of participants included in the present survey.

Overall, 50.8% of the participants were of the male gender, and their mean age was 48.2 ± 5.9 years (30.0% aged 50 years old or more), with average seniority as OPs of 16.3 ± 10.1 years (75.0% of them, with a seniority of 10 years or more). Of these, the large majority had offspring (86.7%) and worked as OPs in healthcare facilities (71.7%) (Table 1).

Table 1. Characteristics of the 120 Italian occupational physicians who participated in the present survey (Italy, 2022).

Variable	No./120	Average ± SD
Gender		
Male	61, 50.8%	
Female	59, 49.2%	
Age (years)		48.2 ± 5.9
Age ≥ 50 years	36, 30.0%	
Offspring	104, 86.7%	
Seniority (years)		16.3 ± 10.3
Seniority ≥ 10 years	90, 75.0%	
Working as Occupational Physician for Healthcare Facilities	86, 71.7%	
General Knowledge Score (%)		74.5% ± 18.2
General Knowledge Score > median (78.6%)	47, 39.2%	

2.2. Assessment of Knowledge Status

Knowledge status was assessed by means of a series of 25 true–false questions, whose internal consistency was good (Cronbach's alpha = 0.873). After percent normalization, the corresponding cumulative score (general knowledge score, or GKS) was generally high (74.5% ± 18.2; actual range 28.6–100%; median 78.6%). A skewed distribution was identified at visual inspection (Figure 2), and the Gaussian distribution was rejected by the D'Agostino–Pearson test (K2 = 22.17, $p < 0.001$).

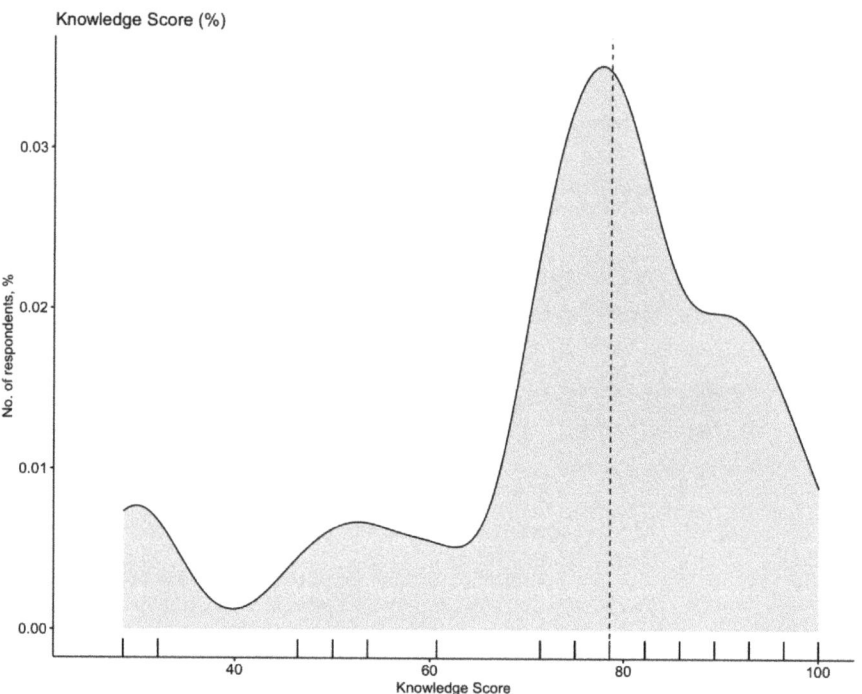

Figure 2. Density plots on general knowledge score (GKS) for participants fulfilling all inclusion criteria (No. 120, 5.9% of the original sample). Average GKS was estimated to be 74.5% ± 18.2 (actual range 28.6–100%; median 78.6%), with a non-Gaussian distribution as confirmed by D'Agostino–Pearson test (K2 = 22.17, $p < 0.001$).

Detailed results of the knowledge test are reported in Table A2. More precisely, substantial uncertainties were associated with items represented by Q19, as only 37.5% of respondents were aware that no RSV vaccine has been to date commercially made available; and Q23, as only 47.5% of participants had any understanding that mRNA vaccines against SARS-CoV-2 vaccines can be employed also in women with a previous history of deep vein thrombosis. Interestingly, even though a large share of participants had a proper understanding of official recommendations that allow the use of vaccines in pregnancy (Q16, 91.7%), similar knowledge gaps affected the recommendations for the delivery of the Tdap vaccine to all pregnant women (Q15, 54.2%) and for avoiding live-attenuated vaccines in pregnancy (Q17, 54.2%).

Moreover, a substantial share of participants exhibited some uncertainties regarding the role of vaccine additives in human health (Q01, 66.7% of correct answers) and the potential resurgence of secondary cases with epidemic potential after vaccinations with live-attenuated vaccines (Q21, 67.5%). Around a third of respondents also exhibited knowledge gaps about the potential vaccine-related induction of encephalitis lethargica (Q04, 66.7%), subacute sclerosing panencephalitis (Q03, 67.5%), and autoimmune Hashimoto's thyroiditis (Q06, 63.3%). Conversely, the large majority of participants properly acknowledged the efficacy of vaccines (Q11), understood the role of smallpox vaccination in the progressive eradication of the pathogen (Q10; 95.8% for both statements), and correctly reported that tetanus vaccination should be delivered in all adults every 10 years (Q18, 91.7%). The large majority of respondents also agreed on the lack of secondary effects of childhood immunization on their resistance to infectious diseases (Q12, 93.3%), and that vaccines do not increase the risk of developing autism (Q07, 91.7%), being of substantial value in promoting the control of infectious disease (Q09, 91.7%).

2.3. Risk Perception

Risk perception scores (RPS) for natural infections and vaccine-related side effects were calculated as the mathematical product of perceived severity (potential range 0 to 5) and perceived incidence (potential range 0 to 5) of the assessed condition (Figures A1 and A2). Briefly, the greatest RPS on natural infections was associated with SARS-CoV-2 (52.7% ± 32.9), followed by rubella (50.3% ± 26.7), varicella (49.4% ± 27.6), seasonal influenza (45.3% ± 31.6), measles (41% ± 26.3), parotitis (40.8% ± 27.5), pertussis (37.8% ± 28.3), hepatitis B (35.1% ± 22.0), diphtheria (27.6% ± 23.3), and tetanus (26.6% ± 22.3).

By arbitrarily assuming seasonal influenza as the reference group, the difference between reported RPS was significant only for tetanus (mean difference in favor of seasonal influenza, 18.71, 95%CI 9.31 to 28.11, $p < 0.001$), diphtheria (mean difference 17.71, 95%CI 8.31 to 27.11, $p < 0.001$), and hepatitis B (mean difference 10.21, 95%CI 8.11 to 19.61, $p = 0.026$) (Table A3). When dealing with reported side effects of vaccinations, the greatest RPS was associated with varicella (25.5% ± 25.7), followed by rubella (21.8% ± 22.4), SARS-CoV-2 immunizations with adenovirus carrier (19.9% ± 19.8), parotitis (19.5% ± 20.0), measles (18.4% ± 19.9), SARS-CoV-2 vaccines based on the mRNA technology (15.7% ± 19.4), hepatitis B vaccine (15.3% ± 16.2), and SARS-CoV-2 vaccines based on the subunit technology (15.2% ± 16.1), while lower estimates were associated with pertussis (13.0% ± 17.0), SIV (12.1% ± 15.0), diphtheria (12.1% ± 16.6), and tetanus (11.4% ± 15.3). When SIV was taken as the reference group, the difference was significant for parotitis (mean difference −7.39, 95%CI −14.09 to 0.70, $p = 0.022$), rubella (mean difference −9.67, 95%CI −16.36 to −2.97 $p = 0.001$), varicella (mean difference −13.33, 95%CI −20.03 to −6.64, $p < 0.001$), and SARS-CoV-2 performed through adenovirus carriers (mean difference −7.79, 95%CI −14.49 to 1.10, $p = 0.013$) (Table A4).

2.4. Attitudes towards Vaccination

When participants were asked about the perceived barriers towards vaccination of pregnant women (Table 2), the most frequently reported one was the inappropriate risk perception by pregnant women (83.3%), followed by their appropriate understanding of official recommendations (79.2%), the fear of side effects (70.8%), the inappropriate understanding of official recommendations by medical professionals (62.5%). Moreover, 45.9% of participants claimed that other medical professionals may not perceive maternal vaccinations as a priority and that vaccination services may be scarcely available given the specificities of pregnant women (37.5%). Only 12.5% of participants reported any complaints about the high costs of vaccines.

Table 2. Perceived barriers towards vaccinations of pregnant women as reported by 120 Italian occupational physicians (Italy, 2022).

Perceived Barriers towards Vaccinations of Pregnant Women (Agree/Totally Agree)	No./120, %
Fear of side effects	85, 70.8%
Costs of vaccinations	15, 12.5%
Not perceived as a priority by other medical professionals	55, 45.9%
Inappropriate risk perception by pregnant women	100, 83.3%
Vaccination services are scarcely available	45, 37.5%
Inappropriate understanding of official recommendations by pregnant women	95, 79.2%
Inappropriate understanding of official recommendations by medical professionals	75, 62.5%

Overall, the majority of participants recommended any of the SARS-CoV-2 vaccines (i.e., mRNA, subunit, or adenovirus-based formulates) in women of childbearing age (74.2%), followed by Tdap (70.8%), SIV (66.7%), and hepatitis B virus vaccine (54.2%) (Table 3). On the contrary, less than 50% of participants actively recommended MPR (45.8%), and varicella (41.7%) immunizations.

Table 3. Vaccinations actively recommended for women of childbearing age by 120 Italian occupational physicians (Italy, 2022).

Vaccines Actively Recommended on Women of Childbearing Age	No./120, %
Seasonal Influenza Virus	80, 66.7%
Diphtheria/Tetanus/Pertussis	85, 70.8%
Measles/Mumps/Rubella	55, 45.8%
Varicella	50, 41.7%
Hepatitis B Virus	65, 54.2%
SARS-CoV-2	89, 74.2%

When participants were asked about their vaccination status (Table 4), 91.7% of them had received a full course for SARS-CoV-2, while 71.7% of them had been reportedly vaccinated against HBV, 65.8% against SIV (at least one time in the previous 5 years). Moreover, 63.3% had received MPR, 61.7% Tdap, and only 16.7% varicella (either in a tetravalent immunization or as an individual vaccination).

Table 4. Vaccination status self-reported by 120 Italian occupational physicians (Italy, 2022).

Previously Vaccinated against ...	No./120, %
Seasonal Influenza Virus [1]	79, 65.8%
Diphtheria/Tetanus/Pertussis [2]	74, 61.7%
Measles/Parotitis/Rubella	76, 63.3%
Varicella	20, 16.7%
Hepatitis B Virus [3]	86, 71.7%
SARS-CoV-2	110, 91.7%

Notes: ([1]) at least 1 time in the previous 5 years; ([2]) at least 1 vaccination shot in the previous 10 years; ([3]) at least 1 vaccination shot in the previous 10 years, or documented antibody titer as >10 UI/mL.

2.5. Univariate Analysis

Overall, a positive correlation between GKS and RPS was identified for the majority of infections reported to the participants, and more precisely: seasonal influenza ($r = 0.341$, $p < 0.001$), pertussis ($r = 0.200$, $p = 0.028$), measles ($r = 0.356$, $p < 0.001$), parotitis ($r = 0.238$, $p = 0.009$), varicella ($r = 0.196$, $p = 0.032$), hepatitis B virus ($r = 0.406$, $p < 001$), and SARS-CoV-2 ($r = 0.428$, $p < 0.001$). In other words, a better understanding of vaccine-related issues was associated with a greater risk perception of the aforementioned disorders, and vice versa (Table A5).

Conversely, SIV ($r = -0.352$, $p < 0.001$), vaccines for diphtheria ($r = -0.450$, $p < 0.001$), tetanus ($r = -0.367$, $p < 0.001$), pertussis ($r = -0.379$, $p < 0.001$), hepatitis B virus ($r = -0.191$, $p = 0.037$), as well as SARS-CoV-2 vaccines based on mRNA ($r = -0.354$, $p < 0.001$), adenoviral carriers ($r = -0.314$, $p < 0.001$), and subunit technology ($r = -0.314$, $p < 0.001$), were negatively correlated with RPS, and a positive correlation between GKS and RPS was only reported for SARS-CoV-2 vaccines based on adenovirus carriers ($r = 0.239$, $p < 0.009$). Therefore, a better GKS meant a reduced risk perception of side effects following the delivery of SIV, and vaccinations against diphtheria, tetanus, pertussis, hepatitis B virus, and SARS-CoV-2 based on mRNA and subunit technology, while individuals exhibiting a better knowledge status were more frequently concerned about SARS-CoV-2 vaccines based on adenovirus carriers. Moreover, as shown in Figure 3, participants recommending the uptake of SIV, Tdap, and SARS-CoV-2 vaccines consistently had greater GKS compared to those who did not (i.e., SIV 81.7% ± 12.4 vs. 60.1% ± 19.5, Mann–Whitney [M-W] U = 2725.0, $p < 0.001$; Tdap 80.0% ± 14.4 vs. 61.3% ± 19.9, M-W U = 2458.0, $p < 0.001$; SARS-CoV-2 79.4% ± 14.3 vs. 60.6% ± 21.1, M-W U = 2194.5, $p < 0.001$).

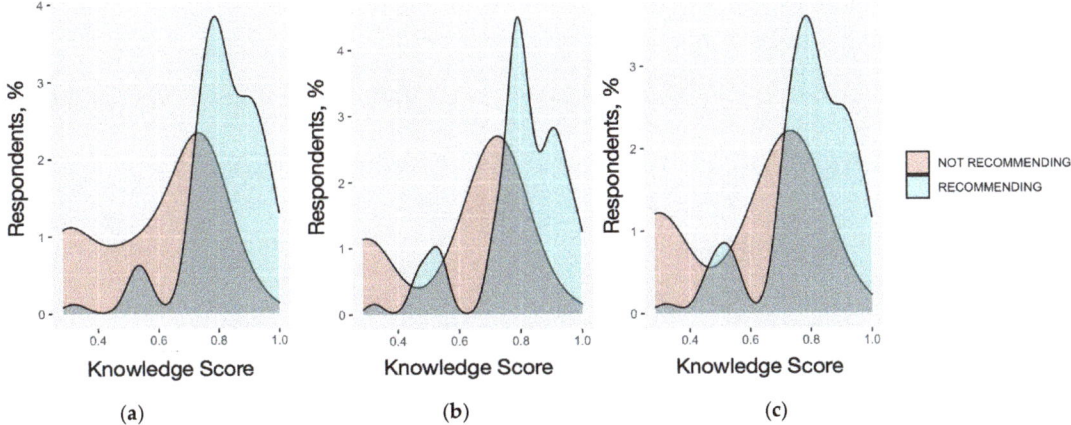

Figure 3. Density plots on General Knowledge Score (GKS). Estimates were broken down by the reported attitude towards the following vaccinations: (**a**) SIV (Seasonal Influenza Virus), (**b**) Tdap, and (**c**) SARS-CoV-2. Briefly, estimates were substantially greater among individuals reporting a positive attitude than among those not recommending the assessed vaccination (i.e., SIV 81.7% ± 12.4 vs. 60.1% ± 19.5, Mann–Whitney [M-W] U = 2725.0, $p < 0.001$; Tdap 80.0% ± 14.4 vs. 61.3% ± 19.9, M-W U = 2458.0, $p < 0.001$; SARS-CoV-2 79.4% ± 14.3 vs. 60.6% ± 21.1, M-W U = 2194.5, $p < 0.001$).

When the outcome variables of actively promoting SIV, Tdap, and SARS-CoV-2 vaccines were compared to the individual characteristics of respondents (Table 5), a positive attitude towards SIV was positively associated with a better knowledge status (55.0% of individuals reporting a favorable attitude versus 7.5% among those not favorable to the reported vaccine, $p < 0.001$), having been previously vaccinated against seasonal influenza (82.5% vs. 32.5%, $p < 0.001$), and reporting higher RPS on influenza (62.5% vs. 25.0%, $p < 0.001$). On the contrary, working as an occupational physician in healthcare facilities (63.7% vs. 87.5%, $p = 0.012$) and reporting higher RPS on the vaccine (25.0% vs. 75.0%, $p < 0.001$) were more frequently reported among individuals not favorable to the vaccine than among those promoting the intervention.

Table 5. Association between the individual attitude towards seasonal influenza vaccine (SIV), diphtheria, tetanus, and pertussis formulate (Tdap), and SARS-CoV-2 vaccination among 120 Italian occupational physicians (Italy, 2022). Note: RPS = risk perception score.

	SIV		
	Favorable (No./80, %)	Not Favorable (No./40, %)	*p* value
Male Gender	45, 56.3%	16, 40.0%	0.138
Age ≥ 50 years	24, 30.0%	12, 30.0%	1.000
Any Offspring	69, 86.3%	35, 87.5%	1.000
Higher Knowledge status	44, 55.0%	3, 7.5%	<0.001
Working as Occupational Physician for Healthcare facilities	51, 63.7%	35, 87.5%	0.012
Vaccinated against SIV	66, 82.5%	13, 32.5%	<0.001
Higher RPS vs. SIV	50, 62.5%	10, 25.0%	<0.001
Higher RPS vs. SIV vaccine	20, 25.0%	30, 75.0%	<0.001

Table 5. Cont.

	SIV		
	Tdap		
	Favorable (No./85, %)	Not Favorable (No./35, %)	p value
Male Gender	50, 58.8%	11, 31.4%	0.011
Age ≥ 50 years	24, 28.2%	12, 34.3%	0.661
Any Offspring	74, 87.1%	30, 85.7%	1.000
Higher Knowledge status	44, 51.8%	3, 8.6%	<0.001
Working as Occupational Physician for Healthcare facilities	61, 71.8%	25, 71.4%	1.000
Vaccinated with Tdap	51, 60.0%	23, 65.7%	0.705
Higher RPS vs. diphtheria	45, 52.9%	5, 14.3%	<0.001
Higher RPS vs. diphtheria vaccine	15, 17.6%	10, 28.6%	0.275
Higher RPS vs. tetanus	40, 47.1%	10, 28.6%	0.096
Higher RPS vs. tetanus vaccine	15, 17.6%	15, 42.9%	0.008
Higher RPS vs. pertussis	55, 64.7%	5, 14.3%	<0.001
Higher RPS vs. pertussis vaccine	34, 40.0%	20, 57.1%	0.130
	SARS-CoV-2		
	Favorable (No./89, %)	Not Favorable (No./31, %)	p value
Male Gender	43, 48.3%	16, 51.6%	0.914
Age ≥ 50 years	20, 22.5%	16, 51.6%	0.005
Any Offspring	77, 86.5%	27, 87.1%	1.000
Higher Knowledge status	45, 50.6%	2, 6.5%	<0.001
Working as Occupational Physician for Healthcare facilities	65, 73.0%	21, 67.7%	0.740
Vaccinated against SARS-CoV-2	88, 98.9%	22, 71.0%	<0.001
Higher RPS vs. SARS-CoV-2	48, 54.5%	12, 37.5%	0.148
Higher RPS vs. SARS-CoV-2 vaccine (mRNA)	34, 38.2%	21, 67.7%	0.008
Higher RPS vs. SARS-CoV-2 vaccine (adenoviral carrier)	39, 43.8%	21, 67.7%	0.037
Higher RPS vs. SARS-CoV-2 vaccine (subunit)	43, 48.3%	17, 54.8%	0.677

Similarly, a positive attitude toward the Tdap vaccine was positively associated with male gender (58.8% vs. 31.4%, $p = 0.011$), reporting a higher knowledge status (51.8% vs. 8.6%, $p < 0.001$), and having a higher RPS on diphtheria (52.9% vs. 14.3%, $p < 0.001$) and pertussis (64.7% vs. 14.3%, $p < 0.001$), while it was negatively associated with higher RPS on tetanus vaccine (17.6% vs. 42.9%, $p = 0.008$).

A favorable attitude towards SARS-CoV-2 vaccine was negatively associated with belonging to older age groups (22.5% among respondents of 50 years or more vs. 51.6% of respondents not favorable to SARS-CoV-2 vaccines) and reporting higher RPS on mRNA (38.2% vs. 67.7%, $p = 0.008$) and adenoviral (43.8% vs. 67.7%, $p = 0.037$) SARS-CoV-2 vaccines. Conversely, having a better knowledge status (50.6% vs. 6.5%, $p < 0.001$), and having been vaccinated against SARS-CoV-2 were positively associated with a favorable attitude (98.9% vs. 71.0%, $p < 0.001$).

2.6. Multivariable Analysis

Multivariable analysis was modeled including the variables that in univariate analysis were significantly associated ($p < 0.05$) with the active promotion among female workers of childbearing age of SIV (Model 1), Tdap (Model 2), and SARS-CoV-2 vaccines (Model 3), and more precisely (Table A6):

(a) Model 1: GKS > median value; having been working as OP in healthcare facilities; having been vaccinated against seasonal influenza; RPS towards SIV and seasonal influenza > median values.
(b) Model 2: being of male gender; GKS > median value; RPS on diphtheria and pertussis > median values; reporting RPS on the vaccine for tetanus > median value.
(c) Model 3: being older than 50 years at the time of the survey; reporting a GKS > median value, having been vaccinated against SARS-CoV-2, reporting RPS values for SARS-CoV-2 vaccines based on mRNA formulates and adenoviral vectors > median.

As shown in Table 6, a favorable attitude towards SIV was more frequently reported among participants exhibiting a better knowledge status (adjusted Odds Ratios [aOR] 102.24, 95% Confidence Interval [95%CI] 9.68 to 1080.26), and having been vaccinated against SIV (aOR 4.90, 95%CI 1.19 to 20.14). On the contrary, it was less frequently reported by participants who reportedly worked as OPs in healthcare facilities (aOR 0.03, 95%CI 0.01 to 0.43) and who reported higher RPS on the vaccine (aOR 0.04, 95%CI 0.01 to 0.35).

Table 6. Multivariable analysis of factors associated with a better individual attitude towards seasonal influenza vaccine (SIV), diphtheria, tetanus, and pertussis formulate (Tdap), and SARS-CoV-2 vaccination among 120 occupational physicians participating in the survey. The assessed models included the favorable attitude towards the individual vaccine as the outcome variable, and assessed as explanatory variables all factors that in univariate analysis were associated ($p < 0.05$) with the corresponding outcomes.

	SIV	Tdap	SARS-CoV-2
	Adjusted Odds Ratio (95% Confidence Intervals)		
Male Gender	-	10.22 (2.60; 40.24)	-
Age $\geq$ 50 years	-	-	0.62 (0.19; 1.99)
Higher Knowledge status	102.24 (9.68; 1080.26)	12.34 (2.62; 58.22)	14.76 (2.74; 79.69)
Working as Occupational Physician for Healthcare facilities	0.03 (0.01; 0.43)	-	-
Vaccinated against . . .			
SIV	4.90 (1.19; 20.14)	-	-
SARS-CoV-2	-	-	7.66 (0.72; 81.12)
Higher RPS vs. the pathogen			
SIV	1.04 (0.23; 4.71)	-	-
diphtheria	-	2.38 (0.36; 15.84)	-
pertussis	-	10.38 (1.47; 73.47)	-
Higher RPS vs. the vaccination			
SIV	0.04 (0.01; 0.35)	-	-
tetanus	-	0.34 (0.10; 1.17)	-
SARS-CoV-2, mRNA	-	-	0.14 (0.02; 1.17)
SARS-CoV-2, adenoviral vector	-	-	2.59 (0.31; 21.45)

Similarly, a better knowledge status was associated with a favorable attitude towards SARS-CoV-2 vaccine (aOR 14.76, 95%CI 2.74 to 79.69), while male gender of respondents (aOR 10.22, 95%CI 2.60 to 40.24), scoring a GKS > median value (aOR 12.34, 95%CI 2.62 to 58.22), and higher risk perception of pertussis (aOR 10.38, 95%CI 1.47 to 73.47) were characterized as explanatory variables for a positive attitude towards Tdap.

3. Discussion

In our cross-sectional study, we assessed the KAP of a small sample of Italian OPs (120 respondents in total) about vaccinations and vaccination policies in female workers of childbearing age. As HCWs, OPs can reasonably represent a model for the general population, but because of their exclusive role in the occupational settings, they are also potentially instrumental in overcoming vaccine hesitancy (delay in acceptance or refusal of vaccines irrespective of their actual availability) [49–51] across workplaces and in high-risk occupational groups [52]. Consequently, when OPs improperly share false beliefs among the workers they care for, they may even become detrimental to the global efforts to achieve and maintain high vaccination rates, not only for "new" vaccines such as SARS-CoV-2 [1,2,36,53] but also for more conventional ones such ad Tdap and SIV [36,48,54,55]. In our study, the majority of respondents exhibited a relatively good performance on the knowledge test (74.5% ± 18.2) and a somehow discrete positive attitude towards SIV (66.7%), Tdap (70.8%), and SARS-CoV-2 (74.2%). It is often believed that the attitudes towards vaccines of medical professionals (including OPs) should not be negative and that they cannot be affected by substantial vaccine hesitancy. Even though these results are obviously desirable, they cannot be taken for granted [17,56–58].

In our study, the aforementioned vaccinations were associated with quite distinctive predictive variables. On the one hand, a better knowledge status was consistently characterized as a predictive variable (aOR 12.34, 95%CI 2.62 to 58.22 for Tdap, aOR 14.76, 95%CI 2.74 to 79.69 for SARS-CoV-2), particularly for promoting SIV (aOR 102.24, 95%CI 9.68 to 1080.26). On the other hand, the promotion of assessed vaccines was associated with the self-reported immunization of the respondents only for SIV (aOR 4.90, 95%CI 1.19 to 20.14). In this regard, participants working as OPs for healthcare facilities and reporting higher RPS towards the vaccine exhibited a negative attitude towards the promotion of SIV among female workers of childbearing age (aOR 0.03, 95%CI 0.01 to 0.43 and aOR 0.04, 95%CI 0.01 to 0.35, respectively). On the contrary, a positive attitude to Tdap was positively associated with male gender (aOR 10.22, 95%CI 2.60 to 40.24) and higher risk perception of pertussis infection (aOR 10.38, 95%CI 1.47 to 73.47).

Our estimates are therefore somewhat consistent with most of the available KAP studies on immunizations [2,6,7,29,33,53,59–66], where the domain of knowledge has been often acknowledged as a main predictor for attitudes and practices of medical professionals. It should be stressed that similar results have been repetitively but not consistently reported in occupational studies, particularly in those performed on OPs [1,2,6,7,36,53]. Particularly when dealing with KAP studies on biological risk in occupational settings, knowledge represents a key factor that should be specifically addressed. As previously stressed by Betsch et al. in a sample of German professionals [1], OPs are not spared by substantial knowledge gaps and misunderstanding of biological risk agents. Similar estimates were reported from several Italian studies [2,7,53,67], and a likely explanation for these knowledge gaps may be tentatively identified in the core curriculum of OPs. Until recently, despite the underlying legal framework, and the substantial burden represented by pathogens such as HBV, HCV, and HIV, the formal education and the medical training of Italian OPs have often prioritized other topics (e.g., work-related musculoskeletal diseases, occupational pulmonary diseases, occupational neoplasia) over biological risk [15,37,39,68]. In other words, despite their professional role, scientific background, and medical training, not only may OPs fail to overcome the gaps between official recommendations and vaccine objectors [1,2,7,67,69], but their knowledge gaps could even lead to a certain degree of vaccine hesitancy [2,6,7,53,59].

In addition, the negative attitude towards the promotion of SIV among female workers of childbearing age could be explained in terms of potential false beliefs, particularly on the actual efficacy and safety profile of the available vaccines [29,32,70,71]. During the previous decade, the reporting of three deaths within 48 h of vaccination with the Fluad® vaccine led to a sustained reduction in vaccination rates between 2014 and 2017 [72,73], also among medical professionals [72,74], with a sustained lack of trust in this preventive intervention [29,53]. Even in our study, SIV was associated with an RPS that exceeded other immunizations, notably including varicella and rubella immunizations. Both vaccines are represented by live-attenuated pathogens: even though reactivation of vaccine strains is usually acknowledged as somewhat unusual for both varicella and rubella, for the safety of mother and children, their delivery is usually avoided in pregnant women [19,75–79]. Moreover, the reported mismatch between antigens contained in the SIV and the circulating pathogens in several winter seasons has presumptively led to the diffuse underscoring of the actual preventive role of SIV [46,80,81]. Nonetheless, we cannot rule out that a certain disregard for SIV could be associated with the misunderstanding of the actual aims of this intervention. While vaccines included in Tdap are aimed to avoid the clinical syndromes associated with the natural infection of the primary pathogens, the primary aim of SIV is avoiding complications of the natural infection, likewise with SARS-CoV-2 immunization [24,74,82,83]. Interestingly, the effectiveness of SIV in avoiding sick leave in certain settings, such as healthcare facilities, although proven [84], has been inconsistently reported in several Italian studies [53,83,84]. In other words, some professionals may have failed to properly appreciate the actual cost-benefit ratio of this medical intervention, particularly in individuals such as pregnant women, where the clinician should not only target the health and safety of the patient (i.e., the pregnant woman) but care also for the unborn child. Not coincidentally, being an occupational physician in medical facilities was a negative predictor for a positive attitude towards SIV [26,33,85–88].

The inappropriate attitude of participating OPs towards SIV is particularly unsatisfactory when keeping in mind that vaccination of pregnant women remains globally low [85], and that there is a certain base of evidence that the failure of HCW to recommend, offer, promote, and perform influenza vaccination represents a substantial barrier to antenatal influenza vaccination [85–87]. A more effective contribution of OPs in overcoming usual barriers to maternal vaccination would be therefore both appreciable and necessary, as previously recommended for other medical professionals interacting with pregnant women [26,33,85,88–91].

In our study, the eventual promotion of the SARS-CoV-2 vaccine among pregnant women was remarkable (74.2%) and quite similar to the overall acceptance of mRNA formulates in a precedent report on Italian OPs (89.8% of 166 professionals) [7]. Moreover, the overall risk perception for these vaccines was comparable to other assessed immunizations, with the notable exception of adenovirus-based formulates. In this regard, a worse acceptance of these formulates was reported even in the aforementioned preliminary report (i.e., 51.2% vs. 89.8%) [7]. In fact, participating OPs appeared to be up-to-date in terms of general recommendations towards SARS-CoV-2 vaccines, with the notable exception of the exemption for women previously reporting cases of deep vein thrombosis. During the first SARS-CoV-2 vaccination campaign, several claims of an increased risk of deep vein thrombosis after SARS-CoV-2 vaccination shots urged for a critical reappraisal of these vaccines in groups potentially at high-risk, including individuals with previous episodes of deep vein thrombosis, women using birth control pills or hormone replacement therapy, and pregnant women [92–96]. Still, most of the reported cases were actually associated with adenovirus-based formulates [92,93,97], while mRNA vaccines and subunit vaccines have shown a safer profile [92,95,96]. Even though SARS-CoV-2 immunizations performed by means of an adenovirus carrier were discontinued during 2021, the overall attitude towards this immunization was actually associated with a quite higher RPS than that reported for mRNA formulates (19.9% ± 19.8 vs. 15.7% ± 19.4) and for SARS-CoV-2 vaccines based on the subunit technology (15.2% ± 16.1). The similar appraisal of mRNA and subunit vaccines—at least in this specific sample—may contribute to our understanding of the unsatisfying uptake of subunit formulates during vaccination campaigns in 2021 and 2022. Even though substantial vaccine hesitancy had previously affected similarly designed vaccines targeting hepatitis B and *Neisseria meningitidis* ACWY [31,98–101], subunit formulates have been initially welcome as "more conventional" drugs that could contribute to overcoming most of the concerns about the innovative mRNA technology [102]. However, according to an official report from the Italian National Health Service, by 26 September 2022, a total of 140,689,960 doses of SARS-CoV-2 vaccines had been delivered among Italian residents; of these, only 0.03% were represented by subunit formulates [103]. In other terms, our results seemingly suggest that interventions improving the understanding of actual guidelines among OPs may also improve their acceptance and proactive attitude towards SARS-CoV-2 vaccines even in pregnant women.

Limits and Strengths. Despite its potential significance, our study is affected by several limitations and is not generalizable because of shortcomings affecting the sampling strategy and generalizability of the sample.

In the first place, our sample was quite small, as it included a total of 120 OPs, which is around 1.5% of all Italian occupational physicians at the time of the survey (n = 7826), and only 5.9% of the potential recipients. Therefore, the sample is not likely to be representative of all OPs. Moreover, because of the limited number of sampled professionals, and the similarly limited response rate across the targeted and invited OPs, the present study was also affected by reduced statistical power, urging for a very cautious appraisal of the results we were able to collect. More precisely, assuming as a reference the acceptance of influenza (68.5%), Tdap (52.7%), and SARS-CoV-2 (90.4%) by Italian OPs from some similarly designed studies [7,36,53], a Type I error of 5% (0.05), and a power of 95%, a minimum sample size ranging between 133 for SARS-CoV-2, 332 for SIV, and 383 for Tdap could be calculated [7]. In other words, the present study only collected one-third of the sample size it would have required in order to gather sufficient statistical power. Still, as the specific topic of immunization of childbearing-age women in occupational settings has been assessed in only a limited fashion, particularly in Italy, and available evidence has been mostly collected from healthcare workers [7,29,104–107], our preliminary results could provide some insight for potential interventions aimed to improve the overall delivery of vaccines by OPs.

Second, our research was designed as an internet-based survey, whose implicit limits have been previously addressed [108–110]. Similarly designed studies are acknowledged as reliable and cost-effective, but they are also affected by an extensive double "self-selection" of participating individuals. On the one hand, as participating individuals are recruited through social media platforms, the sample will only include individuals familiar with new media [36,109,111–113]. In turn, this could lead to the oversampling of individuals more accustomed to sharing personal information through internet access, usually more frequently reported among younger age groups. In effect, our sample included a reduced share of respondents aged 50 years or older (30.0% of the total sample), and these figures are quite inconsistent with the Italian medical workforce [114,115]. On the other hand, this sampling strategy would lead to the oversampling of subjects having greater knowledge and/or interest in the assessed topic [29,32,116,117], while not participating could be understood as a negative attitude or a lack of knowledge about the targeted topic [109], and that may impair the overall reliability and generalizability of collected results. Nonetheless, our study deliberately targeted a relatively homogenous subgroup of medical professionals (i.e., OPs) in order to mitigate as much as possible the potential self-selection of the participants and minimize or even rule out the eventual effect of individual factors such as occupational background and educational level.

Thirdly, we cannot rule out that some of the respondents did not fully adhere to our selection criteria, further compromising the actual representativity of the sample. In order to cope with this potential shortcoming, our study only included participants that were drawn from discussion groups, whose participation was limited to individuals having previously received a specific invitation from the manager and answered specific "selection" questions [118]. Moreover, we do not know how often sampled participants are usually requested to contribute to workers' vaccinations, and more specifically to the vaccination practice of pregnant women [7,29,36,53,104–107].

Fourth, even though the core of this study, i.e., the knowledge test, was based on a reliable model and characterized by a high degree of internal consistency [1,119], we cannot rule out that some of the items assessed might have been affected by some degree of social desirability bias, whereby some participants reported some answers in terms of "common sense", prioritizing more "socially appropriate" answers over their true understanding of certain topics. Interestingly, such potential bias has been repeatedly identified in previous KAP studies on OPs [1,2,36,53,108], including some surveys performed with a quite similar sample. Therefore, we cannot rule out that our results could have ultimately overstated the share of individuals having an effective understanding of vaccine-associated issues, but also actually acknowledging the reported and assessed vaccinations as recommended and promoted in pregnant women and women of childbearing age. In order to attempt a certain quantification of participants affected by social desirability bias, the knowledge test specifically reported the still commercially unavailable maternal RSV vaccination [118,120]. Interestingly, only 37.5% of participants correctly ruled out this option, suggesting the need for a critical appraisal of overall results from the knowledge test and individual attitudes towards reported vaccines.

Finally, our study deliberately assessed the KAP of recruited participants on a selected set of immunizations, but women of childbearing age could be targeted by other interventions of some occupational interest, including but not limited to vaccines for *Neisseria meningitidis* and *Mycobacterium tuberculosis* (i.e., BCG) for healthcare workers, Hepatitis A virus, typhoid vaccines, and tick-borne encephalitis vaccine for workers traveling to parts of the world where these pathologies are common, and even rabies vaccines for professionals involved in laboratory and veterinary practice [30,31,121–127]. Moreover, workplaces may represent an appropriate setting for improving the acceptance of immunizations with a more limited occupational interest, such as pneumococcus, and mostly human papillomavirus (HPV) vaccines. In effect, the pneumococcal vaccine is currently indicated only for individuals having certain chronic medical conditions or other risk factors, and routine medical surveillance by OPs may provide an ideal opportunity for reaching potential recipients and/or addressing their vaccine hesitancy [128,129]. Similarly, OPs could contribute to the shared effort for improving HPV vaccination rates. HPV is not only the current most common sexually transmitted disease in the world but it is also acknowledged as the main risk factor for cervical cancer in women with an estimated 570,000 new cases per year [130–133]. According to the current guidelines, the HPV vaccine is currently recommended for everyone through age 26 years if not adequately vaccinated when younger, and OPs, during medical surveillance, could properly identify and address women that can potentially benefit from catch-up vaccination [134]. According to the total worker health approach, future interventions should be therefore tailored in order to include a more extensive list of assessed vaccinations, not strictly limited to the interventions associated with occupational settings [135,136].

4. Materials and Methods

4.1. Study Design

The present study was designed as a cross-sectional questionnaire-based study according to the STROBE statement (see STROBE checklist as Supplementary File S1) and performed between 1 April 2022 and 30 April 2022. The study was delivered across seven private Facebook group pages and four closed forums focusing on occupational medicine, whose applications were officially limited to OPs. According to the built-in statistics of the parent social media, by 1 April 2022, the group pages had a total of 2034 members. Still, no information could be retrieved about cross-membership and the number of actual, active users.

In order to share the study with the group members, the chief researcher (MR) preventively contacted the administrators of the groups, requesting preventive authorization for posting an invitation link to the questionnaire. Users who clicked on the invitation texts were then provided with a page reporting (a) the full study information; (b) the informed consent (authors' translation of the informed consent is available as Supplementary File S2); and (c) a web link to the first page of the survey (Google Forms; Google LLC; Menlo Park, California, CA, USA).

On the first page of the survey, participants were initially asked whether they (a) were or not living and working in Italy and (b) were working as an OP at the time of the survey. Only participants sharing two positive answers to these checkpoint items received the full questionnaire, while in all other cases, the survey was closed, and no further data were retained. The questionnaire was compiled anonymously: personal data (e.g., name, IP address, email address), and all personal information unnecessary to the survey were not requested, saved, or tracked.

4.2. Questionnaire and Availability of Data and Material

The questionnaire was originally formulated in Italian, being designed as a follow-up to an instrument originally validated in obstetrics and gynecology [29]. The final questionnaire included the following sections:

1. Individual characteristics: age, seniority as OPs, gender, and whether they (a) had any professional experience as an occupational physician with any healthcare provider (yes vs. no) and (b) had any child.
2. Knowledge test: participants received a 31-item questionnaire on vaccination in pregnancy [29] that was based on previous KAP studies in occupational settings [137,138]. Briefly, the questionnaire included a series of true/false items based on the current understanding and guidelines on vaccinations in pregnancy, specifically focusing on (a) general issues about vaccinations and (b) official recommendations on SARS-CoV-2, SIV, and Tdap. GKS was calculated as the sum of correctly and incorrectly marked recommendations: for all correct answers, +1 was added to a sum score, while a missing/"don't know" answer or a wrong indication added 0 to the cumulative score.
3. Risk perception: participants were initially asked to rate by means of a fully labeled 5-point Likert scale (range: 1, "of no significant concern in daily practice", to 5, "of very high concern in daily practice") the perceived severity (C) and the perceived frequency (I) of a series of vaccine-preventable disorders in pregnant women: seasonal influenza, tetanus, diphtheria, pertussis, measles, parotitis, rubella, varicella, hepatitis B, SARS-CoV-2. Similarly, participants were then asked to rate how they perceived a series of vaccinations (i.e., against seasonal flu, tetanus, diphtheria, pertussis, measles, parotitis, rubella, varicella, hepatitis B virus, SARS-CoV-2 delivered as mRNA formulate, adenoviral vector-based formulates, and subunit vaccine) when delivered to pregnant women in terms of the perceived severity (C) and frequency (I) of their side effects.

As previously suggested by Yates, a quantitative estimate of perceived risk can be defined as the mathematical product of the perceived probability of an event and its expected consequences [1,139], and the corresponding RPS for vaccines and natural infection was therefore calculated as:

$$RPS = I \times C$$

4. Attitudes and practices: we initially inquired of participants whether they had previously received any of the following vaccinations: seasonal influenza virus, Tdap or dT, MPR, varicella (either as a single formulate or within an MPR-V vaccine), hepatitis B virus, SARS-CoV-2 (any). Similarly, participants were asked whether, during the last 12 months, they had recommended any of the aforementioned vaccines in women of childbearing age. Finally, we reported a series of potential barriers towards vaccinations in women of childbearing age (i.e., fear of side effects; costs of vaccinations; not being perceived as a priority by other medical professionals; inappropriate risk perception by pregnant women; vaccination services are scarcely available; inappropriate understanding of official recommendations by pregnant women; inappropriate understanding of official recommendations by medical professionals), and participants were asked to rate their perceived significance through a 5-point Likert scale ranging from 1 (not agreeing at all) to 5 (totally agreeing).

All questions were self-reported and not externally validated. The internal consistency or reliability of each of the sections of the questionnaire was assessed with the Cronbach alpha test, the results of which were interpreted in accordance with the literature. An English translation of the questionnaire is available on request to the study Authors.

4.3. Ethical Approval

Before giving their consent to the survey, participants were briefed that the principles and guidelines of the Helsinki Declaration would be followed across all steps of this study. More precisely, data were gathered anonymously and handled confidentially, being stored for a limited timeframe, in order to only allow aggregate data analysis. Participation was strictly voluntary, and no monetary or other compensation was offered to the participants. Moreover, only subjects who had expressed consent for study participation were able to provide the questionnaire for data analysis. As individuals cannot be identified based on the presented material, this study caused no plausible harm or stigma to participants. The study was deliberately designed with an anonymous, observational approach, and it did not include clinical data. Moreover, demographic data were deliberately limited to very generic items (i.e., age, seniority, and gender). According to Italian law (Gazzetta Ufficiale no. 76, dated 31 March 2008; Supplementary File S3), a preliminary evaluation by an ethical committee was not required.

4.4. Data Analysis

Cumulative scores (RPS, GKS) were initially normalized to percent value, being then dichotomized by median value as "high" (i.e., >median) and "low" (≤median) groups. All continuous variables were reported as mean ± standard deviation. After visual inspection, their distributions were assessed by means of the D'Agostino–Pearson K2 test and compared through the Student's t-test for unpaired data or ANOVA for K2 test p value > 0.100 (i.e., normally distributed variable), or through the Mann–Whitney or Kruskal–Wallis test for K2 test p value < 0.100 (i.e., not normally distributed variable). According to the distribution of variables, their correlation was then assessed by Pearson's correlation coefficient (i.e., normally distributed variables) or through Spearman's ranks test (i.e., not normally distributed variable).

In order to properly characterize explanatory variables of the outcome variables represented by a somewhat positive attitude towards recommending SIV, Tdap, and SARS-CoV-2 vaccine, a multivariable analysis was modeled as follows. Firstly, univariate analysis of all of the categorical variables was performed in respect of the aforementioned outcome variables through a chi-squared test in order to test variables to be included in the multivariable analysis. All variables that at univariate analysis were significantly ($p < 0.05$) associated with a somewhat positive attitude towards recommending SIV, Tdap, and SARS-CoV-2 vaccines were then included in a stepwise binary logistic regression analysis model in order to calculate multivariate odds ratios (aOR) and their respective 95% confidence intervals (95%CI). We opted for a more restrictive stepwise approach over an a priori modeling as in a small dataset the latter could find many false associations that happen only by chance [140]. All statistical analyses were performed by means of IBM SPSS Statistics 26.0 for Macintosh (IBM Corp. Armonk, NY, USA).

5. Conclusions

OPs are called upon to play a dual key role, i.e., reconciling the right to work and protecting and promoting workers' health at the same time. Despite a generally favorable attitude towards vaccines among our OP respondents, the results of our study suggest substantial knowledge gaps and a need for better training in the area of immunization of pregnant women. Because of the low response to the survey, however, these results remain preliminary.

Supplementary Materials: The following supporting information can be downloaded at: https://www.mdpi.com/article/10.3390/women3020019/s1, File S1: STROBE checklist; File S2: Authors' translation of the informed consent; File S3: Author's translation of the Gazzetta Ufficiale no. 76, dated 31 March 2008.

Author Contributions: Conceptualization, M.R., A.B., and F.M; Data curation, M.R.; Formal analysis, M.R. and A.B.; Funding acquisition, M.P.C.; Investigation, M.R. and F.M.; Methodology, M.R.; Project administration, F.M.; Resources, A.B.; Software, M.R. and A.B.; Validation, M.R. and F.M.; Writing—original draft, A.B., M.P.C., and F.M.; Writing—review and editing, A.B: and M.P.C. All authors have read and agreed to the published version of the manuscript.

Funding: This research received no external funding.

Institutional Review Board Statement: The study was conducted according to the guidelines of the Declaration of Helsinki. A preventive ethical review and approval were waived for this study because of its anonymous, observational design and due to the lack of clinical data about patients that could configure the present research as a clinical trial. Participants were also guaranteed that retrieved data would be stored only for the time required by data analysis. The study, therefore, did not configure itself as a clinical trial, and a preliminary evaluation by an ethical committee was not required, according to Italian law (Gazzetta Ufficiale no. 76, dated 31 March 2008).

Informed Consent Statement: Informed consent was obtained from all subjects involved in the study

Data Availability Statement: Data are available on request.

Conflicts of Interest: The authors declare no conflict of interest.

Appendix A

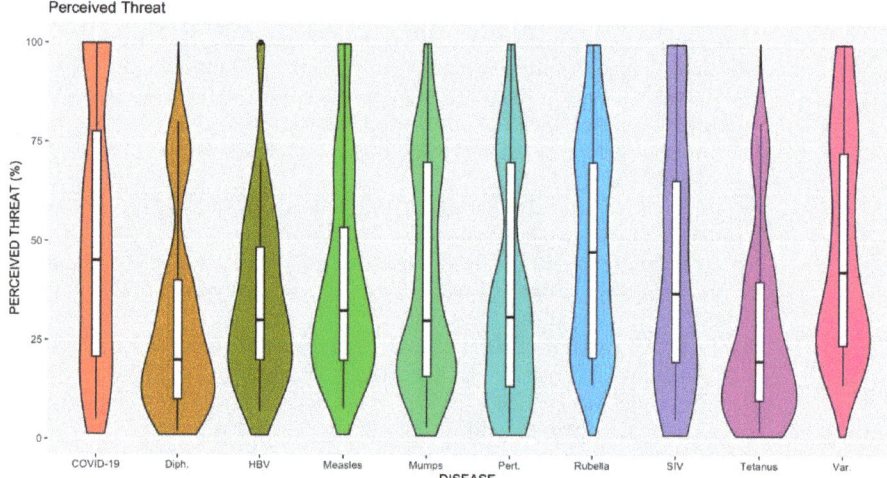

Figure A1. Risk Perception Score (RPS) towards a selected series of vaccine-preventable diseases in pregnant women. Notes: Diph. = diphtheria; HBV = hepatitis B virus; Pert. = pertussis; SIV = Seasonal influenza vaccine; Var. = varicella.

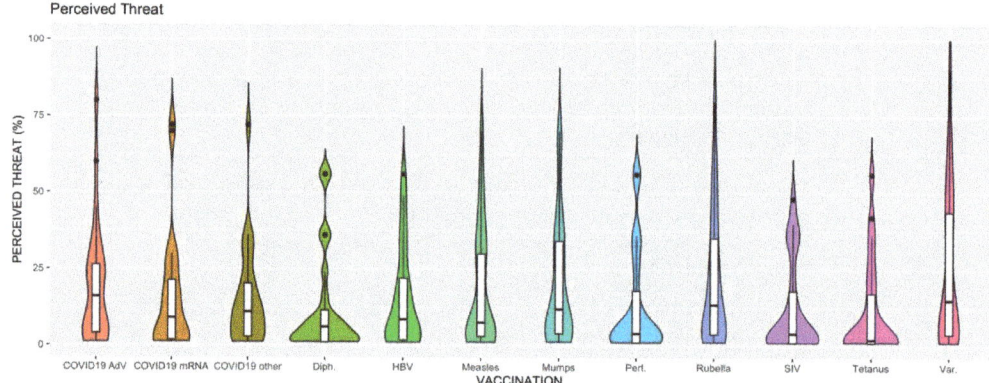

Figure A2. Risk Perception Score (RPS) towards a selected series of vaccines to be performed in pregnant women. Notes: AdV = adenoviral vector; mRNA = mRNA-based vaccine; Diph. = diphtheria; HBV = hepatitis B virus; Pert. = pertussis; SIV = Seasonal influenza vaccine; Var. = varicella.

Table A1. Summary of shortcuts and acronyms employed across the manuscript.

Acronyms	Meaning
95%CI	95% Confidence Interval
aOR	Adjusted Odds Ratio
BMI	Body Mass Index
COVID-19	Coronavirus Disease 2019
GKS	General Knowledge Score
HAV	Hepatitis A Virus
HBV	Hepatitis B Virus
HPV	Human Papillomavirus
ICOH	International Commission on Occupational Health
ISS	Italian National Institute of Health (in Italian, Istituto Superiore di Sanità)
KAP	Knowledge, Attitudes, Practices
MPR	Measles-Parotitis-Rubella vaccine
NHS	National Health Service
NIP	(Italian) National Immunization Plan
OPs	Occupational Physicians
PPE	Personal Protective Equipment
RPS	Risk Perception Score
RSV	Respiratory Syncytial Virus
SARS-CoV-2	Severe acute respiratory syndrome coronavirus 2
SIV	Seasonal Influenza Virus
STROBE	STrengthening the Reporting of Observational studies in Epidemiology
Tdap	trivalent formulation tetanus-diphtheria-acellular pertussis
VPDs	Vaccine-Preventable Disease

Table A2. Knowledge Test in 120 occupational physicians participating in a survey on vaccinations in pregnant women (Italy, 2022).

Statement	Correct Answer	No./120, %
Q01. Addictive used in vaccines are not dangerous for human health	TRUE	80, 66.7%
Q02. Multiple sclerosis may be elicited by HBV recombinant vaccine	FALSE	105, 87.5%
Q03. Subacute sclerosing panencephalitis can be elicited by the measles vaccine	FALSE	81, 67.5%
Q04. Encephalitis lethargica can be elicited by vaccines against influenza (in particular, against pandemic influenza)	FALSE	80, 66.7%
Q05. Some vaccinations increase the risk of developing diabetes	FALSE	100, 83.3%
Q06. Some vaccinations increase the risk of developing autoimmune disorders including Hashimoto's thyroiditis	FALSE	76, 63.3%
Q07. Some vaccinations increase the risk of developing autism (e.g., vaccine against measles)	FALSE	110, 91.7%
Q08. Some vaccinations increase the risk of developing allergies	FALSE	85, 70.8%
Q09. Vaccines are of limited value in controlling infectious diseases as etiological drugs are extensively available	FALSE	110, 91.7%
Q10. Without vaccination programs, smallpox would still exist	TRUE	115, 95.8%
Q11. The efficacy of vaccines has been extensively proven	TRUE	115, 95.8%

Table A2. Cont.

Statement	Correct Answer	No./120, %
Q12. Children would exhibit greater resistance to infectious diseases if they received a more limited number of vaccines	FALSE	100, 93.3%
Q13. A substantial share of vaccines is delivered too early to properly activate the immune system	FALSE	105, 87.5%
Q14. The proper development of the immune system could be impaired by the delivery of a large number of vaccines	FALSE	85, 70.8%
Q15. According to the current National Vaccination Plan, shots with combined vaccine Diphtheria-Tetanus-Pertussis (Tdap) to all pregnant women	TRUE	65, 54.2%
Q16. According to the current National Vaccination Plan, vaccines should be avoided during pregnancy, in general	FALSE	110, 91.7%
Q17. According to the current National Vaccination Plan, live-attenuated vaccines should be avoided during pregnancy	TRUE	65, 54.2%
Q18. According to the current National Vaccination Plan, tetanus vaccination shots should be delivered to all adults every 10 years	TRUE	110, 91.7%
Q19. A vaccine preventing Respiratory Syncytial Virus (RSV) is currently recommended for pregnant women	FALSE	45, 37.5%
Q20. According to the current National Vaccination Plan, seasonal influenza vaccine should be avoided in pregnant women during the third trimester	FALSE	97, 80.8%
Q21. Vaccines against measles, parotitis, and rubella (with and without varicella) can elicit secondary cases with epidemic potential	FALSE	81, 67.5%
Q22. According to our current understanding, mRNA vaccines against SARS-CoV-2 can elicit impairment of fertility	FALSE	95, 79.2%
Q23. According to our current understanding, mRNA vaccines against SARS-CoV-2 should be avoided in women with a previous history of deep vein thrombosis	FALSE	57, 47.5%
Q24. According to the current guidelines, combined delivery of SARS-CoV-2 and Seasonal Influenza vaccines in pregnant women is a potential option.	TRUE	100, 83.3%
Q25. Pregnant women should avoid all occupational settings with a well-defined biological risk.	TRUE	104, 86.7%

Table A3. Comparison between perceived Risk Perception Score (RPS, potential range 0 to 100) on natural infections in pregnant women for selected pathogens as reported by 120 occupational physicians participating in the present survey (Italy, 2022) (Note: 95%CI = 95% confidence interval; ANOVA = analysis of the variance).

Pathogen	RPS (95%CI)	Mean Difference (95%CI)	p Value (ANOVA, Dunnet's Post Hoc Test)
Seasonal influenza Virus	45.29 (39.59 to 50.99)	REFERENCE	REFERENCE
Tetanus	26.58 (23.37 to 31.80)	18.71 (9.31 to 28.11)	<0.001
Diphtheria	27.58 (23.37 to 31.80)	17.71 (8.31 to 27.11)	<0.001
Pertussis	37.79 (32.69 to 42.89)	7.50 (−1.90 to 16.90)	0.185
Measles	41.00 (36.25 to 45.75)	4.29 (−5.11 to 13.69)	0.774
Parotitis	40.75 (35.78 to 45.72)	4.54 (−4.86 to 13.94)	0.722
Rubella	50.33 (45.50 to 55.16)	−5.04 (−14.44 to 4.36)	0.614
Varicella	49.42 (44.42 to 54.41)	−4.13 (−13.52 to 5.27)	0.806
Hepatitis B	35.08 (31.11 to 39.06)	10.21 (0.81 to 19.61)	0.026
SARS-CoV-2	52.71 (46.76 to 58.65)	−7.42 (−16.81 to 1.98)	0.195

Table A4. Comparison between perceived Risk Perception Score (RPS, potential range 0 to 100) on vaccinations for pregnant women as reported by 120 occupational physicians participating in the present survey (Italy, 2022) (Note: 95%CI = 95% confidence interval; ANOVA = analysis of the variance).

Pathogen	RPS (95%CI)	Mean Difference (95%CI)	p Value (ANOVA, Dunnet's Post Hoc Test)
Seasonal Influenza Vaccine	12.13 (9.42 to 14.83)	REFERENCE	REFERENCE
Tetanus	11.38 (8.61 to 14.14)	0.75 (−5.94 to 7.44)	0.999
Diphtheria	12.13 (9.12 to 15.13)	0.00 (−6.69 to 6.69)	1.000
Pertussis	12.96 (9.88 to 16.03)	−0.83 (−7.53 to 5.86)	0.999
Measles	18.44 (14.85 to 22.04)	−6.32 (−13.01 to 0.38)	0.075
Parotitis	19.52 (15.89 to 23.14)	−7.39 (−14.09 to −0.70)	0.022
Rubella	21.79 (17.75 to 25.83)	−9.67 (−16.36 to 2.97)	0.001
Varicella	25.46 (20.81 to 30.11)	−13.33 (−20.03 to −6.64)	<0.001
Hepatitis B	15.29 (12.35 to 18.23)	−3.17 (−9.86 to 3.53)	0.775
SARS-CoV-2 mRNA	15.67 (12.16 to 19.18)	−3.54 (−10.24 to 3.15)	0.660
Adenoviral carrier	19.92 (16.34 to 23.50)	−7.79 (−14.49 to −1.10)	0.013
Subunit vaccine	15.17 (12.25 to 18.08)	−3.04 (−9.74 to 3.65)	0.811

Table A5. Correlation of Risk Perception Score (RPS) on diseases and corresponding vaccinations, and General Knowledge Score in 120 Italian occupational physicians participating in the survey on vaccines in pregnant women. The correlation was assessed by means of Spearman's rank test.

	RPS (Disease) vs. GKS	RPS (Vaccination) vs. RPS (Disease)	RPS (Vaccination) vs. GKS
Seasonal Influenza Virus	r = 0.341 $p < 0.001$	r = −0.157 $p = 0.088$	r = −0.352 $p < 0.001$
Diphtheria	r = 0.072 $p = 0.473$	r = 0.008 $p = 0.931$	r = −0.450 $p < 0.001$
Tetanus	r = 0.041 $p = 0.655$	r = −0.136 $p = 0.139$	r = −0.367 $p < 0.001$
Pertussis	r = 0.200 $p = 0.028$	r = 0.152 $p = 0.097$	r = −0.379 $p < 0.001$
Measles	r = 0.356 $p < 0.001$	r = 0.121 $p = 0.186$	r = −0.061 $p = 0.509$
Parotitis	r = 0.237 $p = 0.009$	r = 0.146 $p = 0.111$	r = −0.079 $p = 0.391$
Rubella	r = 0.177 $p = 0.053$	r = 0.208 $p = 0.022$	r = −0.056 $p = 0.541$
Varicella	r = 0.196 $p = 0.032$	r = 0.135 $p = 0.141$	r = −0.010 $p = 0.918$
Hepatitis B Virus	r = 0.406 $p < 0.001$	r = 0.164 $p = 0.074$	r = −0.191 $p = 0.037$
SARS-CoV-2	r = 0.428 $p < 0.001$	-	-
mRNA vaccine	-	r = −0.054 $p = 0.558$	r = −0.354 $p < 0.001$

Table A5. Cont.

	RPS (Disease) vs. GKS	RPS (Vaccination) vs. RPS (Disease)	RPS (Vaccination) vs. GKS
Adenoviral-based vaccines	-	r = 0.239 p = 0.009	r = −0.294 p = 0.001
Subunit	-	r = 0.155 p = 0.091	r = −0.314 p < 0.001

Table A6. Summary of the categorical variables that were included as explanatory ones in the logistic regression models (Model 1: outcome variable, somehow positive attitude towards Seasonal Influenza Vaccine, SIV; Model 2: outcome variable, somehow positive attitude towards tetanus-diphtheria-pertussis [Tdap] vaccine; Model 3: outcome variable, somehow positive attitude towards SARS-CoV-2 vaccines) (Note: RPS = risk perception score).

	Model 1	Model 2	Model 3
Male Gender	Not included	Included	Not included
Age ≥ 50 years	Not included	Not included	Included
Any Child in the household	Not included	Not Included	Not included
Higher Knowledge status	Included	Included	Included
Working as Occupational Physician for Healthcare facilities	Included	Not included	Not included
Vaccinated (SIV)	Included	-	-
Vaccinated (Tdap)	-	Not included	-
Vaccinated (SARS-CoV-2)	-	-	Included
Higher RPS vs. seasonal influenza	Included	-	-
Higher RPS vs. diphtheria	-	Included	-
Higher RPS vs. tetanus	-	Not included	-
Higher RPS vs. pertussis	-	Included	-
Higher RPS vs. SARS-CoV-2	-	-	Not included
Higher RPS vs. SIV	Included	-	-
Higher RPS vs. diphtheria vaccine	-	Not included	-
Higher RPS vs. tetanus vaccine	-	Included	-
Higher RPS vs. pertussis vaccine	-	Not included	-
Higher RPS vs. SARS-CoV-2 vaccine (mRNA)	-	-	Included
Higher RPS vs. SARS-CoV-2 vaccine (adenoviral carrier)	-	-	Included
Higher RPS vs. SARS-CoV-2 vaccine (subunit)	-	-	Not Included

References

1. Betsch, C.; Wicker, S. Personal Attitudes and Misconceptions, Not Official Recommendations Guide Occupational Physicians' Vaccination Decisions. *Vaccine* **2014**, *32*, 4478–4484. [CrossRef] [PubMed]
2. Riccò, M.; Cattani, S.; Casagranda, F.; Gualerzi, G.; Signorelli, C. Knowledge, Attitudes, Beliefs and Practices of Occupational Physicians towards Vaccinations of Health Care Workers: A Cross Sectional Pilot Study in North-Eastern Italy. *Int. J. Occup. Med. Environ. Health* **2017**, *30*, 775–790. [CrossRef] [PubMed]
3. Peretti-Watel, P.; Seror, V.; Cortaredona, S.; Launay, O.; Raude, J.; Verger, P.; Beck, F.; Legleye, S.; L'Haridon, O.; Ward, J. A Future Vaccination Campaign against COVID-19 at Risk of Vaccine Hesitancy and Politicisation. *Lancet* **2020**, *20*, 769–770. [CrossRef]

4. Verger, P.; Dubé, E. Restoring Confidence in Vaccines in the COVID-19 Era. *Expert Rev. Vaccines* **2020**, *19*, 991–993. [CrossRef]
5. Verger, P.; Scronias, D.; Dauby, N.; Adedzi, K.A.; Gobert, C.; Bergeat, M.; Gagneur, A.; Dubé, E. Attitudes of Healthcare Workers towards COVID-19 Vaccination: A Survey in France and French-Speaking Parts of Belgium and Canada, 2020. *Euro Surveill.* **2021**, *26*, 2002047. [CrossRef] [PubMed]
6. Riccò, M.; Gualerzi, G.; Ranzieri, S.; Ferraro, P.; Bragazzi, N.L. Knowledge, Attitudes, Practices (KAP) of Italian Occupational Physicians towards Tick Borne Encephalitis. *Trop. Med. Infect. Dis.* **2020**, *5*, 117. [CrossRef] [PubMed]
7. Riccò, M.; Ferraro, P.; Peruzzi, S.; Balzarini, F.; Ranzieri, S. Mandate or Not Mandate: Knowledge, Attitudes, and Practices of Italian Occupational Physicians towards SARS-CoV-2 Immunization at the Beginning of Vaccination Campaign. *Vaccines* **2021**, *9*, 889. [CrossRef]
8. Accurti, V.; Gambitta, B.; Iodice, S.; Manenti, A.; Boito, S.; Dapporto, F.; Leonardi, M.; Molesti, E.; Fabietti, I.; Montomoli, E.; et al. SARS-CoV-2 Seroconversion and Pregnancy Outcomes in a Population of Pregnant Women Recruited in Milan, Italy, between April 2020 and October 2020. *Int. J. Environ. Res. Public Health* **2022**, *19*, 16720. [CrossRef]
9. Gabutti, G.; Cetin, I.; Conversano, M.; Costantino, C.; Durando, P.; Giuffrida, S. Experts' Opinion for Improving Pertussis Vaccination Rates in Adolescents and Adults: A Call to Action. *Int. J. Environ. Res. Public Health* **2022**, *19*, 4412. [CrossRef]
10. van Beukering, M.D.M.; Schuster, H.J.; Peelen, M.J.C.S.; Schonewille, M.E.A.; Hajenius, P.J.; Duijnhoven, R.G.; Brand, T.; Painter, R.C.; Kok, M. Working Conditions in Low Risk Nulliparous Women in The Netherlands: Are Legislation and Guidelines a Guarantee for a Healthy Working Environment? A Cohort Study. *Int. Arch. Occup. Environ. Health* **2022**, *95*, 1305–1315. [CrossRef]
11. Esté, J.; Cabrera-rodrí, R. Zika Virus Pathogenesis: A Battle for Immune Evasion. *Vaccines* **2021**, *9*, 294.
12. Loconsole, D.; Metallo, A.; De Robertis, A.L.; Morea, A.; Quarto, M.; Chironna, M. Seroprevalence of Dengue Virus, West Nile Virus, Chikungunya Virus, and Zika Virus in International Travelers Attending a Travel and Migration Center in 2015–2017, Southern Italy. *Vector Borne Zoonotic Dis.* **2018**, *18*, 331–334. [CrossRef] [PubMed]
13. Silva, N.M.; Santos, N.C.; Martins, I.C. Dengue and Zika Viruses: Epidemiological History, Potential Therapies, and Promising Vaccines. *Trop. Med. Infect. Dis.* **2020**, *5*, 150. [CrossRef] [PubMed]
14. Brunelli, L.; Antinolfi, F.; Malacarne, F.; Cocconi, R.; Brusaferro, S. A Wide Range of Strategies to Cope with Healthcare Workers' Vaccine Hesitancy in A North-Eastern Italian Region: Are They Enough? *Healthcare* **2020**, *9*, 4. [CrossRef] [PubMed]
15. Maggiore, U.L.R.; Scala, C.; Toletone, A.; Debarbieri, N.; Perria, M.; D'Amico, B.; Montecucco, A.; Martini, M.; Dini, G.; Durando, P. Susceptibility to Vaccine-Preventable Diseases and Vaccination Adherence among Healthcare Workers in Italy: A Cross-Sectional Survey at a Regional Acute-Care University Hospital and a Systematic Review. *Hum. Vaccin. Immunother.* **2017**, *13*, 470–476. [CrossRef] [PubMed]
16. Dzieciolowska, S.; Hamel, D.; Gadio, S.; Dionne, M. Covid-19 Vaccine Acceptance, Hesitancy, and Refusal among Canadian Healthcare Workers: A Multicenter Survey. *Am. J. Infect. Control.* 2021; in press. [CrossRef]
17. Maltezou, H.C.; Theodoridou, K.; Ledda, C.; Rapisarda, V.; Theodoridou, M. Vaccination of Healthcare Workers: Is Mandatory Vaccination Needed? *Expert Rev. Vaccines* **2019**, *18*, 5–13. [CrossRef]
18. Dini, G.; Toletone, A.; Sticchi, L.; Orsi, A.; Bragazzi, N.L.; Durando, P. Influenza Vaccination in Healthcare Workers: A Comprehensive Critical Appraisal of the Literature. *Hum. Vaccin. Immunother.* **2018**, *14*, 772–789. [CrossRef]
19. Chodick, G.; Ashkenazi, S.; Livni, G.; Lerman, Y. Cost-Effectiveness of Varicella Vaccination of Healthcare Workers. *Vaccine* **2005**, *23*, 5064–5072. [CrossRef]
20. Loulergue, P.; Moulin, F.; Vidal-Trecan, G.; Absi, Z.; Demontpion, C.; Menager, C.; Gorodetsky, M.; Gendrel, D.; Guillevin, L.; Launay, O. Knowledge, Attitudes and Vaccination Coverage of Healthcare Workers Regarding Occupational Vaccinations. *Vaccine* **2009**, *27*, 4240–4243. [CrossRef]
21. Marshall, H.; McMillan, M.; Andrews, R.M.; Macartney, K.; Edwards, K. Vaccines in Pregnancy: The Dual Benefit for Pregnant Women and Infants. *Hum. Vaccin. Immunother.* **2016**, *12*, 848–856. [CrossRef] [PubMed]
22. Kuehn, B.M. Recommended Vaccines Underused During Pregnancy. *J. Am. Med. Assoc.* **2019**, *320*, 1949. [CrossRef] [PubMed]
23. Fortner, K.B.; Nieuwoudt, C.; Reeder, C.F.; Swamy, G.K. Infections in Pregnancy and the Role of Vaccines. *Obstet. Gynecol. Clin. N. Am.* **2018**, *45*, 369–388. [CrossRef] [PubMed]
24. Gall, S.A. Vaccines for Pertussis and Influenza: Recommendations for Use in Pregnancy. *Clin. Obstet. Gynecol.* **2008**, *51*, 486–497. [CrossRef]
25. Bonville, C.A.; Cibula, D.A.; Domachowske, J.B.; Suryadevara, M. Vaccine Attitudes and Practices among Obstetric Providers in New York State Following the Recommendation for Pertussis Vaccination during Pregnancy. *Hum. Vaccin. Immunother.* **2015**, *11*, 713–718. [CrossRef]
26. Naleway, A.L.; Smith, W.J.; Mullooly, J.P. Delivering Influenza Vaccine to Pregnant Women. *Epidemiol. Rev.* **2006**, *28*, 47–53. [CrossRef] [PubMed]
27. Kharbanda, E.O.; Vazquez-Benitez, G.; Lipkind, H.S.; Klein, N.P.; Cheetham, T.C.; Naleway, A.L.; Lee, G.M.; Hambidge, S.; Jackson, M.L.; Omer, S.B.; et al. Maternal Tdap Vaccination: Coverage and Acute Safety Outcomes in the Vaccine Safety Datalink, 2007–2013. *Vaccine* **2016**, *34*, 968–973. [CrossRef]
28. DeSilva, M.; Vazquez-Benitez, G.; Nordin, J.D.; Lipkind, H.S.; Klein, N.P.; Cheetham, T.C.; Naleway, A.L.; Hambidge, S.J.; Lee, G.M.; Jackson, M.L.; et al. Maternal Tdap Vaccination and Risk of Infant Morbidity. *Vaccine* **2017**, *35*, 3655–3660. [CrossRef]

29. Riccò, M.; Vezzosi, L.; Gualerzi, G.; Balzarini, F.; Capozzi, V.A.; Volpi, L. Knowledge, Attitudes, Beliefs and Practices of Obstetrics-Gynecologists on Seasonal Influenza and Pertussis Immunizations in Pregnant Women: Preliminary Results from North-Western Italy. *Minerva Ginecol.* **2019**, *71*, 288–297. [CrossRef]
30. Bonanni, P.; Ferrero, A.; Guerra, R.; Iannazzo, S.; Odone, A.; Pompa, M.; Rizzuto, E.; Signorelli, C. Vaccine Coverage in Italy and Assessment of the 2012–2014 National Immunization Prevention Plan. *Epidemiol. Prev.* **2015**, *39*, 146–158. [CrossRef]
31. Signorelli, C.; Guerra, R.; Siliquini, R.; Ricciardi, W. Italy's Response to Vaccine Hesitancy: An Innovative and Cost Effective National Immunization Plan Based on Scientific Evidence. *Vaccine* **2017**, *35*, 4057–4059. [CrossRef] [PubMed]
32. Napolitano, F.; Napolitano, P.; Angelillo, I.F. Seasonal Influenza Vaccination in Pregnant Women: Knowledge, Attitudes, and Behaviors in Italy. *BMC Infect. Dis.* **2017**, *17*, 1–7. [CrossRef] [PubMed]
33. D'Alessandro, A.; Napolitano, F.; D'Ambrosio, A.; Angelillo, I.F. Vaccination Knowledge and Acceptability among Pregnant Women in Italy. *Hum. Vaccin. Immunother.* **2018**, *14*, 1573–1579. [CrossRef] [PubMed]
34. Esposito, S.; Principi, N. Prevention of Pertussis: An Unresolved Problem. *Hum. Vaccin. Immunother.* **2018**, *14*, 2452–2459. [CrossRef]
35. Meregaglia, M.; Ferrara, L.; Melegaro, A.; Demicheli, V. Parent "Cocoon" Immunization to Prevent Pertussis-Related Hospitalization in Infants: The Case of Piemonte in Italy. *Vaccine* **2013**, *31*, 1135–1137. [CrossRef]
36. Riccò, M.; Vezzosi, L.; Gualerzi, G.; Bragazzi, N.L.; Balzarini, F. Pertussis Immunization in Healthcare Workers Working in Pediatric Settings: Knowledge, Attitudes and Practices (KAP) of Occupational Physicians. Prelim. Results A Web-Based Surv. **2020**, *61*, E66–E75.
37. Durando, P.; Dini, G.; Massa, E.; La Torre, G. Tackling Biological Risk in the Workplace: Updates and Prospects Regarding Vaccinations for Subjects at Risk of Occupational Exposure in Italy. *Vaccines* **2019**, *7*, 141. [CrossRef]
38. Esposito, S.; Durando, P.; Bosis, S.; Ansaldi, F.; Tagliabue, C.; Icardi, G. Vaccine-Preventable Diseases: From Paediatric to Adult Targets. *Eur. J. Intern. Med.* **2014**, *25*, 203–212. [CrossRef]
39. Manzoli, L.; Sotgiu, G.; Magnavita, N.; Durando, P.; Barchitta, M.; Carducci, A.; Conversano, M.; De Pasquale, G.; Dini, G.; Firenze, A.; et al. Evidence-Based Approach for Continuous Improvement of Occupational Health. *Epidemiol. Prev.* **2015**, *39*, 81–85.
40. Ding, H.; Black, C.L.; Ball, S.; Fink, R.V.; Williams, W.W.; Fiebelkorn, A.P.; Lu, P.-J.; Kahn, K.E.; D'Angelo, D.V.; Devlin, R.; et al. Influenza Vaccination Coverage Among Pregnant Women—United States, 2016–2017 Influenza Season. *Morb. Mortal. Wkly. Rep.* **2017**, *66*, 1016–1022. [CrossRef]
41. Sukumaran, L.; McCarthy, N.L.; Kharbanda, E.O.; Weintraub, E.S.; Vazquez-Benitez, G.; McNeil, M.M.; Li, R.; Klein, N.P.; Hambidge, S.J.; Naleway, A.L.; et al. Safety of Tetanus, Diphtheria, and Acellular Pertussis and Influenza Vaccinations in Pregnancy. *Obstet. Gynecol.* **2016**, *48*, 923–930. [CrossRef]
42. Regan, A.K.; Tracey, L.E.; Blyth, C.C.; Richmond, P.C.; Effler, P.V. A Prospective Cohort Study Assessing the Reactogenicity of Pertussis and Influenza Vaccines Administered during Pregnancy. *Vaccine* **2016**, *34*, 2299–2304. [CrossRef] [PubMed]
43. Donders, G.G.G.; Grinceviciene, S.; Haldre, K.; Lonnee-Hoffmann, R.; Donders, F.; Tsiakalos, A.; Adriaanse, A.; de Oliveira, J.M.; Ault, K.; Mendling, W. Isidog Consensus Guidelines on Covid-19 Vaccination for Women before, during and after Pregnancy. *J. Clin. Med.* **2021**, *10*, 2902. [CrossRef] [PubMed]
44. Centers for Disease Control and Prevention (CDC). Safety and Effectiveness of COVID-19 Vaccination during Pregnancy. 2022, CDC, Atlanta, USA. Available online: https://www.cdc.gov/coronavirus/2019-ncov/vaccines/recommendations/pregnancy.html (accessed on 3 May 2023).
45. Giusti, A.; Zambri, F.; Marchetti, F.; Corsi, E.; Preziosi, J.; Sampaolo, L. Interim Guidance on Pregnancy, Childbirth, Breastfeeding and Care of Infants (0–2 Years) in Response to the COVID-19 Emergency. 2021 Italian National Health Institute (ISS), Rome. Available online: https://www.iss.it/documents/5430402/0/Rapporto+ISS+COVID-19+2_2021_EN.pdf/421a0bc6-1933-aa77-6b39-a7860d866a16?t=1615472502820 (accessed on 3 May 2023).
46. Falato, R.; Ricciardi, S.; Franco, G. Influenza Risk Perception and Vaccination Attitude in Medical and Nursing Students during the Vaccination Campaigns of 2007/2008 (Seasonal Influenza) and 2009/2010 (H1N1 Influenza). *Med. Lav.* **2011**, *102*, 208–215. [PubMed]
47. La Torre, G.; Scalingi, S.; Garruto, V.; Siclari, M.; Chiarini, M.; Mannocci, A. Knowledge, Attitude and Behaviours towards Recommended Vaccinations among Healthcare Workers. *Healthcare* **2017**, *5*, 13. [CrossRef]
48. Graves, M.C.; Harris, J.R.; Kohn, M.; Hannon, P.A.; Lichiello, P.A.; Martin, D.P. Employers' Views on Influenza and Tetanus-Diphtheria-Pertussis Vaccination in the Workplace. *J. Occup. Environ. Med.* **2016**, *58*, e157–e158. [CrossRef]
49. Dubé, E.; MacDonald, N.E. How Can a Global Pandemic Affect Vaccine Hesitancy? *Expert Rev. Vaccines* **2020**, *19*, 899–901. [CrossRef]
50. Bloom, B.R.; Marcuse, E.; Mnookin, S. Addressing Vaccine Hesitancy. *Science* **2014**, *344*, 339. [CrossRef]
51. Goldstein, S.; MacDonald, N.E.; Guirguis, S.; Eskola, J.; Liang, X.; Chaudhuri, M.; Dube, E.; Gellin, B.; Larson, H.; Manzo, M.L.; et al. Health Communication and Vaccine Hesitancy. *Vaccine* **2015**, *33*, 4212–4214. [CrossRef]
52. Yaqub, O.; Castle-Clarke, S.; Sevdalis, N.; Chataway, J. Attitudes to Vaccination: A Critical Review. *Soc. Sci. Med.* **2014**, *112*, 1–11. [CrossRef]

63. Riccò, M.; Cattani, S.; Casagranda, F.; Gualerzi, G.; Signorelli, C. Knowledge, Attitudes, Beliefs and Practices of Occupational Physicians towards Seasonal Influenza Vaccination: A Cross-Sectional Study from North-Eastern Italy. *J. Prev. Med. Hyg.* **2017**, *58*, E141–E154. [PubMed]
64. Dorribo, V.; Lazor-Blanchet, C.; Hugli, O.; Zanetti, G. Health Care Workers' Influenza Vaccination: Motivations and Mandatory Mask Policy. *Occup. Med. (Chic. Ill.)* **2015**, *65*, 739–745. [CrossRef]
65. Riphagen-Dalhuisen, J.; Gefenaite, G.; Hak, E. Predictors of Seasonal Influenza Vaccination among Healthcare Workers in Hospitals: A Descriptive Meta-Analysis. *Occup. Environ. Med.* **2012**, *69*, 230–235. [CrossRef] [PubMed]
66. Maltezou, H.C.; Gargalianos, P.; Nikolaidis, P.; Katerelos, P.; Tedoma, N.; Maltezos, E.; Lazanas, M. Attitudes towards Mandatory Vaccination and Vaccination Coverage against Vaccine-Preventable Diseases among Health-Care Workers in Tertiary-Care Hospitals. *J. Infect.* **2012**, *64*, 319–324. [CrossRef]
67. Maltezou, H.C.; Wicker, S.; Borg, M.; Heininger, U.; Puro, V.; Theodoridou, M.; Poland, G.A. Vaccination Policies for Health-Care Workers in Acute Health-Care Facilities in Europe. *Vaccine* **2011**, *29*, 9557–9562. [CrossRef] [PubMed]
68. Maltezou, H.C.; Botelho-Nevers, E.; Brantsæter, A.B.; Carlsson, R.M.; Heininger, U.; Hübschen, J.M.; Josefsdottir, K.S.; Kassianos, G.; Kyncl, J.; Ledda, C.; et al. Vaccination of Healthcare Personnel in Europe: Update to Current Policies. *Vaccine* **2019**, *37*, 7576–7584. [CrossRef] [PubMed]
69. Riccò, M.; Ferraro, P.; Camisa, V.; Satta, E.; Zaniboni, A.; Ranzieri, S.; Baldassarre, A.; Zaffina, S.; Marchesi, F. When a Neglected Tropical Disease Goes Global: Knowledge, Attitudes and Practices of Italian Physicians towards Monkeypox, Preliminary Results. *Trop. Med. Infect. Dis.* **2022**, *7*, 135. [CrossRef] [PubMed]
70. Morrone, T.; Napolitano, F.; Albano, L.; Di, G. Meningococcal Serogroup B Vaccine: Knowledge and Acceptability among Parents in Italy Meningococcal Serogroup B Vaccine: Knowledge and Acceptability among Parents in Italy. *Hum. Vaccines Immunother.* **2017**, *3*, 1921–1927. [CrossRef]
71. Eppes, C.; Wu, A.; Cameron, K.A.; Garcia, P.; Grobman, W. Does Obstetrician Knowledge Regarding Influenza Increase H1N1 Vaccine Acceptance among Their Pregnant Patients? *Vaccine* **2012**, *30*, 5782–5784. [CrossRef]
72. Bert, F.; Olivero, E.; Rossello, P.; Gualano, M.R.; Castaldi, S.; Damiani, G.; D'Errico, M.M.; di Giovanni, P.; Fantini, M.P.; Fabiani, L.; et al. Knowledge and Beliefs on Vaccines among a Sample of Italian Pregnant Women: Results from the NAVIDAD Study. *Eur. J. Public Health* **2019**, *30*, 286–292. [CrossRef]
73. Loubet, P.; Kernéis, S.; Groh, M.; Loulergue, P.; Blanche, P.; Verger, P.; Launay, O. Attitude, Knowledge and Factors Associated with Influenza and Pneumococcal Vaccine Uptake in a Large Cohort of Patients with Secondary Immune Deficiency. *Vaccine* **2015**, *33*, 3703–3708. [CrossRef] [PubMed]
74. Gualano, M.R.; Olivero, E.; Voglino, G.; Corezzi, M.; Rossello, P.; Vicentini, C.; Bert, F.; Siliquini, R. Knowledge, Attitudes and Beliefs towards Compulsory Vaccination: A Systematic Review. *Hum. Vaccin. Immunother.* **2019**, *15*, 918–931. [CrossRef] [PubMed]
75. Zhang, J.; While, A.E.; Norman, I.J. Knowledge and Attitudes Regarding Influenza Vaccination among Nurses: A Research Review. *Vaccine* **2010**, *28*, 7207–7214. [CrossRef]
76. Smith, S.; Sim, J.; Halcomb, E. Nurses' knowledge, attitudes and practices regarding influenza vaccination: An integrative review. *J. Clin. Nurs.* **2016**, *25*, 2730–2744. [CrossRef] [PubMed]
77. La Vecchia, C.; Alicandro, G.; Negri, E.; Scarpino, V.; Coggiola, M.; Spatari, G. Attitudes towards COVID-19 Vaccination and Containment Measures in Italy and the Role of Occupational Physicians. *Med. Del Lav.* **2022**, *113*, e2022018. [CrossRef]
78. Bagnasco, A.; Zanini, M.; Catania, G.; Watson, R.; Hayter, M.; Dasso, N.; Dini, G.; Agodi, A.; Pasquarella, C.; Zotti, C.M.; et al. Predicting Needlestick and Sharps Injuries in Nursing Students: Development of the SNNIP Scale. *Nurs. Open* **2020**, *7*, 1578–1587. [CrossRef] [PubMed]
79. Kirupakaran, J.; Meloche, C.; Upfal, M. Practices and Attitudes of Michigan-Based Occupational Physicians Regarding Adult Immunization. *J. Occup. Environ. Med.* **2018**, *60*, 1034–1041. [CrossRef]
80. La Torre, G.; Semyonov, L.; Mannocci, A.; Boccia, A. Knowledge, Attitude, and Behaviour of Public Health Doctors towards Pandemic Influenza Compared to the General Population in Italy. *Scand. J. Soc. Med.* **2012**, *40*, 69–75. [CrossRef]
81. Albano, L.; Matuozzo, A.; Marinelli, P.; di Giuseppe, G. Knowledge, Attitudes and Behaviour of Hospital Health-Care Workers Regarding Influenza A/H1N1: A Cross Sectional Survey. *BMC Infect. Dis.* **2014**, *14*, 208. [CrossRef]
82. Levi, M.; Bonanni, P.; Biffino, M.; Conversano, M.; Corongiu, M.; Morato, P.; Maio, T. Influenza Vaccination 2014–2015: Results of a Survey Conducted among General Practitioners in Italy. *Hum. Vaccin. Immunother.* **2018**, *14*, 1342–1350. [CrossRef]
83. Levi, M.; Sinisgalli, E.; Lorini, C.; Santomauro, F.; Chellini, M.; Bonanni, P. The "Fluad Case" in Italy: Could It Have Been Dealt Differently? *Hum. Vaccin. Immunother.* **2017**, *13*, 379–384. [CrossRef] [PubMed]
84. Bonanni, P.; Boccalini, S.; Zanobini, P.; Dakka, N.; Lorini, C.; Santomauro, F.; Bechini, A. The Appropriateness of the Use of Influenza Vaccines: Recommendations from the Latest Seasons in Italy. *Hum. Vaccin. Immunother.* **2018**, *14*, 699–705. [CrossRef] [PubMed]
85. van Lier, A.; Ferreira, J.A.; Mollema, L.; Sanders, E.A.M.; de Melker, H.E. Intention to Vaccinate Universally against Varicella, Rotavirus Gastroenteritis, Meningococcal B Disease and Seasonal Influenza among Parents in the Netherlands: An Internet Survey. *BMC Res. Notes* **2017**, *10*, 672. [CrossRef]
86. Taddei, C.; Ceccherini, V.; Niccolai, G.; Porchia, B.R.; Boccalini, S.; Levi, M.; Tiscione, E.; Santini, M.G.; Baretti, S.; Bonanni, P.; et al. Attitude toward Immunization and Risk Perception of Measles, Rubella, Mumps, Varicella, and Pertussis in Health Care Workers Working in 6 Hospitals of Florence, Italy 2011. *Hum. Vaccin. Immunother.* **2014**, *10*, 2612–2622. [CrossRef] [PubMed]

77. Fedeli, U.; Zanetti, C.; Saia, B. Susceptibility of Healthcare Workers to Measles, Mumps Rubella and Varicella. *J. Hosp. Infect.* **2002**, *51*, 133–135. [CrossRef]
78. Lambert, N.; Strebel, P.; Orenstein, W.; Icenogle, J.; Poland, G.A. Rubella. *Lancet* **2015**, *385*, 2297–2307. [CrossRef]
79. Schenk, J.; Abrams, S.; Theeten, H.; van Damme, P.; Beutels, P.; Hens, N. Immunogenicity and Persistence of Trivalent Measles, Mumps, and Rubella Vaccines: A Systematic Review and Meta-Analysis. *Lancet Infect. Dis.* **2021**, *21*, 286–295. [CrossRef]
80. Asma, S.; Akan, H.; Uysal, Y.; Poçan, A.G.; Sucaklı, M.H.; Yengil, E.; Gereklioğlu, Ç.; Korur, A.; Başhan, İ.; Erdogan, A.F.; et al. Factors Effecting Influenza Vaccination Uptake among Health Care Workers: A Multi-Center Cross-Sectional Study. *BMC Infect. Dis.* **2016**, *16*, 192. [CrossRef]
81. Hayward, A.C.; Harling, R.; Wetten, S.; Johnson, A.M.; Munro, S.; Smedley, J.; Murad, S.; Watson, J.M. Effectiveness of an Influenza Vaccine Programme for Care Home Staff to Prevent Death, Morbidity, and Health Service Use among Residents: Cluster Randomised Controlled Trial. *BMJ* **2006**, *333*, 1241. [CrossRef]
82. Osterholm, M.T.; Kelley, N.S.; Sommer, A.; Belongia, E.A. Quantifying the Efficacy of Influenza Vaccines: Authors' Reply. *Lancet Infect. Dis.* **2012**, *12*, 660–661. [CrossRef]
83. Zhai, Y.; Santibanez, T.A.; Kahn, K.E.; Black, C.L.; de Perio, M.A. Paid Sick Leave Benefits, Influenza Vaccination, and Taking Sick Days Due to Influenza-like Illness among U.S. Workers. *Vaccine* **2018**, *36*, 7316–7323. [CrossRef] [PubMed]
84. Gianino, M.M.; Politano, G.; Scarmozzino, A.; Charrier, L.; Testa, M.; Giacomelli, S.; Benso, A.; Zotti, C.M. Estimation of Sickness Absenteeism among Italian Healthcare Workers during Seasonal Influenza Epidemics. *PLoS ONE* **2017**, *12*, e0182510. [CrossRef] [PubMed]
85. Buchy, P.; Badur, S.; Kassianos, G.; Preiss, S.; Tam, J.S. Vaccinating Pregnant Women against Influenza Needs to Be a Priority for All Countries: An Expert Commentary. *Int. J. Infect. Dis.* **2020**, *92*, 1–12. [CrossRef]
86. Dubé, E.; Gagnon, D.; Kaminsky, K.; Green, C.R.; Ouakki, M.; Bettinger, J.A.; Brousseau, N.; Castillo, E.; Crowcroft, N.S.; Driedger, S.M.; et al. Vaccination Against Influenza in Pregnancy: A Survey of Canadian Maternity Care Providers. *J. Obstet. Gynaecol. Can.* **2019**, *41*, 479–488. [CrossRef] [PubMed]
87. Gualano, M.R.; Bert, F.; Voglino, G.; Buttinelli, E.; D'Errico, M.M.; de Waure, C.; di Giovanni, P.; Fantini, M.P.; Giuliani, A.R.; Marranzano, M.; et al. Attitudes towards Compulsory Vaccination in Italy: Results from the NAVIDAD Multicentre Study. *Vaccine* **2018**, *36*, 3368–3374. [CrossRef]
88. Eppes, C.; Wu, A.; You, W.; Cameron, K.A.; Garcia, P.; Grobman, W. Barriers to Influenza Vaccination among Pregnant Women. *Vaccine* **2013**, *31*, 2874–2878. [CrossRef]
89. O'Leary, S.T.; Riley, L.E.; Lindley, M.C.; Allison, M.A.; Crane, L.A.; Hurley, L.P.; Beaty, B.L.; Brtnikova, M.; Collins, M.; Albert, A.P.; et al. Immunization Practices of U.S. Obstetrician/Gynecologists for Pregnant Patients. *Am. J. Prev. Med.* **2018**, *54*, 205–213. [CrossRef]
90. Stark, L.M.; Power, M.L.; Turrentine, M.; Samelson, R.; Siddiqui, M.M.; Paglia, M.J.; Strassberg, E.R.; Kelly, E.; Murtough, K.L.; Schulkin, J. Influenza Vaccination among Pregnant Women: Patient Beliefs and Medical Provider Practices. *Infect. Dis. Obstet. Gynecol.* **2016**, *2016*, 3281975. [CrossRef]
91. Vilca, M.L.; Esposito, S. The Crucial Role of Maternal Care Providers as Vaccinators for Pregnant Women. *Vaccine* **2017**, *36*, 5379–5384. [CrossRef]
92. Willame, C.; Dodd, C.; Durán, C.; Elbers, R.; Gini, R.; Bartolini, C.; Paoletti, O.; Wang, L.; Ehrenstein, V.; Kahlert, J.; et al. Background Rates of 41 Adverse Events of Special Interest for COVID-19 Vaccines in 10 European Healthcare Databases—An ACCESS Cohort Study. *Vaccine* **2023**, *41*, 251–262. [CrossRef]
93. Lee, M.T.; Choi, W.; You, S.H.; Park, S.; Kim, J.Y.; Nam, D.R.; Lee, J.W.; Jung, S.Y. Safety Profiles of MRNA COVID-19 Vaccines Using World Health Organization Global Scale Database (VigiBase): A Latent Class Analysis. *Infect. Dis. Ther.* **2022**, *12*, 443–458. [CrossRef] [PubMed]
94. Barello, S.; Palamenghi, L.; Graffigna, G. Public Reaction towards the Potential Side Effects of a COVID-19 Vaccine: An Italian Cross-Sectional Study. *Vaccines* **2022**, *10*, 429. [CrossRef] [PubMed]
95. Serrao, A.; Agrippino, R.; Brescini, M.; Mormile, R.; Chistolini, A. Thromboembolic Events Following MRNA Vaccines for COVID 19: A Case Series. *J. Thromb. Thrombolysis* **2022**, *53*, 971–973. [CrossRef] [PubMed]
96. Carli, G.; Nichele, I.; Ruggeri, M.; Barra, S.; Tosetto, A. Deep Vein Thrombosis (DVT) Occurring Shortly after the Second Dose of MRNA SARS-CoV-2 Vaccine. *Intern. Emerg. Med.* **2021**, *16*, 803–804. [CrossRef]
97. Durand, J.; Dogné, J.; Cohet, C.; Browne, K.; Gordillo Maranon, M.; Piccolo, L.; Zaccaria, C.; Genov, G. Safety Monitoring of COVID-19 Vaccines: Perspective from the European Medicines Agency. *Clin. Pharmacol. Ther.* **2022**; *Epub Ahead of print*. [CrossRef]
98. Cascini, F.; Pantovic, A.; Al-Ajlouni, Y.; Failla, G.; Ricciardi, W. Attitudes, Acceptance and Hesitancy among the General Population Worldwide to Receive the COVID-19 Vaccines and Their Contributing Factors: A Systematic Review. *EClinicalMedicine* **2021**, *40*, 101113. [CrossRef]
99. Killian, M.; Detoc, M.; Berthelot, P.; Charles, R.; Gagneux-Brunon, A.; Lucht, F.; Pulcini, C.; Barbois, S.; Botelho-Nevers, E. Vaccine Hesitancy among General Practitioners: Evaluation and Comparison of Their Immunisation Practice for Themselves, Their Patients and Their Children. *Eur. J. Clin. Microbiol. Infect. Dis.* **2016**, *35*, 1837–1843. [CrossRef]
100. Mesch, G.S.; Schwirian, K.P. Social and Political Determinants of Vaccine Hesitancy: Lessons Learned from the H1N1 Pandemic of 2009–2010. *Am. J. Infect. Control.* **2015**, *43*, 1161–1165. [CrossRef]

101. Moore, P.J.A.; Millar, B.C.; Moore, J.E. Meningococcal ACWY Vaccine Uptake and Awareness among Student Freshers Enrolled at Northern Ireland Universities. *Int. J. Adolesc. Med. Health* **2017**, *32*, 20160087. [CrossRef]
102. Richmond, P.; Hatchuel, L.; Dong, M.; Ma, B.; Hu, B.; Smolenov, I.; Li, P.; Liang, P.; Han, H.H.; Liang, J.; et al. Safety and Immunogenicity of S-Trimer (SCB-2019), a Protein Subunit Vaccine Candidate for COVID-19 in Healthy Adults: A Phase 1, Randomised, Double-Blind, Placebo-Controlled Trial. *Lancet* **2021**, *397*, 682–694. [CrossRef]
103. AIFA (Italian Medicine Agency) Rapporto Sulla Sorveglianza Dei Vaccini Anti-COVID-19, N.13; AIFA, Rome. 2022. Available online: https://www.aifa.gov.it/web/guest/rapporti-su-sorveglianza-dei-vaccini-covid-19?p_p_id=it_gov_aifa_portlet_GestioneCookies&p_p_lifecycle=1&p_p_state=normal&p_p_mode=view&_it_gov_aifa_portlet_GestioneCookies_javax.portlet.action=saveCookieAIFA (accessed on 1 March 2023).
104. He, Q.; Wang, G.; He, J.; Wang, Y.; Zhang, J.; Luo, B.; Chen, P.; Luo, X.; Ren, J. Knowledge, Attitude and Practice Regarding Occupational Protection against COVID-19 among Midwives in China: A Nationwide Cross-Sectional Study. *Int. J. Disaster Risk Reduct.* **2022**, *79*, 103184. [CrossRef] [PubMed]
105. Tasnim, H.; Amin, M.B.; Roy, N.; Aktarujjaman, M.; Rogers, B.T.; Rosby, R.; Hossain, E. Knowledge, Attitudes, and Practices towards COVID-19 among Pregnant Women in Northern Bangladesh: A Community-Based Cross-Sectional Study. *Behav. Sci.* **2022**, *13*, 2. [CrossRef] [PubMed]
106. Napolitano, F.; Navaro, M.; Vezzosi, L.; Santagati, G.; Angelillo, I.F. Primary Care Pediatricians' Attitudes and Practice towards Hpv Vaccination: A Nationwide Survey in Italy. *PLoS ONE* **2018**, *13*, e0194920. [CrossRef] [PubMed]
107. Di Giuseppe, G.; Pelullo, C.P.; della Polla, G.; Montemurro, M.V.; Napolitano, F.; Pavia, M.; Angelillo, I.F. Surveying Willingness towards SARS-CoV-2 Vaccination of Healthcare Workers in Italy. *Expert Rev. Vaccines* **2021**, *20*, 881–889. [CrossRef]
108. Riccò, M.; Cerviere, M.P.; Marchesi, F.; Bottazzoli, M. Invasive Meningococcal Disease and Meningococcal Serogroup B Vaccination in Adults and Their Offspring: Knowledge, Attitudes, and Practices in Italy (2019). *Vaccines* **2023**, *11*, 508. [CrossRef]
109. Heiervang, E.; Goodman, R. Advantages and Limitations of Web-Based Surveys: Evidence from a Child Mental Health Survey. *Soc. Psychiat. Epidemiol.* **2011**, *46*, 69–76. [CrossRef]
110. Huang, Y.; Xu, S.; Lei, W.; Zhao, Y.; Liu, H.; Yao, D.; Xu, Y.; Lv, Q.; Hao, G.; Xu, Y.; et al. Knowledge, Attitudes, and Practices Regarding Zika: Paper and Internet Based Survey in Zhejiang, China. *JMIR Public Health Surveill.* **2017**, *3*, e81. [CrossRef]
111. Riccò, M.; Ferraro, P.; Peruzzi, S.; Balzarini, F.; Ranzieri, S. Hantaviruses in Agricultural and Forestry Workers: Knowledge, Attitudes and Practices in Italian Physicians. *Trop. Med. Infect. Dis.* **2021**, *6*, 169. [CrossRef]
112. Riccò, M.; Ferraro, P.; Camisa, V.; di Palma, P.; Minutolo, G.; Ranzieri, S.; Zaffina, S.; Baldassarre, A.; Restivo, V. Managing of Migraine in the Workplaces: Knowledge, Attitudes and Practices of Italian Occupational Physicians. *Medicina (B Aires)* **2022**, *58*, 686. [CrossRef]
113. Maietti, E.; Reno, C.; Sanmarchi, F.; Montalti, M.; Fantini, M.P.; Gori, D. Are psychological status and trust in information related to vaccine hesitancy during COVID-19 pandemic? A latent class and mediation analyses in Italy. *Hum. Vaccin. Immunother.* **2022**, *18*, 2157622. [CrossRef]
114. Riccò, M.; Vezzosi, L.; Balzarini, F. Challenges Faced by the Italian Medical Workforce. *Lancet* **2020**, *395*, e55–e56. [CrossRef] [PubMed]
115. Vicarelli, G.; Pavolini, E. Health Workforce Governance in Italy. *Health Policy* **2015**, *119*, 1606–1612. [CrossRef] [PubMed]
116. Hayat, A.M.; Tribble, D.R.; Sanders, J.W.; Faix, D.J.; Shiau, D.; Armstrong, A.W.; Riddle, M.S. Knowledge, Attitudes, and Practice of Travelers' Diarrhea Management among Frontline Providers. *J. Travel Med.* **2011**, *18*, 310–317. [CrossRef]
117. Çiftci, F.; Şen, E.; Demir, N.; Çiftci, O.; Erol, S.; Kayacan, O. Beliefs, Attitudes, and Activities of Healthcare Personnel about Influenza and Pneumococcal Vaccines. *Hum. Vaccin. Immunother.* **2018**, *14*, 111–117. [CrossRef] [PubMed]
118. Riccò, M.; Ferraro, P.; Peruzzi, S.; Zaniboni, A.; Ranzieri, S. Respiratory Syncytial Virus: Knowledge, Attitudes and Beliefs of General Practitioners from North-Eastern Italy (2021). *Pediatr. Rep.* **2022**, *14*, 147–165. [CrossRef]
119. Zingg, A.; Siegrist, M. Measuring People's Knowledge about Vaccination: Developing a One-Dimensional Scale. *Vaccine* **2012**, *30*, 3771–3777. [CrossRef]
120. Baraldi, E.; Checcucci Lisi, G.; Costantino, C.; Heinrichs, J.H.; Manzoni, P.; Riccò, M.; Roberts, M.; Vassilouthis, N. RSV Disease in Infants and Young Children: Can We See a Brighter Future? *Hum. Vaccin. Immunother.* **2022**, *18*, 2079322. [CrossRef]
121. Cuadera, M.K.Q.; Mader, E.M.; Safi, A.G.; Harrington, L.C. Knowledge, attitudes, and practices for tick bite prevention and tick control among residents of Long Island, New York, USA. *Ticks Tick Borne Dis.* **2023**, *14*, 102124. [CrossRef]
122. Coyer, L.; Sogan-Ekinci, A.; Greutélaers, B.; Kuhn, J.; Saller, F.S.; Hailer, J.; Böhm, S.; Brosch, R.; Wagner-Wiening, C.; Böhmer, M.M. Knowledge, Attitudes and Behaviors regarding Tick-Borne Encephalitis Vaccination and Prevention of Tick-Borne Diseases among Primary Care Physicians in Bavaria and Baden-Wuerttemberg, Germany, May-September 2022. *Microorganisms* **2023**, *11*, 961. [CrossRef]
123. Bocquier, A.; Branchereau, M.; Gauchet, A.; Bonnay, S.; Simon, M.; Ecollan, M.; Chevreul, K.; Mueller, J.E.; Gagneux-Brunon, A.; Thilly, N. PrevHPV Study Group. Promoting HPV vaccination at school: A mixed methods study exploring knowledge, beliefs and attitudes of French school staff. *BMC Public Health* **2023**, *23*, 486. [CrossRef]
124. Marano, C.; Moodley, M.; Melander, E.; de Moerlooze, L.; Nothdurft, H.D. Multinational Survey Shows Low Awareness of Tick-Borne Encephalitis and Rabies among Travellers to Endemic Regions. *J. Travel Med.* **2018**, *26*, S1–S2. [CrossRef]

125. Olson, S.; Hall, A.; Riddle, M.S.; Porter, C.K. Travelers' Diarrhea: Update on the Incidence, Etiology and Risk in Military and Similar Populations—1990–2005 versus 2005–2015, Does a Decade Make a Difference? *Trop. Dis. Travel Med. Vaccines* **2019**, *5*, 1. [CrossRef] [PubMed]
126. Tan, E.M.; St. Sauver, J.L.; Sia, I.G. Impact of Pre-Travel Consultation on Clinical Management and Outcomes of Travelers' Diarrhea: A Retrospective Cohort Study. *Trop. Dis. Travel Med. Vaccines* **2018**, *4*, 16. [CrossRef] [PubMed]
127. Riccò, M.; Zaniboni, A.; Satta, E.; Baldassarre, A.; Cerviere, M.P.; Marchesi, F.; Peruzzi, S. Management and Prevention of Traveler's Diarrhea: A Cross-Sectional Study on Knowledge, Attitudes, and Practices in Italian Occupational Physicians (2019 and 2022). *Trop. Med. Infect. Dis.* **2022**, *7*, 370. [CrossRef]
128. Cafiero-Fonseca, E.T.; Stawasz, A.; Johnson, S.T.; Sato, R.; Bloom, D.E. The Full Benefits of Adult Pneumococcal Vaccination: A Systematic Review. *PLoS ONE* **2017**, *12*, e0186903. [CrossRef] [PubMed]
129. Gualano, M.R.; Santoro, P.E.; Borrelli, I.; Rossi, M.F.; Amantea, C.; Tumminello, A.; Daniele, A.; Beccia, F.; Moscato, U. Employee Participation in Workplace Vaccination Campaigns: A Systematic Review and Meta-Analysis. *Vaccines* **2022**, *10*, 1898. [CrossRef]
130. la Torre, G.; de Waure, C.; Chiaradia, G.; Mannocci, A.; Capri, S.; Bamfi, F.; Ricciardi, W. Guidance for Future HTA Applications to Vaccines: The HPV Lesson. *Hum. Vaccin.* **2011**, *7*, 900–904. [CrossRef]
131. de Waure, C.; Quaranta, G.; Ianuale, C.; Panatto, D.; Amicizia, D.; Apprato, L.; Campanella, P.; Colotto, M.; de Meo, C.; di Nardo, F.; et al. Knowledge, Attitudes and Behaviors of the Italian Population towards Neisseria Meningitidis, Streptococcus Pneumoniae and HPV Diseases and Vaccinations: A Cross-Sectional Multicentre Study. *Public Health* **2016**, *141*, 136–142. [CrossRef]
132. Bogani, G.; Raspagliesi, F.; di Donato, V.; Brusadelli, C.; Guerrisi, R.; Pinelli, C.; Casarin, J.; Ghezzi, F.; del Fabro, A.; Ditto, A.; et al. Spotlight on the Role of Human Papillomavirus Vaccines. *Gynecol. Oncol.* **2021**, *160*, 346–350. [CrossRef]
133. Monti, M.; D'aniello, D.; Scopelliti, A.; Tibaldi, V.; Santangelo, G.; Colagiovanni, V.; Giannini, A.; di Donato, V.; Palaia, I.; Perniola, G.; et al. Relationship between Cervical Excisional Treatment for Cervical Intraepithelial Neoplasiaand Obstetrical Outcome. *Minerva Obstet. Gynecol.* **2021**, *73*, 233–246. [CrossRef]
134. Meites, E.; Szilagyi, P.G.; Chesson, H.W.; Unger, E.R.; Romero, J.R.; Markowitz, L.E. Human Papillomavirus Vaccination for Adults: Updated Recommendations of the Advisory Committee on Immunization Practices. *Morb. Mortal. Wkly. Rev.* **2019**, *68*, 698–702. [CrossRef] [PubMed]
135. Pronk, N. Total Worker Health ®: An Emerging Innovation in Workplace Health and Well-Being. *ACSM's Health Fit. J.* **2020**, *24*, 42–44. [CrossRef]
136. di Prinzio, R.R.; Nigri, A.G.; Zaffina, S. Total Worker Heath Strategies in Italy: New Challenges and Opportunities for Occupational Health and Safety Practice. *J. Health Soc. Sci.* **2021**, *6*, 313–318.
137. Riccò, M.; Vezzosi, L.; Cella, C.; Pecoraro, M.; Novembre, G.; Moreo, A.; Ognibeni, E.M.; Schellenberg, G.; Maranelli, G. Tetanus Vaccination Status in Construction Workers: Results from an Institutional Surveillance Campaign. *Acta Biomed.* **2019**, *90*, 269–278. [CrossRef]
138. Riccò, M.; Vezzosi, L.; Balzarini, F.; Bragazzi, N.L. Inappropriate Risk Perception for SARS-CoV-2 Infection among Italian HCWs in the Eve of COVID-19 Pandemic. *Acta Biomed.* **2020**, *91*, 1–2. [CrossRef]
139. Yates, F.J.; Stone, E.R. The Risk Construct. In *Risk-Taking Behaviour*; Yates, F.J., Ed.; John Wiley & Sons: Chichester, UK, 1992; pp. 1–25. ISBN 0471922501.
140. Bursac, Z.; Gauss, C.H.; Williams, D.K.; Hosmer, D.W. Purposeful Selection of Variables in Logistic Regression. *Source Code Biol. Med.* **2008**, *3*, 17. [CrossRef]

Disclaimer/Publisher's Note: The statements, opinions and data contained in all publications are solely those of the individual author(s) and contributor(s) and not of MDPI and/or the editor(s). MDPI and/or the editor(s) disclaim responsibility for any injury to people or property resulting from any ideas, methods, instructions or products referred to in the content.

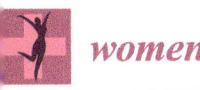

Article

Determinants of Antenatal Education and Breastfeeding Uptake in Refugee-Background and Australian-Born Women

Tam Anh Nguyen [1], Mohammed Mohsin [2,3], Batool Moussa [2], Jane Fisher [4], Nawal Nadar [2], Fatima Hassoun [2], Batoul Khalil [2], Mariam Youssef [2], Yalini Krishna [2], Megan Kalucy [2] and Susan Rees [2,*]

[1] Faculty of Medicine & Health, University of New South Wales, Sydney, NSW 2052, Australia; tamanhalice@gmail.com
[2] Discipline of Psychiatry and Mental Health, School of Clinical Medicine, Faculty of Medicine & Health, University of New South Wales, Sydney, NSW 2052, Australia; m.mohsin@unsw.edu.au (M.M.); b.moussa@unsw.edu.au (B.M.); n.nadar@unsw.edu.au (N.N.); f.hassoun@unsw.edu.au (F.H.); b.khalil@unsw.edu.au (B.K.); m.yousif@unsw.edu.au (M.Y.); yalini.krishna@unsw.edu.au (Y.K.); m.kalucy@unsw.edu.au (M.K.)
[3] Mental Health Research Unit, Liverpool Hospital, NSW Health, Sydney, NSW 2170, Australia
[4] Global and Women's Health Unit, Public Health and Preventive Medicine, Monash University, Clayton, VIC 3800, Australia; jane.fisher@monash.edu
* Correspondence: s.j.rees@unsw.edu.au

Abstract: Despite the well-established benefits of antenatal education (ANE) and breastfeeding for mothers, there is a paucity of evidence about the uptake of ANE and breastfeeding amongst women from refugee backgrounds or its associations with sociodemographic factors. The current study is a cross-sectional survey at two time points examining the prevalence of ANE attendance, breastfeeding, and intimate partner violence (IPV) amongst 583 women refugees resettled in Australia and a control group of 528 Australian-born women. Multi-logistic regression was used to explore bivariate associations between ANE attendance, breastfeeding, IPV, and sociodemographic characteristics (parity, maternal employment, and education). Refugee-background women compared to Australian-born women have lower ANE utilization (20.4% vs. 24.1%), higher rates of breastfeeding on hospital discharge (89.3% vs. 81.7%), and more IPV reports (43.4% vs. 25.9%). Factors such as nulliparity, higher level of education, and employment predict higher rates of ANE and breastfeeding adoption. In contrast, IPV is a risk factor for ANE underutilization. Further, of the women from refugee backgrounds who accessed ANE services, 70% attended clinics designed for women from non-English-speaking backgrounds. These findings support the need to ensure effective screening and interventions for IPV during antenatal care and to better understand the role of culture as a protective or risk factor for breastfeeding initiation.

Keywords: antenatal education; intimate partner violence; breastfeeding; refugee; employment; women

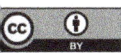

1. Introduction

In Australia, antenatal education (ANE) is considered an important component of antenatal care. ANE is offered in group classes to women at most public and many private hospitals [1]. These educational programs typically focus on education to develop knowledge, skills, and confidence in understanding pregnancy, the birth process, and the hospital setting. The broad goal is to prepare the woman, her partner, and her family, if appropriate, for childbirth and early parenting [1]. Women who attend ANE classes are associated with better adjustment to parenthood [2], lower rates of negative birth outcomes, reduced maternal stress, and use of interventions (including cesarean section and epidural anesthesia) [3,4]. Furthermore, it has been identified that to improve health outcomes, culture- or language-specific ANE programs should be offered for women from mainly non-English-speaking or immigrant backgrounds [5]. Multicultural health workers play a vital role in facilitating referrals to these specialized services and promoting community development [6].

Despite better health equity and universal healthcare coverage provision in high-income countries (HICs), such as Medicare in Australia, which provides free antenatal care amongst other health services [6], women who arrive as migrants (both forced and economic) have lower rates of participation in antenatal care, where pregnancy-related screening and monitoring occur and social factors relevant to the pregnancy are discussed [7–11]. Poor, late, or lack of antenatal appointment attendance has been linked to negative birth outcomes in both groups of women [7,10]. While being of refugee background poses a risk factor for both adverse post-partum health outcomes and antenatal services underutilization [7], there exists a scarcity of empirical research on the impact and outcomes of ANE, as distinct from the general antenatal services participation, among refugee-background women in comparison to women born in HICs. In addition to immigration status, data from North America, Australia, and Europe have revealed that low income, low socioeconomic status (SES), and limited educational attainment contribute to lower antenatal services utilization and engender maternal health inequity [12,13]. Given this well-established association between socioeconomic factors and health outcomes, as well as the fact that women from refugee backgrounds often have lower SES compared to their native-born counterparts [14,15], it is imperative to explore the disparities between these two cohorts and factors contributing to their health trajectories.

As part of routine antenatal care, intimate partner violence (IPV) screening is typically conducted as an essential component of risk assessment [6]. In the antenatal setting, IPV often remains inadequately acknowledged, despite its higher prevalence than other obstetric risks such as pre-eclampsia or gestational diabetes [16]. Intimate partner violence is defined as any behavior by a current or former intimate partner that involves physical, sexual, financial, or psychological harm [17,18]. According to the World Health Organization (WHO), one-third of women worldwide have been subjected to IPV in their lifetime [19], with the highest rate observed in regions of Oceania and Sub-Saharan Africa (29–32%) and the lowest reported in central Europe (16%) [20]. IPV during pregnancy increases the risk of miscarriage, stillbirth, pre-term labor, and low-birth-weight neonates [16,21]. The evidence also suggests that IPV perpetrated primarily against the mother has has developmental effects on the child, such as increased risk of insulin resistance, psychiatric disorders, low intellectual capability, and cognitive impairment [22]. Predisposing factors include IPV-related prenatal insults such as stress, substance abuse, inadequate nutritional intake, poor antenatal services utilization, and infective agents. During infancy, witnessing IPV and associated parental stress can have negative effects on socio-emotional development [22–26]. Women from refugee backgrounds experience higher rates of psychological and/or physical IPV during pregnancy compared to women born in the host country, with reported prevalence of 44.4% and 25.8%, respectively [27]. Whilst general perinatal care routinely includes IPV screening in most Australian jurisdictions, refugee-background women are more likely to experience barriers and challenges accessing that care. Furthermore, lack of trust and differences in expectations and communication styles from those of healthcare providers, may result in the underreporting of IPV [27,28].

Promoting early and exclusive breastfeeding is a central feature of ANE. Early and long-term breastfeeding, including exclusive breastfeeding for six months and non-exclusive continuation for two years, is recommended due to its numerous health benefits for both babies and mothers [29]. Early initiation of breastfeeding has been linked to a two-fold reduction in the mortality of infants across countries [30]. Breastfed babies demonstrate greater immunity, with lower odds of infectious morbidities such as gastrointestinal diseases, respiratory infections, otitis media, and urinary tract infections [31]. With respect to the child's long-term outcomes, breastfeeding improves cognitive function and performance on intelligence tests [32], and it protects against type 2 diabetes [29,33]. For mothers, breastfeeding is associated with decreased risk of maternal depression, breast and ovarian cancer [29], endometrial cancer, osteoporosis [34], and strokes amongst postmenopausal women [35]. Additionally, there is strong evidence of positive maternal–infant bonding associated with breastfeeding [34]. The current evidence shows that while breastfeeding is initiated in 98% of infants soon after birth [36], the duration of exclusive breastfeeding at 6 months can drop to lower than 20% in HICs, with a critically low 1% reported in an Australian national survey [33,36,37]. In comparison, low/middle-income countries (LMICs) reported slightly higher rates of exclusive breastfeeding at 6 months (36%) [33,37]. In conflict-affected countries, the median prevalence of exclusive breastfeeding has been reported to be 25% across 56 studies [37]. However, one study found that although breastfeeding rates are low when refugee-background women initially settle in HICs, those rates increase for each additional year living in the host country [38].

A variety of maternal sociodemographic factors, including age, socioeconomic status, education, and employment, have been shown to exert a notable influence on the likelihood of breastfeeding [39–41]. However, the individual effects and levels of significance of these determinants vary across HICs [42–45], suggesting the presence of country-specific confounders intertwined with cultural nuances, economic circumstances, and social infrastructure. Since SES is linked to employment status and educational attainment to the disadvantages of those with lower SES [46,47], future social interventions should have a special focus on women from low SES backgrounds. There is also a need to consider culturally specific programs for refugee-background populations, as they are often subject to discriminatory practices in both education and the workplace [15]. The literature provides mixed findings about the association between IPV and breastfeeding. IPV during pregnancy may affect breastfeeding directly, through physical stress hindering breastmilk release, or indirectly, via psychological barriers such as self-doubt, body negativity, male partner coercion, and depression [48]. While studies from Spain and the United States found an association between IPV and lower rates of breastfeeding [38,49,50], studies from Australia and Sweden reported no association [51,52]. On the other hand, almost all studies from LMICs, particularly in Asia and Africa, report associations between IPV and reduced rates of breastfeeding [26,53,54], as well as shortened duration of breastfeeding [55].

Aim

To inform future analyses, this study aimed to present preliminary findings on the effects of intimate partner violence and sociodemographic factors on ANE attendance and early breastfeeding in two cohorts: refugee-background women resettled in Australia and Australian-born women. These findings will provide valuable insights for policymakers and healthcare providers in developing comprehensive strategies to enhance the health and well-being of refugee mothers and children. The study proposed the following hypotheses: (1) refugee-background women would have lower ANE attendance rates and higher prevalence of IPV; and (2) individuals who were exposed to IPV and did not attend any ANE classes would have lower rates of breastfeeding on discharge from hospital. These hypotheses were formulated to guide the analysis and interpretation of the study's findings.

2. Results

2.1. Participants

A total of 1111 eligible women were interviewed at both T1 and T2, including 528 (47.6%) women born in Australia and 583 (52.5%) women who migrated from conflict-affected countries, referred to as refugee-background women in this paper (Table 1). The mean age of Australian-born women in our study was 29.1 (SD, 5.4) years, and the mean age of refugee-background women was 29.8 (SD, 5.4) years (Table 1). In total, 57% of the Australian-born women had completed a university degree or other post-school qualification, compared to 50.8% of women from refugee backgrounds. It can be assumed that some women from the latter group may have gained their qualifications from their country of origin. While the levels of education were similar between the two groups, there was a substantial disparity in the rates of employment. At T1, 60.0% of the Australian-born women were employed, while the employment rate was only 26.8% for refugee-background women. Among the Australian-born women, 34.2% were categorized as nulliparous, and this rate was 30.2% for refugee-background women.

Table 1. Sociodemographic characteristics, intimate partner violence, and antenatal education visits for women born in Australia and women born in conflict-affected countries.

Variable	Australian-Born (n = 528)		Refugee-Background (n = 583)	
	N	%	N	%
Age groups [T1]				
<25 years old	115	21.8	102	17.5
25–34 years old	321	60.8	362	62.1
≥35 years old	92	17.4	119	20.4
Mean Age (SD)		29.1 (5.4)		29.8 (5.4)
Education [T1]				
No post-school qualification	225	42.6	287	49.2
Diploma and vocational education	136	25.8	99	17.0
University degree	167	31.6	197	33.8
Employment status [T1]				
Unemployed	211	40.0	427	73.2
Employed	317	60.0	156	26.8
Intimate partner violence [T1]				
No	391	74.1	330	56.6
Yes	137	25.9	253	43.4
N	528	100	583	100
Intimate partner violence [T2]				
No	385	72.9	327	56.1
Yes	143	27.1	256	43.9
N	528	100	583	100
Parity [T1]				
Multiparous	347	65.8	407	69.8
Nulliparous	180	34.2	176	30.2
N	527	100	583	100
Antenatal education [T2]				
No	400	75.9	464	79.6
Yes	127	24.1	119	20.4
Total	527	100	583	100
Number of antenatal education classes [T2]				
1–2 times	94	75.2	52	46.4
1–4 times	11	8.8	17	13.2
1–6 times	15	12.0	21	18.8
>6 times	3	2.4	22	19.6
Not stated	2	1.6	0	0
N	125	100	112	100
# Designated classes [T2]				
Arabic and Sudanese pregnancy care classes	NA		47	56.0
Multicultural antenatal classes			24	28.6
Others			11	13.0
Not stated			2	2.4
N			84	100
Breastfeeding on discharge [T2]				
No	96	18.3	62	10.7
Yes	430	81.7	520	89.3
N	526	100	582	100
Duration of breastfeeding [T2]				
<1 months	187	36.9	195	34.9
≥1 months	320	63.1	364	65.1
Total	507	100	559	100

SD: Standard deviation. NA: Not applicable to Australian-born women. N: Total number of interview answers.
Designated classes: This question was directed to women born in conflict-affected countries only.

Refugee-background women reported higher rates of any IPV compared to Australian-born women at both time points. At T1, 25.9% of Australian-born women reported experiences of IPV in the past 12 months, whilst amongst women of refugee backgrounds, the rate of IPV experience was 43.4% (Table 1). Moreover, these rates increased slightly from T1 to T2 in both groups, with an additional 1.2% of Australian-born women reporting IPV at T2 (27.1%) and an additional 0.5% of refugee-background women reporting IPV (43.9%) at T2.

Australian-born women had higher ANE utilization compared to refugee-background women when measured by whether they had attended any ANE class (24.1% vs. 20.4%) (Table 1). Of the 119 refugee-background women who reported having attended ANE, up to 70.6% (84 out of 119) visited designated culture-specific or multicultural ANE classes.

Women from refugee backgrounds had higher breastfeeding rates compared to Australian-born women (89.3% vs. 81.7%, respectively). Both groups reported similar breastfeeding patterns: 34.9% of refugee-background women did not breastfeed or did for less than 1 month vs. 36.9% of Australian-born women; 65.1% of refugee-background women breastfed for more than 1 month vs. 63.1% of Australian-born women (Table 1).

2.2. Factors Associated with Antenatal Education Engagement

Results from bivariate analyses, presented in Table 2, show that the prevalence of ANE visits amongst Australian-born women was significantly higher for those who obtained post-school qualification ($p = 0.001$), were employed ($p = 0.001$), were nulliparous ($p = 0.001$), and reported no experiences of IPV during the perinatal period ($p = 0.006$). A similar trend between these factors and ANE attendance rates was also observed in refugee-background women. However, only higher educational attainment was statistically significant ($p = 0.003$).

Table 2. Association of sociodemographic characteristics and intimate partner violence with antenatal education (ANE) visits for women born in Australia and women born in conflict-affected countries.

Sociodemographic Characteristics, IPV and Parity	Australian-Born (n = 528)			Refugee-Background (n = 583)		
	N	ANE n	ANE %	N	ANE n	ANE %
All	527	127	24.1	583	119	20.4
Age [T1]						
<25 years old	114	27	23.7	102	24	23.5
25–34 years old	321	78	24.3	362	78	21.5
≥35 years old	92	22	23.9	119	17	14.3
p			0.990			0.162
Education [T1]						
No post-school qualification	225	33	14.7	287	42	14.6
Diploma and vocational education	135	41	30.4	99	24	24.2
University degree	167	53	31.7	197	53	26.9
p			0.001			0.003
Employment status [T1]						
Unemployed	211	28	13.3	427	83	19.4
Employed	316	99	31.3	156	36	23.1
p			0.001			0.335
Intimate partner violence [T1]						
No	391	106	27.1	330	75	22.7
Yes	136	21	15.4	253	44	17.4
p			0.006			0.113
Parity [T1]						
Multiparous	347	27	7.8	407	42	10.3
Nulliparous	179	99	55.3	176	77	43.8
p			0.001			0.001

Adjusting for age, employment status, and other sociodemographic factors, adjusted odd ratios (AORs) from multiple logistic analyses, presented in Table 3, further predicted that for both groups, women with a post-school level of education were twice as likely to attend ANE classes (University degree—Australian-born, AOR: 2.69, 95% CI, 1.45–5.00, $p < 0.01$. Refugee-background, AOR: 2.61, 95% CI, 1.43–4.74, $p < 0.01$). Furthermore, nulliparous women in both groups were more likely to attend ANE classes (Australian-born, AOR: 14.57, 95% CI, 8.67–24.55, $p < 0.01$. Refugee-background, AOR: 6.45, 95% CI, 4.13–10.09, $p < 0.01$). Employment status and IPV exposure were not found to be significantly associated with ANE visits for any group of women (Table 3).

Table 3. Associations of sociodemographic characteristics and intimate partner Violence (IPV) with Antenatal Education attendance: Adjusted odds ratios (AORs) with 95% confidence interval (95% CI) from logistic regression analysis for women born in Australia and women born in conflict-affected countries.

Significant Factors #	Outcome Variables	
	Antenatal Education (no = 0, yes = 1)	
	Australian-Born	Refugee-Background
	AOR (95% CI)	
Education [T1]		
No post-school qualification (RC)	1.00	1.00
Diploma and vocational education	2.01 (1.08–3.73) *	1.38 (0.75–2.56)
University degree	2.69 (1.45–5.00) **	1.81 (1.08–3.04) *
Employment status [T1]		
Unemployed (RC)	1.00	1.00
Employed	1.06 (0.58–1.93) **	0.76 (0.45–1.28)
Any IPV [baseline]		
No IPV (RC)	1.00	1.00
Any IPV	0.54 (0.29–1.02)	0.91 (0.57–1.45)
Parity		
Multiparous (RC)	1.00	1.00
Nulliparous	14.57 (8.67–24.55) **	6.45 (4.13–10.09) **

Factors included in multiple logistic regression model were found to be statistically significant ($p < 0.05$) in bivariate analysis. RC, reference category; AOR, adjusted odds ratio; 95% CI, 95% confidence interval; * $p < 0.05$; ** $p < 0.01$.

2.3. Factors Associated with Breastfeeding Status

Results presented in Table 4 indicate that for both Australian-born and refugee-background women, the prevalence of breastfeeding at discharge was significantly higher for those who obtained post-school qualifications and were employed ($p < 0.05$). For both groups of women, the association of breastfeeding status with age and IPV exposure was not found to be statistically significant ($p > 0.05$). A positive association between ANE utilization and breastfeeding rates was observed in both groups of women. However, the data showed that this association was not statistically significant ($p > 0.05$).

AORs from multiple logistic analyses presented in Table 5 revealed that, amongst refugee-background women, none of the predictors were statistically significant ($p > 0.05$). However, Australian-born women with post-school level of education are three times more likely to be breastfeeding at discharge (diploma and vocational education—AOR: 3.26, 95% CI, 1.72–6.18, $p < 0.01$. University degree—AOR: 2.61, 95% CI, 1.43–4.74, $p < 0.01$).

Table 4. Association of sociodemographic characteristics, intimate partner violence, and antenatal education visits with breastfeeding rates for women born in Australia and women born in conflict-affected countries.

Variable	Australian-Born (n = 528)			Refugee-Background (n = 583)		
	N	Breastfeeding		N	Breastfeeding	
		n	%		n	%
All	526	430	81.7	582	520	89.3
Age [T1]						
<25 years old	113	83	82.3	102	89	87.3
25–34 years old	321	263	81.9	362	327	90.3
≥35 years old	92	74	80.4	118	104	88.1
p			0.934			0.601
Education [T1]						
No post-school qualification	224	161	72.3	286	247	86.4
Diploma and vocational education	135	121	89.6	99	89	89.9
University degree	167	147	88.0	197	184	93.4
p			0.001			0.047
Employment status [T1]						
Unemployed	210	161	76.7	426	373	87.6
Employed	316	269	85.1	156	147	94.2
p			0.014			0.021
Intimate partner violence [T1]						
No	391	318	81.3	330	297	90.0
Yes	135	112	83.0	252	223	88.5
p			0.672			0.559
Parity [T1]						
Multiparous	346	276	79.8	406	360	88.7
Nulliparous	179	153	85.8	176	160	90.9
p			0.109			0.421
Antenatal Education [T2]						
No	399	321	80.5	463	408	88.1
Yes	127	109	85.8	119	112	94.1
p			0.172			0.059

Table 5. Associations of sociodemographic characteristics and intimate partner violence (IPV) with breastfeeding at discharge: adjusted odds ratios (AOR) with 95% confidence interval (95% CI) from logistic regression analysis for women born in Australia and women born in conflict-affected countries.

Significant Factors #	Outcome Variables	
	Breastfeeding (no = 0, yes = 1)	
	Australian-Born	Refugee-Background
	AOR (95% CI)	
Education [T1]		
No post-school qualification (RC)	1.00	1.00
Diploma and vocational education	3.26 (1.72–6.18) **	1.27 (0.60–2.68)
University degree	2.61 (1.43–4.74) **	1.86 (0.93–3.71)
Employment status [T1]		
Unemployed (RC)	1.00	1.00
Employed	1.32 (0.80–2.19)	1.89 (0.87–4.09)

Factors included in multiple logistic regression model were found to be statistically significant ($p < 0.05$) in bivariate analysis. RC, reference category; AOR, adjusted odds ratio; 95% CI, 95% confidence interval; ** $p < 0.01$.

3. Materials and Method

Ethics approval: The longitudinal WATCH cohort study was approved by the South Western Sydney Local Health District Human Research Ethics Committee (HC13049) and Monash Health Ethics Committee. Participants gave written informed consent and were remunerated for their time. The study included extensive training of research staff derived from the same cultural and language backgrounds as the target populations, followed by tests of interview competence (rater reliability). Staff received training for IPV, sensitive interview techniques, research methods, and the use of World Health Organization diagnostic measures for IPV. The study also followed the WHO protocol for ensuring the safety of participants who may have experienced IPV and applied a recognized approach for designing and testing measures that are not in English.

3.1. Study Design

This study analyzed the baseline (T1) and first-follow-up (T2) data of 1335 women who participated in the Women Aware with Their Children (WATCH) study. The baseline survey was undertaken between January 2015 and March 2016, and follow-up occurred approximately six months after the birth of the child. The study design and methods are fully described in previous papers [27,56].

The primary study was undertaken at three large public hospital antenatal clinics, two in Sydney and one in Melbourne. Women from refugee-background were systematically invited to participate in the study as part of the refugee cohort if they were identified to be from Arabic-speaking, Sudanese, or Sri Lankan Tamil backgrounds. These three groupings ensured a good representation of the global refugee intake entering Australia at the time of data collection. The criteria for participation were not limited to the type of visa held. Women born in Australian-born were recruited at the same time and from the same hospitals using a randomized selection process. Data for the current analysis are from two time points (T1 is the first trimester of pregnancy, and T2 is 6 months post-partum). Finally, the present study consisted of 1111 women who participated in the primary interviews.

3.2. Data Collection and Measures

All data for this secondary study, including the demographics, were obtained from the WATCH study database for the specific and planned research analysis of IPV, ANE attendance, and breastfeeding.

Recruitment and the baseline interview (T1) occurred at, or close to, the participant's first appointment at the antenatal clinic (most occurred between 12 and 20 weeks of gestation). Follow-up interviews (T2) were conducted at home, either in person or by telephone, approximately 6 months after the birth of the index child. At baseline (T1), the response rate was 84.8% (1335 women out of 1574); at T2, the retention rate was 83.2% (1111 out of 1335 interviewed at T1) [56]. The analytical sample of this secondary study included 1111 out of 1335 women who participated in the interviews.

Measures related to IPV were included at both T1 and T2 interviews. At T2, standardized Local Health District measures related to pregnancy and childbirth were added: antenatal care uptake, antenatal clinic visits, and breastfeeding status.

Measures were subjected to rigorous assessment of cultural and linguistic accuracy in the languages used, including standard translation, back-translation, and assessment and refinements by groups of linguistic and cultural experts [27,56].

3.2.1. Sociodemographic Characteristics

Items recording age, marital status, level of education and qualification, household composition, employment, and housing status were consistent with the Australian National Census. These items can be benchmarked against the Australian population. Countries of birth for inclusion in the study (all Arabic-speaking countries, Sudan, and Sri Lanka) were identified by clinic records, requests for an interpreter, or culturally recognizable surnames, and country of birth was checked again at the time of recruitment. Many people arrive from conflict-affected settings on visas other than special humanitarian visas, which are therefore not accurate reflections of being a refugee. For this analysis, we have included all recruited women who were born in conflict-affected countries, whom, in this paper, we refer to as refugee-background women.

3.2.2. Parity

Parity was assessed during the baseline survey. For this study, women having no previous births reported at baseline were categorized as 'nulliparous women', and women having had at least one previous birth were categorized as 'multiparous women'.

3.2.3. Intimate Partner Violence

IPV was assessed using items from the WHO Violence Against Women questionnaire, which asks about physical, psychological, and sexual violence perpetrated by the current or most recent partner in the past 12 months [56]. For this study, women were assigned to two IPV categories: (1) No IPV; (2) Any IPV (either psychological and/or physical IPV; psychological IPV includes jealousy or anger if she talks to other men, accusations of being unfaithful, not permitting meetings with female friends, limiting contact with family, insisting on knowing the woman's whereabouts, humiliating her in front of others, threatening harm to her or someone close to her; physical abuse includes pushing, shaking, throwing items, slapping, twisting arm, punching, kicking, dragging, strangling, burning, threats with a knife, gun, or other weapon, and attacks with a knife, gun, or other weapon).

3.2.4. Antenatal Education Attendance

Survey answers were collected regarding whether the participant attended any ANE sessions (yes/no), as well as the number of antenatal classes attended, and whether they attended ANE classes specifically offered for women from mainly non-English-speaking backgrounds, including ANE offered at the Blacktown Hospital site for women from Sudanese and Arabic-speaking backgrounds.

3.2.5. Breastfeeding

Women were asked at T2, "Were you breastfeeding on discharge? After discharge, how long did you breastfeed up to this point?" These are standard questions asked by NSW Health (Australia's largest public health system) on discharge after the birth of the child.

3.3. Statistical Analysis

Descriptive statistics of participants' characteristics (age, educational attainment, employment status, parity, prevalence of IPV, ANE visits, and breastfeeding status) of those who attended both T1 and T2 surveys were explored for both groups of women. Bivariate (cross-tabular) and multiple logistic regression analyses were performed to examine the association of sociodemographic factors, parity, and IPV exposure with ANE visits. Potential risk factors for ANE visits found to be statistically significant ($p < 0.05$) in bivariate analysis were included in multiple logistic regression analyses. The aim of multiple logistic regression analysis was to estimate the relative contributions of each significant risk factor to ANE visits. Further, we also performed bivariate and multiple logistic regression analysis to explore the association of sociodemographic factors, IPV exposure, and ANE visits with breastfeeding status at discharge. Results of bivariate analyses are presented as percentages and means; chi-square (χ^2) was applied to examine the significant differences across sub-groups. The adjusted odds ratios (AORs) from logistic regression analysis with their 95% confidence intervals (95% CI) are shown to express the relative contributions of each potential risk factor to likelihood of ANE visits and breastfeeding status, adjusted for the effects of other variables in the model. All the analyses were carried out separately for both Australian-born and refugee-background women. The analyses were conducted with SPSS v. 27 [57].

4. Discussion

Despite the known benefits of maternal awareness and agency associated with ANE, there remains a critical gap in evidence regarding the prevalence of ANE uptake and its impact on maternal and child outcomes, particularly amongst women from refugee backgrounds. This population may encounter unique challenges, including increased susceptibility to complications related to prior trauma, IPV, and psychosocial adversity [56,58]. Our study is large and methodically rigorous, enabling us to compare the prevalence of and associations between ANE attendance, IPV exposure, early breastfeeding rates, and various other sociodemographic factors. The uniqueness of our study lies in its focus on women from refugee backgrounds who resettled in Australia, allowing us to make meaningful comparisons regarding their experiences in antenatal care to those of women born in Australian. The study follows a cohort design, and data for this analysis were drawn from two relevant time points (the first trimester of pregnancy and the post-partum period). The findings provide important insights for antenatal clinicians and policymakers.

4.1. Antenatal Education

ANE attendance was similar for both groups when measured categorically by any attendance. The rates for the utilization of ANE amongst Australian-born women were significantly lower (24.1%) compared to findings from past studies in both Australia (89%) [59] and the U.K. (53.1%) [60]. Rates of ANE attendance can vary by country of birth [11] and psychosocial factors [61], suggesting that the lower rates in our study may be attributed to the recruitment of women living in lower-socioeconomic-status areas of Sydney and Melbourne [61]. Women from refugee backgrounds attending ANE participated in a higher number of antenatal classes: 19.6% of women from refugee backgrounds visited ANE classes more than 6 times, with an average of 1–4 visits. Directly comparing the number of classes attended by Australian-born and refugee-background women was challenging due to the disparity in the number of classes offered. Australian-born women attending the standard programs had access to approximately six classes in our study. In contrast, women from mainly non-English-speaking backgrounds, including refugee-background women, were offered up to 21 classes. The notable number of ANE classes attended by women from refugee backgrounds is, regardless of comparison, indicative of a positive experience. We posit that the high number of attendances per person reflects the culturally sensitive and supportive nature of the specialized ANE programs run for mainly non-English-speaking-background women (attended by 70.6% of the sample). Although further research is required to fully explore this observation, our finding is a novel and noteworthy finding regarding the pivotal role of culturally and linguistically specific ANEs in enhancing healthcare accessibility. Notably, the Arabic and Sudanese Pregnancy Care Clinic at Blacktown Hospital in Sydney, which was one of our recruitment sites and is the site for a current qualitative study [27], is a prominent example (attended by 58% of the sample). The emergence of such specialized clinics catering to the unique needs of diverse populations holds the potential to close healthcare gaps and promote culturally responsive services.

4.2. Social Determinants

Antenatal services are predominantly attended by women with higher levels of education and from the middle-to-upper socioeconomic strata across various developed nations, namely Canada and the United States [62,63], South Korea [64], and Belgium [65]. Regardless of immigration background, women attaining higher levels of education typically exhibit greater health literacy and autonomy in navigating their pregnancy [66,67]. As such, our study confirms that maternal educational level is the universal and most predictive determinant of ANE utilization, encompassing both women from refugee backgrounds and native Australians. Higher parity has a negative effect on ANE attendance, and this resonates with previously published literature on adequate antenatal care attendance [68–70]. First-time mothers may be encouraged or motivated to learn to care for themselves and their unborn child, whereas parous women may not perceive the ANE as a necessity, given that they are well "experienced" with previous pregnancies, especially if they were uncomplicated [71]. The higher uptake of ANE amongst employed women in the Australian-born cohort, as observed in our study, aligns with similar findings in a recent study in Belgium [65] and in older literature across HICs [72,73]. However, a recent study in the United Arab Emirates did not find any direct associations between employment status and antenatal visits [74], suggesting that contemporary work-related issues may engender barriers to attending clinic appointments [75]. These issues may encompass limited work time flexibility, including insufficient time off for medical visits, and greater job demands hindering a women's ability to prioritize their health [76]. Women occupying higher professional and executive roles are more likely to face these challenges [76], a factor for which our study did not examine. The recruitment of women from a lower-SES region in Sydney and Melbourne, therefore, may have resulted in a sample of women having fewer occupational demands and better attendance to health needs [67]. While the association between employment and ANE attendance amongst refugee-background women is weak and statistically insignificant in our study, it suggests a potential association worth further exploration. Nonetheless, there is limited contemporary research on the specific impact of working during pregnancy and consideration of workplace culture in HICs, including the magnitude of workplace modification to cater to the unique needs of pregnant women. Our study highlights the potential benefits of employment during pregnancy and emphasizes the need to further explore work-related factors that can facilitate healthcare-seeking behavior.

Health services and support provided in HICs are typically less accessible or culturally sensitive, particularly for women facing social and economic marginalization, including those from refugee backgrounds [15,77]. Our study reinforces the significance of sociodemographic factors in predicting ANE attendance and underscores the need to address barriers to healthcare access that are influenced by economic disadvantage, lower educational levels, and visa status. This exploration will be instrumental for the design of targeted health interventions for women from culturally diverse backgrounds.

4.3. Intimate Partner Violence

We report a high number of pregnant Australian women, refugee-background and Australian-born, have experienced IPV. Data in Roman-Galvez and colleagues' systematic review [78] showed that the highest range of any kind of IPV during pregnancy (including sexual, physical and emotional) was reported in Australia (15.4–40%), along with Portugal and the USA. Our study confirms this broad range in findings, suggesting that specific subpopulations in the same region can be at increased risk of experiencing IPV during pregnancy [21]. General rates are lower when compared to another study focusing on any IPV in women of refugee backgrounds (79.8%) [79], highlighting the urgent need to address the alarming risk faced by this population, which can engender severe and lethal consequences. IPV during pregnancy is associated with serious negative outcomes for maternal and child health [80,81]. The most described adverse physical health impacts associated with IPV in the literature include maternal death, pregnancy complications, and stillbirth [16,21]. While our protocol measured IPV experience within the last 12 months, we were unable to assess whether women in our study were exposed to IPV during their pregnancy. Nevertheless, IPV-related trauma can directly impair a women's functioning before, during, and after birth. The risk is particularly high for women from conflict-affected countries who face unique risk factors, including trauma before arrival in the settlement country [27], lack of social support, and increased dependency on their intimate partners after the resettlement [82]. Further, our study shows a slight increase in IPV rates from the women's first trimester to six months post-partum in both groups. This concerning finding postulates either new perpetrations during or after the pregnancy or underreporting of IPV at T1, and it emphasizes the need to strengthen IPV screening tools and intervention programs during antenatal care. To prevent detrimental harm to the women and their babies in the perinatal period, there is a dire need for awareness and interventions for IPV amongst pregnant women, with a focus on women arriving in Australia from conflict-affected settings.

This study is unique in that it explores the relationship between perinatal IPV and the utilization of antenatal education. To the best of our knowledge, this is the only study that investigates this relationship, comparing the correlations in two distinctive cohorts of Australian-born and women from conflict-affected countries. The findings from our study suggest that women who have experienced any form of IPV by a former or current partner, whether it occurred before or during pregnancy, were significantly more likely to receive inadequate ANE by way of lower attendance compared to women who reported no IPV. This association was observed regardless of the women's background.

Although a causal link is unable to be established from this preliminary analysis, IPV may prevent women from accessing ANE, either because of a coercive and controlling partner hindering a woman's attendance, psychological distress and impaired functioning, or financial hardship. For example, previous studies have reported IPV to be significantly associated with depression, anxiety, and suicidal ideation and related poor functioning [18,83,84]. Further studies show that IPV reduces decision-making power and creates financial barriers [85]. Despite underreporting, minority or migrant women, including refugee-background women, experience higher rates of IPV during pregnancy [86], a factor that is consistent with our findings of IPV prevalence. Women from refugee backgrounds may have lower socioeconomic status, fewer social supports, and higher rates of mental disorders, including depression. Moreover, refugee-background women may also experience specific factors that may further lower the likelihood of attending ANE: for example, lack of trust in authorities, trauma related to war and conflict, and poor English language skills [27]. This supposition supports the finding that women experiencing IPV are less likely to attend ANE. Of great interest is that women from refugee backgrounds who did attend ANE, regardless of IPV status, attended several classes, indicating that they enjoyed or benefited from the experience. We also note the significance of 70.6% of our refugee background cohort having attended an ANE designed for women from mainly non-English-speaking backgrounds, a service that may resonate with refugee-background women because of the qualitatively described appreciation of cultural and linguistical familiarity provided by such ANE programs at the hospitals from which the participants were recruited. This is a current area of inquiry for our team.

Our findings confirm the importance of antenatal services such as ANE as sites for IPV identification, prevention, and intervention, as well as the need for specialized assessments and ANE programs for women from refugee backgrounds.

4.4. Breastfeeding

We report a positive correlation between ANE attendance during pregnancy and early breastfeeding on discharge. Although the association was not statistically significant in either cohort, the positive health correlates of breastfeeding for women and their babies reinforce the inherent value of reporting an association. These findings are also consistent with previous studies that have examined the effect of utilizing antenatal services and breastfeeding education on the rates of early breastfeeding initiation and continuation [41,87–93]. Knowledge about breastfeeding gained through maternal health services, such as ANE, may help mothers to overcome concerns related to breastfeeding [94,95] and encourage them to favor breastfeeding over other types of infant feeding [96].

We found that despite higher IPV prevalence and lower ANE attendance, women from refugee backgrounds were slightly more likely to initiate breastfeeding soon after birth. However, it should be noted that the rates of breastfeeding initiation in both cohorts still remain lower when compared to a national survey conducted in Australia, which reported a prevalence of 98% for breastfeeding initiation, of which 93% of infants were exclusively breastfed [36]. Cultural views and norms related to breastfeeding are important to understand as factors that may impact breastfeeding, in addition to any information provided during ANE. A study found that mothers may make the decision about breastfeeding long before conception, based on cultural beliefs [97]. For example, breastfeeding for 2 years is recommended in the holy book (Qur'an) in Islam, and therefore, the desire to breastfeed amongst Middle Eastern women is deeply rooted in their cultural values and the belief that they will receive support from the woman's partner and her community [98]. The evidence shows that breastfeeding is more widely practiced in LMICs than it is in most HICs [33] and that women from LMICs who migrated to HICs may not change their breastfeeding patterns [99]. Not all non-Western cultures, however, continue to breastfeed at higher rates after migration. It should be acknowledged that we did not measure either group's adherence to the recommended duration of exclusive breastfeeding for 6 months' duration. However, it is worth noting that the rates of discontinuing breastfeeding within the first month were significantly high, reaching 34.9–36.9%. An Australian study showed that Vietnamese refugee-background women had higher ANE attendance rates but lower rates of breastfeeding compared to Australian-born women, mostly due to cultural traditions [100]. Another study in California also reported a lack of interest in obtaining information on breastfeeding amongst Southeast Asian women from refugee backgrounds attending ANE [101]. Our study highlights the importance of understanding cultural differences and the need for ANE content to be adapted for the specific population. We recommend that ANE is delivered by bicultural or bilingual workers from relevant backgrounds to ensure diverse cultural practices and norms of the target demographics are reflected.

This study goes some way to addressing the paucity of evidence on ANE and its association with socioeconomic factors, IPV, and breastfeeding practices. With increasing numbers of economic and humanitarian migrants entering Australia, our study suggests the need for ANE programs that are specific to culturally diverse groups. There is a critical need to adopt trauma-informed approaches when caring for expecting mothers, taking into consideration the impact of IPV and conflict-related trauma, during both pregnancy and the post-partum period. All women should be screened for IPV in the antenatal setting, and those who disclose IPV should be provided with additional support to access ANE classes. When appropriate, referral to culturally appropriate and accessible domestic violence services should also be provided. Furthermore, to address barriers to disclosure amongst women with difficulties reporting their partners, future ANE planning should include access to IPV wraparound services. Given the high prevalence of IPV amongst pregnant women attending ANE in our study, all healthcare providers in the ANE setting should receive training consistent with a trauma-informed approach. This will enable them to identify signs of IPV and respond appropriately.

4.5. Strength and Limitations

We performed a large, rigorous, systematically recruited study of women at two time points in the perinatal period. The study included measures for ANE, IPV, breastfeeding rates on discharge, and sociodemographic characteristics. One of the notable strengths of the study is the data for both a population with refugee backgrounds and one that is Australian-born, which is rare to find in the current literature. The IPV questions relate to the current or most recent relationship in the past 12 months, which means that we cannot assume the presence of current IPV at the time of the interview or during the pregnancy. Despite using two time points, the study is cross-sectional, and associations are indicative but cannot demonstrate causation. It should be acknowledged that some findings reported in our study did not reach statistical significance. However, despite these limitations, the findings provide valuable preliminary insights and associations that contribute to the existing knowledge on the topic of obstetric health among refugee women in high-income countries. The study prompts the need for future research to validate and confirm our findings.

5. Conclusions

Our findings confirm a higher prevalence of IPV and lower ANE uptake among women from refugee backgrounds compared with women born in Australia. These results warrant attention to ANE access and support for refugee-background women (who were exposed to war-related conflict and have resettled in developed countries). In both groups of women, higher education and nulliparity are better predictors of ANE attendance than employment, although all are highly associated with increased rates of ANE class attendance. Women exposed to any kind of IPV (emotional, sexual, or physical IPV) tend to have lower ANE attendance rates. Although it is not statistically significant, poor ANE utilization reduced breastfeeding rates. The novel and summary finding is that being from refugee backgrounds, a single report of IPV, lower educational attainment, and unemployment define subpopulations of women at higher risk for lower utilization of ANE and/or lower likelihood of breastfeeding. This indicates that checking sociodemographic and psychosocial information at the antenatal clinic and subsequent screening and support for higher-risk women may help avert negative pregnancy and childbirth outcomes.

Author Contributions: Conceptualization, S.R., J.F., N.N.; Investigation, N.N., B.M., F.H., B.K., M.Y., Y.K.; Formal analysis, T.A.N., M.M., S.R.; Writing—original draft, T.A.N., S.R.; Writing—review and editing, T.A.N., S.R., M.M., J.F., M.K., N.N., B.M., F.H., B.K., M.Y., Y.K.; Supervision, S.R., M.K.; Funding acquisition, S.R., J.F. All authors have read and agreed to the published version of the manuscript.

Funding: This research was funded by the National Health and Medical Research Council, Australia, grant numbers GNT1086774 and GNT1164736.

Institutional Review Board Statement: The study was conducted in accordance with the Declaration of Helsinki and approved by the South Western Sydney Local Health District Human Research Ethics Committee (HC13049) and Monash Health Ethics Committee.

Informed Consent Statement: Written informed consent has been obtained from the patient(s) to publish this paper.

Data Availability Statement: Data are available upon reasonable request from the corresponding author.

Acknowledgments: We acknowledge the women participants in the WATCH study, Anggy Duarte for managing data entry, and Gordana Sobacic at Southwest Sydney Local Health District for administrative support.

Conflicts of Interest: The authors declare no conflict of interest.

References

1. Svensson, J.; Barclay, L.; Cooke, M. Effective antenatal education: Strategies recommended by expectant and new parents. *J. Perinat. Educ.* **2008**, *17*, 33–42. [CrossRef] [PubMed]
2. Pilcher, H.; Hughes, A.J. Parent's perceptions of antenatal groups in supporting them through the transition to parenthood. *MIDIRS Midwifery Dig.* **2014**, *24*. Available online: https://nottingham-repository.worktribe.com/output/996665 (accessed on 21 July 2016).
3. Sandall, J.; Soltani, H.; Gates, S.; Shennan, A.; Devane, D. Midwife-led continuity models versus other models of care for childbearing women. *Cochrane Database Syst. Rev.* **2016**, *4*, CD004667. [CrossRef] [PubMed]
4. Hong, K.; Hwang, H.; Han, H.; Chae, J.; Choi, J.; Jeong, Y.; Lee, J.; Lee, K.J. Perspectives on antenatal education associated with pregnancy outcomes: Systematic review and meta-analysis. *Women Birth* **2021**, *34*, 219–230. [CrossRef]
5. Yelland, J.; Riggs, E.; Small, R.; Brown, S. Maternity services are not meeting the needs of immigrant women of non-English speaking background: Results of two consecutive Australian population based studies. *Midwifery* **2015**, *31*, 664–670. [CrossRef]
6. Australian Government Department of Health. Pregnancy Care Guidelines. Available online: https://www.health.gov.au/resources/publications/pregnancy-care-guidelines (accessed on 7 October 2022).
7. Sturrock, S.; Williams, E.; Greenough, A. Antenatal and perinatal outcomes of refugees in high income countries. *J. Perinat. Med.* **2020**, *49*, 80–93. [CrossRef]
8. Boerleider, A.W.; Wiegers, T.A.; Manniën, J.; Francke, A.L.; Devillé, W.L.J.M. Factors affecting the use of prenatal care by non-western women in industrialized western countries: A systematic review. *BMC Pregnancy Childbirth* **2013**, *13*, 81. [CrossRef]
9. Small, R.; Roth, C.; Raval, M.; Shafiei, T.; Korfker, D.; Heaman, M.; McCourt, C.; Gagnon, A. Immigrant and non-immigrant women's experiences of maternity care: A systematic and comparative review of studies in five countries. *BMC Pregnancy Childbirth* **2014**, *14*, 152. [CrossRef]
10. Higginbottom, G.M.A.; Morgan, M.; Alexandre, M.; Chiu, Y.; Forgeron, J.; Kocay, D.; Barolia, R. Immigrant women's experiences of maternity-care services in Canada: A systematic review using a narrative synthesis. *Syst. Rev.* **2015**, *4*, 13. [CrossRef]
11. Heaman, M.; Bayrampour, H.; Kingston, D.; Blondel, B.; Gissler, M.; Roth, C.; Alexander, S.; Gagnon, A. Migrant women's utilization of prenatal care: A systematic review. *Matern. Child Health J.* **2013**, *17*, 816–836. [CrossRef]

12. Dawson, P.; Auvray, B.; Jaye, C.; Gauld, R.; Hay-Smith, J. Social determinants and inequitable maternal and perinatal outcomes in Aotearoa New Zealand. *Womens Health* **2022**, *18*, 17455065221075913. [CrossRef] [PubMed]
13. Downe, S.; Finlayson, K.; Walsh, D.; Lavender, T. 'Weighing up and balancing out': A meta-synthesis of barriers to antenatal care for marginalised women in high-income countries. *BJOG* **2009**, *116*, 518–529. [CrossRef] [PubMed]
14. Nielsen, S.S.; Hempler, N.F.; Krasnik, A. Issues to consider when measuring and applying socioeconomic position quantitatively in immigrant health research. *Int. J. Environ. Res. Public Health* **2013**, *10*, 6354–6365. [CrossRef] [PubMed]
15. Misztal, B.A. Migrant women in Australia. *J. Intercult. Stud.* **1991**, *12*, 15–34. [CrossRef]
16. Román-Gálvez, R.M.; Martín-Peláez, S.; Fernández-Félix, B.M.; Zamora, J.; Khan, K.S.; Bueno-Cavanillas, A. Worldwide Prevalence of Intimate Partner Violence in Pregnancy. A Systematic Review and Meta-Analysis. *Front. Public Health* **2021**, *9*, 738459. [CrossRef]
17. Dicola, D.; Spaar, E. Intimate Partner Violence. *Am. Fam. Physician* **2016**, *94*, 646–651.
18. Rees, S.; Silove, D.; Chey, T.; Ivancic, L.; Steel, Z.; Creamer, M.; Teesson, M.; Bryant, R.; McFarlane, A.C.; Mills, K.L.; et al. Lifetime prevalence of gender-based violence in women and the relationship with mental disorders and psychosocial function. *JAMA* **2011**, *306*, 513–521. [CrossRef]
19. World Health Organization. Violence against Women. Available online: https://www.who.int/en/news-room/fact-sheets/detail/violence-against-women (accessed on 16 October 2022).
20. Sardinha, L.; Maheu-Giroux, M.; Stöckl, H.; Meyer, S.R.; García-Moreno, C. Global, regional, and national prevalence estimates of physical or sexual, or both, intimate partner violence against women in 2018. *Lancet* **2022**, *399*, 803–813. [CrossRef]
21. World Health Organization. Global and Regional Estimates of Violence against Women: Prevalence and Health Effects of Intimate Partner Violence and Non-Partner Sexual Violence. Available online: https://apps.who.int/iris/handle/10665/85239 (accessed on 18 October 2022).
22. Mueller, I.; Tronick, E. Early Life Exposure to Violence: Developmental Consequences on Brain and Behavior. *Front. Behav. Neurosci.* **2019**, *13*, 156. [CrossRef] [PubMed]
23. Murray, A.L.; Kaiser, D.; Valdebenito, S.; Hughes, C.; Baban, A.; Fernando, A.D.; Madrid, B.; Ward, C.L.; Osafo, J.; Dunne, M.; et al. The Intergenerational Effects of Intimate Partner Violence in Pregnancy: Mediating Pathways and Implications for Prevention. *Trauma Violence Abus.* **2020**, *21*, 964–976. [CrossRef]
24. Kim, D.R.; Bale, T.L.; Epperson, C.N. Prenatal programming of mental illness: Current understanding of relationship and mechanisms. *Curr. Psychiatry Rep.* **2015**, *17*, 5. [CrossRef] [PubMed]
25. Bale, T.L. Epigenetic and transgenerational reprogramming of brain development. *Nat. Rev. Neurosci.* **2015**, *16*, 332–344. [CrossRef] [PubMed]
26. Ariyo, T.; Jiang, Q. Intimate partner violence and exclusive breastfeeding of infants: Analysis of the 2013 Nigeria demographic and health survey. *Int. Breastfeed. J.* **2021**, *16*, 15. [CrossRef] [PubMed]
27. Rees, S.J.; Fisher, J.R.; Steel, Z.; Mohsin, M.; Nadar, N.; Moussa, B.; Hassoun, F.; Yousif, M.; Krishna, Y.; Khalil, B.; et al. Prevalence and Risk Factors of Major Depressive Disorder Among Women at Public Antenatal Clinics From Refugee, Conflict-Affected, and Australian-Born Backgrounds. *JAMA* **2019**, *2*, e193442. [CrossRef] [PubMed]
28. Cha, S.; Masho, S.W. Intimate partner violence and utilization of prenatal care in the United States. *J. Interpers. Violence* **2014**, *29*, 911–927. [CrossRef]
29. World Health Organization. Infant and Young Child Feeding. Available online: https://www.who.int/news-room/fact-sheets/detail/infant-and-young-child-feeding (accessed on 16 October 2022).
30. Acharya, P.; Khanal, V. The effect of mother's educational status on early initiation of breastfeeding: Further analysis of three consecutive Nepal Demographic and Health Surveys. *BMC Public Health* **2015**, *15*, 1069. [CrossRef]
31. Frank, N.M.; Lynch, K.F.; Uusitalo, U.; Yang, J.; Lönnrot, M.; Virtanen, S.M.; Hyöty, H.; Norris, J.M.; Rewers, M.; Bautista, K.; et al. The relationship between breastfeeding and reported respiratory and gastrointestinal infection rates in young children. *BMC Pediatr.* **2019**, *19*, 339. [CrossRef]
32. Horta, B.L.; Loret de Mola, C.; Victora, C.G. Breastfeeding and intelligence: A systematic review and meta-analysis. *Acta Paediatr.* **2015**, *104*, 14–19. [CrossRef]
33. Victora, C.G.; Bahl, R.; Barros, A.J.; França, G.V.; Horton, S.; Krasevec, J.; Murch, S.; Sankar, M.J.; Walker, N.; Rollins, N.C. Breastfeeding in the 21st century: Epidemiology, mechanisms, and lifelong effect. *Lancet* **2016**, *387*, 475–490. [CrossRef]
34. Allen, J.; Hector, D. Benefits of breastfeeding. *NSW Public Health Bull.* **2005**, *16*, 42–46. [CrossRef]
35. Jacobson, L.T.; Hade, E.M.; Collins, T.C.; Margolis, K.L.; Waring, M.E.; Van Horn, L.V.; Silver, B.; Sattari, M.; Bird, C.E.; Kimminau, K.; et al. Breastfeeding History and Risk of Stroke Among Parous Postmenopausal Women in the Women's Health Initiative. *J. Am. Heart Assoc.* **2018**, *7*, e008739. [CrossRef] [PubMed]
36. Netting, M.J.; Moumin, N.A.; Knight, E.J.; Golley, R.K.; Makrides, M.; Green, T.J. The Australian Feeding Infants and Toddler Study (OzFITS 2021): Breastfeeding and Early Feeding Practices. *Nutrients* **2022**, *14*, 206. [CrossRef] [PubMed]
37. Rabbani, A.; Padhani, Z.A.; Siddiqui, F.A.; Das, J.K.; Bhutta, Z. Systematic review of infant and young child feeding practices in conflict areas: What the evidence advocates. *BMJ Open* **2020**, *10*, e036757. [CrossRef] [PubMed]
38. Martin-de-las-Heras, S.; Velasco, C.; Luna-del-Castillo, J.; Khan, K. Breastfeeding avoidance following psychological intimate partner violence during pregnancy: A cohort study and multivariate analysis. *BJOG: Int. J. Obstet. Gynaecol.* **2019**, *126*, 778–783. [CrossRef] [PubMed]

39. Oakley, L.L.; Renfrew, M.J.; Kurinczuk, J.J.; Quigley, M.A. Factors associated with breastfeeding in England: An analysis by primary care trust. *BMJ Open* **2013**, *3*, e002765. [CrossRef] [PubMed]
40. Magnano San Lio, R.; Maugeri, A.; La Rosa, M.C.; Cianci, A.; Panella, M.; Giunta, G.; Agodi, A.; Barchitta, M. The Impact of Socio-Demographic Factors on Breastfeeding: Findings from the "Mamma & Bambino" Cohort. *Medicina* **2021**, *57*, 103. [CrossRef]
41. Cohen, S.S.; Alexander, D.D.; Krebs, N.F.; Young, B.E.; Cabana, M.D.; Erdmann, P.; Hays, N.P.; Bezold, C.P.; Levin-Sparenberg, E.; Turini, M.; et al. Factors Associated with Breastfeeding Initiation and Continuation: A Meta-Analysis. *J. Pediatr.* **2018**, *203*, 190–196.e121. [CrossRef]
42. Dubois, L.; Girard, M. Social determinants of initiation, duration and exclusivity of breastfeeding at the population level: The results of the Longitudinal Study of Child Development in Quebec (ELDEQ 1998-2002). *Can. J. Public Health* **2003**, *94*, 300–305. [CrossRef]
43. Tarrant, M.; Fong, D.Y.; Wu, K.M.; Lee, I.L.; Wong, E.M.; Sham, A.; Lam, C.; Dodgson, J.E. Breastfeeding and weaning practices among Hong Kong mothers: A prospective study. *BMC Pregnancy Childbirth* **2010**, *10*, 27. [CrossRef]
44. Bick, D.E.; MacArthur, C.; Lancashire, R.J. What influences the uptake and early cessation of breast feeding? *Midwifery* **1998**, *14*, 242–247. [CrossRef]
45. Heck, K.E.; Braveman, P.; Cubbin, C.; Chávez, G.F.; Kiely, J.L. Socioeconomic status and breastfeeding initiation among California mothers. *Public Health Rep.* **2006**, *121*, 51–59. [CrossRef] [PubMed]
46. Doku, D.T.; Acacio-Claro, P.J.; Koivusilta, L.; Rimpelä, A. Health and socioeconomic circumstances over three generations as predictors of youth unemployment trajectories. *Eur. J. Public Health* **2019**, *29*, 517–523. [CrossRef] [PubMed]
47. Bartley, M.; Owen, C. Relation between socioeconomic status, employment, and health during economic change, 1973–1993. *BMJ* **1996**, *313*, 445–449. [CrossRef]
48. Normann, A.K.; Bakiewicz, A.; Kjerulff Madsen, F.; Khan, K.S.; Rasch, V.; Linde, D.S. Intimate partner violence and breastfeeding: A systematic review. *BMJ Open.* **2020**, *10*, e034153. [CrossRef] [PubMed]
49. Silverman, J.G.; Decker, M.R.; Reed, E.; Raj, A. Intimate partner violence around the time of pregnancy: Association with breastfeeding behavior. *J. Womens Health* **2006**, *15*, 934–940. [CrossRef]
50. Sipsma, H.L.; Magriples, U.; Divney, A.; Gordon, D.; Gabzdyl, E.; Kershaw, T. Breastfeeding behavior among adolescents: Initiation, duration, and exclusivity. *J. Adolesc. Health* **2013**, *53*, 394–400. [CrossRef] [PubMed]
51. James, J.P.; Taft, A.; Amir, L.H.; Agius, P. Does intimate partner violence impact on women's initiation and duration of breastfeeding? *Breastfeed. Rev.* **2014**, *22*, 11–19. [PubMed]
52. Finnbogadóttir, H.; Thies-Lagergren, L. Breastfeeding in the context of domestic violence-a cross-sectional study. *J. Adv. Nurs.* **2017**, *73*, 3209–3219. [CrossRef]
53. Metheny, N.; Stephenson, R. Is intimate partner violence a barrier to breastfeeding? An analysis of the 2015 Indian National Family Health Survey. *J. Fam. Violence* **2020**, *35*, 53–64. [CrossRef]
54. Islam, M.J.; Baird, K.; Mazerolle, P.; Broidy, L. Exploring the influence of psychosocial factors on exclusive breastfeeding in Bangladesh. *Arch. Womens Ment. Health* **2017**, *20*, 173–188. [CrossRef]
55. Ribeiro, M.R.C.; Batista, R.F.L.; Schraiber, L.B.; Pinheiro, F.S.; Santos, A.M.D.; Simões, V.M.F.; Confortin, S.C.; Aristizabal, L.Y.G.; Yokokura, A.; Silva, A. Recurrent Violence, Violence with Complications, and Intimate Partner Violence Against Pregnant Women and Breastfeeding Duration. *J. Womens Health* **2021**, *30*, 979–989. [CrossRef] [PubMed]
56. Rees, S.; Mohsin, M.; Moussa, B.; Fisher, J.; Steel, Z.; Nadar, N.; Hassoun, F.; Khalil, B.; Youssef, M.; Krishna, Y. Cohort profile: Intimate partner violence and mental health among women from refugee background and a comparison group of Australian-born–the WATCH cohort study. *BMJ Open* **2022**, *12*, e051887. [CrossRef] [PubMed]
57. IBMCorp. *IBM SPSS Statistics for Windows*; Version 27.0; IBM Corp Released: Armonk, NY, USA, 2020.
58. Correa-Velez, I.; Ryan, J. Developing a best practice model of refugee maternity care. *Women Birth* **2012**, *25*, 13–22. [CrossRef] [PubMed]
59. Shand, A.W.; Lewis-Jones, B.; Nielsen, T.; Svensson, J.; Lainchbury, A.; Henry, A.; Nassar, N. Birth outcomes by type of attendance at antenatal education: An observational study. *Aust. N. Z. J. Obstet. Gynaecol.* **2022**, *62*, 859–867. [CrossRef]
60. Kacperczyk-Bartnik, J.; Bartnik, P.; Symonides, A.; Sroka-Ostrowska, N.; Dobrowolska-Redo, A.; Romejko-Wolniewicz, E. Association between antenatal classes attendance and perceived fear and pain during labour. *Taiwan. J. Obstet. Gynecol.* **2019**, *58*, 492–496. [CrossRef] [PubMed]
61. Trinh, L.T.; Rubin, G. Late entry to antenatal care in New South Wales, Australia. *Reprod. Health* **2006**, *3*, 8. [CrossRef]
62. Heaman, M.I.; Martens, P.J.; Brownell, M.D.; Chartier, M.J.; Thiessen, K.R.; Derksen, S.A.; Helewa, M.E. Inequities in utilization of prenatal care: A population-based study in the Canadian province of Manitoba. *BMC Pregnancy Childbirth* **2018**, *18*, 430. [CrossRef]
63. Gregory, E.J.; DeFranco, E. Risk Factors Affecting Rising Rate of No Prenatal Care in US Births Between 2012–2016 [27C]. *Obstet. Gynecol.* **2020**, *135*, 36S. [CrossRef]
64. Kim, M.K.; Lee, S.M.; Bae, S.-H.; Kim, H.J.; Lim, N.G.; Yoon, S.-J.; Lee, J.Y.; Jo, M.-W. Socioeconomic status can affect pregnancy outcomes and complications, even with a universal healthcare system. *Int. J. Equity Health* **2018**, *17*, 2. [CrossRef]
65. Beeckman, K.; Louckx, F.; Putman, K. Determinants of the number of antenatal visits in a metropolitan region. *BMC Public Health* **2010**, *10*, 527. [CrossRef]

66. Leppälä, S.; Lamminpää, R.; Gissler, M.; Vehviläinen-Julkunen, K. Prenatal care adequacy of migrants born in conflict-affected countries and country-born parturients in Finland. *J. Migr. Health* **2022**, *6*, 100122. [CrossRef] [PubMed]
67. Barrett, N.M.; Burrows, L.; Atatoa-Carr, P.; Smith, L.T.; Masters-Awatere, B. Holistic antenatal education class interventions: A systematic review of the prioritisation and involvement of Indigenous Peoples' of Aotearoa New Zealand, Australia, Canada and the United States over a 10-year period 2008 to 2018. *Arch. Public Health* **2022**, *80*, 169. [CrossRef] [PubMed]
68. Simkhada, B.; Teijlingen, E.R.; Porter, M.; Simkhada, P. Factors affecting the utilization of antenatal care in developing countries: Systematic review of the literature. *J. Adv. Nurs.* **2008**, *61*, 244–260. [CrossRef] [PubMed]
69. Okedo-Alex, I.N.; Akamike, I.C.; Ezeanosike, O.B.; Uneke, C.J. Determinants of antenatal care utilisation in sub-Saharan Africa: A systematic review. *BMJ Open* **2019**, *9*, e031890. [CrossRef] [PubMed]
70. Seidu, A.-A. Factors associated with early antenatal care attendance among women in Papua New Guinea: A population-based cross-sectional study. *Arch. Public Health* **2021**, *79*, 70. [CrossRef]
71. Pell, C.; Meñaca, A.; Were, F.; Afrah, N.A.; Chatio, S.; Manda-Taylor, L.; Hamel, M.J.; Hodgson, A.; Tagbor, H.; Kalilani, L.; et al. Factors affecting antenatal care attendance: Results from qualitative studies in Ghana, Kenya and Malawi. *PLoS ONE* **2013**, *8*, e53747. [CrossRef]
72. Murphy, J.F.; Dauncey, M.; Newcombe, R.; Garcia, J.; Elbourne, D. Employment in pregnancy: Prevalence, maternal characteristics, perinatal outcome. *Lancet* **1984**, *1*, 1163–1166. [CrossRef]
73. Stengel, B.; Saurel-Cubizolles, M.J.; Kaminski, M. Pregnant immigrant women: Occupational activity, antenatal care and outcome. *Int. J. Epidemiol.* **1986**, *15*, 533–539. [CrossRef]
74. Ali, N.; Elbarazi, I.; Alabboud, S.; Al-Maskari, F.; Loney, T.; Ahmed, L.A. Antenatal Care Initiation Among Pregnant Women in the United Arab Emirates: The Mutaba'ah Study. *Front. Public Health* **2020**, *8*, 211. [CrossRef]
75. Alkomos, M.F.; Mendez, D.; Mazzei-Pifano, D.; Shafeek, F.; Rodriguez, C.; Ali, F.; Banks, C.; Melki, G.; Michael, P. Patients' reasons for missing scheduled clinic appointments and their solutions at a major urban-based academic medical center. *J. Community Hosp. Intern. Med. Perspect.* **2020**, *10*, 426–430. [CrossRef]
76. Dixon, J.; Banwell, C.; Strazdins, L.; Corr, L.; Burgess, J. Flexible employment policies, temporal control and health promoting practices: A qualitative study in two Australian worksites. *PLoS ONE* **2019**, *14*, e0224542. [CrossRef] [PubMed]
77. King, M.; Smith, A.; Gracey, M. Indigenous health part 2: The underlying causes of the health gap. *Lancet* **2009**, *374*, 76–85. [CrossRef] [PubMed]
78. Román-Gálvez, R.M.; Martín-Peláez, S.; Martínez-Galiano, J.M.; Khan, K.S.; Bueno-Cavanillas, A. Prevalence of Intimate Partner Violence in Pregnancy: An Umbrella Review. *Int. J. Environ. Res. Public Health* **2021**, *18*, 707. [CrossRef] [PubMed]
79. Delkhosh, M.; Merghati Khoei, E.; Ardalan, A.; Rahimi Foroushani, A.; Gharavi, M.B. Prevalence of intimate partner violence and reproductive health outcomes among Afghan refugee women in Iran. *Health Care Women Int.* **2019**, *40*, 213–237. [CrossRef]
80. Dadras, O.; Nakayama, T.; Kihara, M.; Ono-Kihara, M.; Seyedalinaghi, S.; Dadras, F. The prevalence and associated factors of adverse pregnancy outcomes among Afghan women in Iran; Findings from community-based survey. *PLoS ONE* **2021**, *16*, e0245007. [CrossRef]
81. Mishkin, K.E.; Ahmed, H.M.; Maqsood, S.S. Factors associated with experiencing lifetime intimate partner violence among pregnant displaced women living in refugee camps in Erbil, Iraq. *Glob. Public Health* **2022**, *17*, 1–10. [CrossRef]
82. Sabri, B.; Nnawulezi, N.; Njie-Carr, V.P.S.; Messing, J.; Ward-Lasher, A.; Alvarez, C.; Campbell, J.C. Multilevel Risk and Protective Factors for Intimate Partner Violence Among African, Asian, and Latina Immigrant and Refugee Women: Perceptions of Effective Safety Planning Interventions. *Race Soc. Probl.* **2018**, *10*, 348–365. [CrossRef]
83. Sharps, P.W.; Laughon, K.; Giangrande, S.K. Intimate partner violence and the childbearing year: Maternal and infant health consequences. *Trauma. Violence Abuse* **2007**, *8*, 105–116. [CrossRef]
84. Fisher, J.; Tran, T.D.; Biggs, B.; Dang, T.H.; Nguyen, T.T.; Tran, T. Intimate partner violence and perinatal common mental disorders among women in rural Vietnam. *Int. Health* **2013**, *5*, 29–37. [CrossRef]
85. Taillieu, T.L.; Brownridge, D.A. Violence against pregnant women: Prevalence, patterns, risk factors, theories, and directions for future research. *Aggress. Violent Behav.* **2010**, *15*, 14–35. [CrossRef]
86. Halpern-Meekin, S.; Costanzo, M.; Ehrenthal, D.; Rhoades, G. Intimate Partner Violence Screening in the Prenatal Period: Variation by State, Insurance, and Patient Characteristics. *Matern. Child Health J.* **2019**, *23*, 756–767. [CrossRef] [PubMed]
87. Kavle, J.A.; LaCroix, E.; Dau, H.; Engmann, C. Addressing barriers to exclusive breast-feeding in low- and middle-income countries: A systematic review and programmatic implications. *Public Health Nutr.* **2017**, *20*, 3120–3134. [CrossRef] [PubMed]
88. Sharma, I.K.; Byrne, A. Early initiation of breastfeeding: A systematic literature review of factors and barriers in South Asia. *Int. Breastfeed. J.* **2016**, *11*, 17. [CrossRef]
89. Olufunlayo, T.F.; Roberts, A.A.; MacArthur, C.; Thomas, N.; Odeyemi, K.A.; Price, M.; Jolly, K. Improving exclusive breastfeeding in low and middle-income countries: A systematic review. *Matern. Child. Nutr.* **2019**, *15*, e12788. [CrossRef] [PubMed]
90. Lumbiganon, P.; Martis, R.; Laopaiboon, M.; Festin, M.R.; Ho, J.J.; Hakimi, M. Antenatal breastfeeding education for increasing breastfeeding duration. *Cochrane Database Syst. Rev.* **2016**, *12*, CD006425. [CrossRef] [PubMed]
91. Meedya, S.; Fernandez, R.; Fahy, K. Effect of educational and support interventions on long-term breastfeeding rates in primiparous women: A systematic review and meta-analysis. *JBI Database Syst. Rev. Implement. Rep.* **2017**, *15*, 2307–2332. [CrossRef]

92. McFadden, A.; Gavine, A.; Renfrew, M.J.; Wade, A.; Buchanan, P.; Taylor, J.L.; Veitch, E.; Rennie, A.M.; Crowther, S.A.; Neiman, S.; et al. Support for healthy breastfeeding mothers with healthy term babies. *Cochrane Database Syst. Rev.* **2017**, *2*, CD001141. [CrossRef]
93. McFadden, A.; Siebelt, L.; Marshall, J.L.; Gavine, A.; Girard, L.-C.; Symon, A.; MacGillivray, S. Counselling interventions to enable women to initiate and continue breastfeeding: A systematic review and meta-analysis. *Int. Breastfeed. J.* **2019**, *14*, 42. [CrossRef]
94. Medina, F.; Fernández, G. Breastfeeding problems prevention in early breast feeding through effective technique. *Enfermería Glob.* **2013**, *31*, 443–444.
95. Oribe, M.; Lertxundi, A.; Basterrechea, M.; Begiristain, H.; Santa Marina, L.; Villar, M.; Dorronsoro, M.; Amiano, P.; Ibarluzea, J. Prevalence of factors associated with the duration of exclusive breastfeeding during the first 6 months of life in the INMA birth cohort in Gipuzkoa. *Gac. Sanit.* **2015**, *29*, 4–9. [CrossRef]
96. Kinshella, M.-L.W.; Prasad, S.; Hiwa, T.; Vidler, M.; Nyondo-Mipando, A.L.; Dube, Q.; Goldfarb, D.; Kawaza, K. Barriers and facilitators for early and exclusive breastfeeding in health facilities in Sub-Saharan Africa: A systematic review. *Glob. Health Res. Policy* **2021**, *6*, 21. [CrossRef] [PubMed]
97. Earle, S. Factors affecting the initiation of breastfeeding: Implications for breastfeeding promotion. *Health Promot. Int.* **2002**, *17*, 205–214. [CrossRef] [PubMed]
98. Jessri, M.; Farmer, A.P.; Olson, K. Exploring Middle-Eastern mothers' perceptions and experiences of breastfeeding in Canada: An ethnographic study. *Matern. Child Nutr.* **2013**, *9*, 41–56. [CrossRef] [PubMed]
99. Erten, E.Y.; van den Berg, P.; Weissing, F.J. Acculturation orientations affect the evolution of a multicultural society. *Nat. Commun.* **2018**, *9*, 58. [CrossRef]
100. Ward, B.G.; Pridmore, B.R.; Cox, L.W. Vietnamese refugees in Adelaide: An obstetric analysis. *Med. J. Aust.* **1981**, *1*, 72–75. [CrossRef]
101. Mattson, S.; Lew, L. Culturally sensitive prenatal care for Southeast Asians. *J. Obstet. Gynecol. Neonatal Nurs.* **1992**, *21*, 48–54. [CrossRef]

Disclaimer/Publisher's Note: The statements, opinions and data contained in all publications are solely those of the individual author(s) and contributor(s) and not of MDPI and/or the editor(s). MDPI and/or the editor(s) disclaim responsibility for any injury to people or property resulting from any ideas, methods, instructions or products referred to in the content.

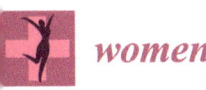

Article

Prenatal, Delivery and Postpartum Care Experiences among Black Women in Mississippi during COVID-19 Pandemic 2020–2021

Praise Ebimaye Tangbe [1,*], Mary Shaw-Ridley [1], Gerri Cannon-Smith [2], Sheila McKinney [1], Nelson Atehortua [1] and Russell Bennett [1]

1. College of Health Sciences, Jackson State University, Jackson, MS 39213, USA
2. Mississippi State Department of Health Consultant, Jackson, MS 39216, USA
* Correspondence: praise.tangbe@gmail.com

Abstract: The COVID-19 pandemic has presented challenges for countries to maintain high-quality, essential maternal health services, altering pregnancy experiences for women. This qualitative study aims to explore the impact of COVID-19 mitigation strategies on self-reported prenatal, delivery, and postpartum care experiences among Black women in Mississippi. Postpartum Black women who gave birth between March 2020 and March 2021 were recruited from a Federally Qualified Health Clinic that serves three Mississippi counties. Using a semi-structured interview guide, 10 postpartum women were interviewed, and their responses were analyzed utilizing the thematic content analysis approach. Major themes identified were stress related to COVID-19, disruption of social life/support, disruption of expected healthcare services, uncertainty and fear about coronavirus, COVID-19 mitigation strategies, and associated poor maternal health outcome. COVID-19 mitigation strategies exacerbated normal maternity-related stress. Postpartum women reported increased anxiety, fear, frustration, emotional stress, and lack of social support resulting in what was described as depression and feelings of loneliness. The results of this qualitative study of 10 Black women who gave birth during COVID-19 suggest the importance of stress-informed care.

Keywords: pregnancy; experiences; concerns; COVID-19 pregnancy script; black women; maternal mental health; attitudes

Citation: Tangbe, P.E.; Shaw-Ridley, M.; Cannon-Smith, G.; McKinney, S.; Atehortua, N.; Bennett, R. Prenatal, Delivery and Postpartum Care Experiences among Black Women in Mississippi during COVID-19 Pandemic 2020–2021. *Women* **2023**, *3*, 295–309. https://doi.org/10.3390/women3020022

Academic Editors: Claudio Costantino, Maiorana Antonio and Mary V. Seeman

Received: 16 February 2023
Revised: 14 May 2023
Accepted: 16 May 2023
Published: 24 May 2023

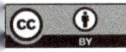

Copyright: © 2023 by the authors. Licensee MDPI, Basel, Switzerland. This article is an open access article distributed under the terms and conditions of the Creative Commons Attribution (CC BY) license (https://creativecommons.org/licenses/by/4.0/).

1. Introduction

Maternal morbidity and mortality are prominent global public health challenges, and the coronavirus pandemic has increased difficulties in delivering optimal prenatal, delivery, and postpartum services [1]. COVID-19 exacerbated maternal health disparities and undermined maternal health [2]. COVID-19 mitigation strategies restricted prenatal care visits, triggering feelings of isolation that may have contributed to higher rates of postpartum depression. Pregnancies of Black women were found to be disproportionately affected [3,4]. Vaccine hesitancy led to relatively low rates of COVID-19 vaccine uptake in this population [5], resulting in increased rates of maternal morbidity and mortality [6]. One study pointed out that Black pregnant women in the United Kingdom showed significantly higher rates of maternal mortality than White mothers [7]. Another similar study showed that pregnant Black women in the U.S. who opted for telehealth prenatal care experienced challenges [4]. They did not receive quality care that included essential tests or necessary in-person visits [4,8], which worsened already existing healthcare inequities [9]. As of April 2021, approximately 86,877 pregnant women in the U.S. were infected with coronavirus and 97 died [5]. Due to the physiological changes in cardiopulmonary systems and immune systems during pregnancy, the severity of COVID-19-related illness increases [10]. Previous coronavirus outbreaks had already suggested that pregnant women and their fetuses are particularly susceptible [11]. Reported complications are stillbirth, preterm birth, and maternal mortality [12]. In addition, there is an increased risk for cesarean section, postpartum hemorrhage, preterm birth, and hypertensive crises [13]. Mitigation strategies such as social distancing, self-isolation, quarantining, and face masks [3] interfere with prenatal care, labor and delivery, and postpartum care [10,14]. The pregnancy experience during COVID-19 may have long-term implications for the health and well-being of mothers and their children [14]. In Mississippi, where maternal morbidity and mortality rates are among the highest in the U.S., there are no known studies on the COVID-19 lived experiences of Black pregnant women despite the burden of maternal morbidity and mortality in this population [15]. Therefore, this qualitative study aims to (a) explore Black women's experiences with prenatal, delivery, and postpartum care during the COVID-19 pandemic, and (b) the effects of mitigation strategies. It hopes to generate themes that will be able to guide maternal stress-informed care during crises such as those experienced during COVID-19.

2. Methods

2.1. Protection of Human Participants

This study received ethics approval from the Jackson State University Institutional Review Board. Additionally, this study required written informed consent and participants' were informed of their right to decline participation at any time during the interview.

2.2. Maternal Healthcare Framework

The Maternal Healthcare Framework (MHCF) was adapted [16] to guide the study design. The model provides the framework for exploring the COVID-19 impact on prenatal, delivery, and postpartum care among Black postpartum women.

- Prenatal care experiences: The pandemic led to limited access to healthcare facilities, which caused limitations and restrictions in prenatal visits [17]. Black postpartum women express their lived experiences with prenatal care during the coronavirus pandemic.
- Delivery care: COVID-19 impacted hospitals by restricting visitation to hospitalized patients to support mandated social distancing. According to [18], most maternity wards allowed solely the woman's partner in the delivery room. Therefore, a critical element of the MHCF is to have mothers reflect on and describe their childbirth (delivery) experience during the COVID-19 pandemic.
- Postpartum care support: There is a realization that the COVID-19 mitigation strategies were important to curb the spread of coronavirus, but the lack of social support was a non-intended outcome. Most hospitals took precautions by prohibiting visits during postpartum hospital stay [18]. Moreover, the implemented stay-in-place measures prevented visits by family members and friends and limited face-to-face care management by caregivers. These restrictions placed mothers with newborns in an emotionally harmful, psychologically vulnerable space that increased risk of postpartum depression. Therefore, postpartum mothers expressed their lived experiences with the coronavirus pandemic and postpartum care support.

The MHCF model situates prenatal, delivery, and postpartum care experiences of Black women within a culture (both societal and hospital) that has COVID-19 mitigation strategies/behaviors in place (see Figure 1).

2.3. Study Design

We conducted a cross-sectional qualitative study using a narrative approach to explore participants' experiences with prenatal, delivery, and postpartum care services during the COVID-19 pandemic (March 2020–March 2021).

2.4. Population and Sample

Using convenience sampling, participants were (a) women between ages 18 and 45 years; (b) postpartum women who gave birth between March 2020 and March 2021; (c) people self-identifying as Black or African American in Mississippi; (d) postpartum women who spoke and understand English. Participants were separated into three age groups (18 to 24, 25 to 34, and 35 to 45) because, in the U.S., the prevalence of preterm birth is higher among women < 20 years of age (young maternal age) and women between the ages of 35 and 45 (advanced maternal age) compared to women in their mid-twenties to early thirties. Moreover, in this qualitative study, the saturation points guided determination of the final sample size [19,20]. Therefore, data saturation was reached with ten participants' responses.

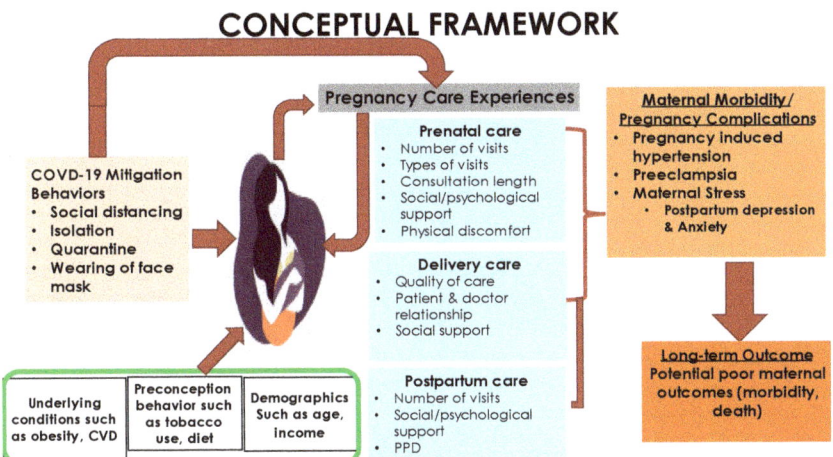

Figure 1. Maternal Healthcare Framework (MHCF). Source: The Maternal Healthcare Framework © 2022 Praise Ebimaye Tangbe was adapted from "Chronic Disease Management: What will it take to improve care for chronic illness?" by Wagner E. H., 1998, *Effective clinical practices*, vol 1 [16].

2.5. Instrumentation

The researcher developed pregnancy experience instrument is based on the WRISK survey [21]. In a two-round process, the researchers developed an interview guide that was validated for content validity, face validity, and readability by a panel of three qualitative research experts. In addition, the instrument was pilot-tested with three Black postpartum women (from the same clinic where participants were recruited) to evaluate study procedures and develop appropriate probes for study interviews. The instrument consists of two sections: demographic profile and a semi-structured interview guide with three parts (prenatal care, delivery care, and postnatal care support).

Demographic Profile. The first section consists of eight items, representing the participant demographics: age, marital status, education level, employment status, income, insurance status, gestational age, and number of pregnancies.

Pregnancy Experiences. The second section of the instrument is organized into three parts consisting of six items that assess prenatal care during COVID-19, eight items that assess delivery care during COVID-19, and seven items that assess postpartum care support during COVID-19.

2.6. Recruitment Strategy

Recruitment occurred between 1 December and 15 December 2021 (fifth wave of COVID-19 during the omicron variant surge). We recruited women receiving postpartum care support from a Jackson Metropolitan area Family Health Center (FQHC). The site is a Federally Qualified Health Center that serves about 2900 low-income rural and urban pregnant and postpartum women in three counties (Madison, Humphreys, and Yazoo). During the first wave of the pandemic, the Family Health Center strictly enforced the CDC COVID-19 mitigation guidelines [3] in care facilities. For example, prenatal and postpartum visitations were moved from in-person to virtual; the Women Infant Children

(WIC) program weekly meetings were temporarily canceled; and wearing of face masks, regular hand washing/sanitation, and staying 6 feet apart were made compulsory in the facility. Eventually, the researcher and the clinic physicians disseminated recruitment cards during reinstated WIC weekly program meetings and doctor's appointments. Interested postpartum women contacted the primary investigator by phone. Postpartum women were screened via phone using a three-item screening eligibility tool. Eligible women were enrolled in the study and scheduled for an interview (face-to-face on site or virtual) one week later.

2.7. Data Collection Procedures

Interviews were conducted in person and virtually for five weeks, from 1 February 2022 to 7 March 2022. A team of two trained interviewers including the researcher were available to conduct the interviews. Each participant consented prior to the beginning of the interview. The researcher discussed the details of the study with the participants before proceeding with the interview. For interviews via Zoom, informed consent was emailed to each enrolled participant one week before the interview date. Moreover, participants were required to consent to audio recordings. One interviewer asked the interview questions, and the other took notes and observed participants' responses during the conversation, such as tone of voice, non-verbal body languages, and important notes about the interview. Each interviews lasted approximately 30 to 45 min. Two interviews were conducted in person, and eight interviews were conducted virtually. Each participant received a 20-dollar gift card incentive upon completion of the interview.

2.8. Data Analysis

2.8.1. Quantitative

The Statistical Package for Social Sciences (SPSS) version 27 was used to analyze the demographic data. Descriptive statistics were used to report demographic information.

2.8.2. Qualitative

Data were transcribed using the online Rev transcription services. The transcripts were then entered into an Excel spreadsheet. Next, thematic content analysis was employed to analyze the presence, meanings, and relationships across the dataset that provided answers to the research questions. We identified these patterns through (a) data collection familiarization, (b) coding data, (c) applying templates of codes, (d) connecting codes and identifying themes, and (e) validating themes.

First stage (data collection and familiarization). We reviewed transcripts to become familiar with the dataset. This process helped identify meaningful units characterizing participants' prenatal, delivery, and postpartum experiences during COVID-19.

Second stage (coding the data). Members of the data-analysis team independently reviewed the text and developed codes. We then met several times to determine preliminary codes by reviewing highlighted meaningful units. Once the frequently used words and phrases were identified and the phenomenon was captured, the codes were categorized based on their differences and similarities in addressing participants' responses.

Third stage (applying template of codes). The Codebook was developed utilizing Microsoft Spreadsheet. Preliminary codes were inserted in the Excel spreadsheet. Each interview question included a set of codes with supporting participants' responses on prenatal, delivery, and postpartum care experiences.

Fourth stage (connecting codes and identifying themes). The codes were categorized into themes and patterns in the data. The themes permitted comparison of pregnancy experiences (prenatal, delivery, and postpartum) during COVID-19.

Fifth stage (corroborating and validating themes). This stage included the process of clustering the themes that were identified from the coded text. The aim was to identify the essence of each theme and to establish that they were representative of the preliminary assigned code. We conducted several iterations of reviewing text, codes, and themes, then agreed on succinct and easily understandable words/phrases for each theme before moving to the interpretive phase of the analysis.

3. Results
3.1. Demographic Characteristics of Participants

The results are discussed in two sections. First, the demographic characteristics of the participants are presented. Secondly, major findings from the thematic content analysis are presented in a qualitative style format. Table 1 shows the demographic profile of the participants.

Table 1. Demographic Characteristics of Participants ($N = 10$).

Variables	Frequency
Age-group	
18–24 years old	3
25–34 years old	5
35–45 years old	2
Marital Status	
Married	6
Single	4
Education Level	
Associate degree	3
College degree	2
High school degree	4
Vocational training	1
Employment Status	
Unemployed (not looking for job)	1
Unemployed (looking for job)	3
Working full-time	4
Working part-time	1
Student	1
Household Income	
$10,000–$19,999	1
$20,000–$29,999	3
$30,000–$39,999	1
$40,000–$59,999	5
Insurance Status	
Medicaid	4
Other (marketplace)	2
Private	4
Delivery Status	
Late preterm	2
Past-due	2
Due date	6
Pre-existing Health Conditions	
ADHD	1
High blood pressure	1
Incompetence pelvic	1
None	7

Note. $N = 10$.

3.2. Participants' Interview Responses

The five major themes that emerged about prenatal care, delivery care, and postpartum support are the following: stress related to COVID-19, disruption of social life/support, disruption of expected healthcare services, uncertainty and fear about coronavirus, COVID-19 mitigation strategies-associated poor maternal health outcome.

Table 2 shows the five derived themes with supporting quotes. The study results show how a sample of Black postpartum women characterized the prenatal, delivery care, and postpartum support experiences during the COVID-19 pandemic.

Table 2. Themes and Supporting Quotes.

Themes	Supporting Quotes
Stress related to COVID-19	"Somehow stressed, emotional stress of thinking of the uncertainty of what the virus would do to the child." "It was tough, even though I enjoyed lockdown but just being confined to the house with a newborn Umm and still having to like work from home, it was tough. There was moment of frustrations." "The COVID-19 restrictions when going to the hospital, it was a little bit stressful." "I was kind of nervous about everything", "it was a little bit stressful." "It was a bit stressful you know with the sleepless nights and then trying to get better take care of the baby and do everything by yourself without people around, It was a little you know exhausting." "I think it was a little more stressful because I had three kids to take care of, and the mask I was wearing also made it stressful. very uncomfortable and stressful because at every point in time, we also have to maskup, you're sleeping and somebody comes into your room, you have to wake up and mask up." "Umm stressful, anxious and frustrated and "I was moody, very moody but not a bad temper but kind of snappy." "Frustrated and stressed and COVID was around and I had to deliver during COVID and I had to dislike wearing face mask." "Wearing masks are stressful and uncomfortable and when you're pregnant, especially when you start getting to the second and third trimester it's very, when walking you know, sometimes you feel breathless."
Disruption of social life/support	"They had to limit people coming into the room to just one person to know like I know before the pandemic, you will have your maybe your parents your spouse, but you just have to have only one person present. It was out, personally I wasn't happy with it because you Know, I like that experience I wanted family and my spouse to be present but it just had to it was one or the other." "It was bad to not have, like in during pre-COVID you could have as many people in the room as you want to, but during the COVID I am with one person and you know not having your mom or sister around when you deliver was kind of tough." "I feel very much separated, being away from family and friends." "I didn't like the experience that much people where not allow to be with me during delivery, I actually wanted my step mom to be with me because this is my first child." "I felt a little I guess alone because people didn't visit that much and I couldn't visit as well." "I could only choose one person to be with me, but when I delivered him, it was his dad and my mom. It was just weird because I just remember everything, even my friends who have kids you know before COVID, everybody was just in the hospital, you know celebrating the baby and stuff, mine was just so different because you know you can't invite people because of COVID." "Umm not being able to go anywhere and not being able to have anyone come around, and whenever somebody kind of bring something they would leave it on the doorstep, so I feel like I have to play by yourself and like people had to avoid me at all costs, so I felt very isolated." "It was a little sad, because due to social distancing I couldn't go visit people and that made me sad." "At home, I felt a little I guess alone because people didn't visit that much." "I feel very much separated, being away from family and friends."

Table 2. Cont.

Themes	Supporting Quotes
Disruption of expected healthcare services	"I like the way they handle their social distancing procedures but the waiting period was a long one." "What I can say is that they won't allow you to have your baby until like 39 weeks. They stopped inducing; before COVID-19 they can induce people Okay, but now because of COVID-19, they do not induce people; they want you to get ready, maybe baby almost you know. they will want you to come to the hospital for delivery when you are sure is your due day. This was because they don't want too much people to be in the hospital at the same time." "It was a long wait, the doctor I was seeing had a lot of patients, a patients was about to have a baby so he had to go there, so I either wait or reschedule." "They made it in way that once you put to birth within 24 h you are to leave for another person to come in. It was a really tough one." "They limit their appointment time or the number of people who are present during each appointment. Just to reduce like exposure to other people may have COVID." "I guess unavailability of scheduling by not been able to get a visit within the week I needed to come because of the COVID it may have been delayed, so I will be coming two weeks after." "So I was really concern I don't want to get COVID while pregnant. My prenatal appointment was cancelled by the Doctor and rescheduled for another date." "It was just really the delivery part and about like being sent home too early, because of COVID guidelines. I came to the hospital on 25th night, gave birth to my child on the 26th and I was back home on the 27th. I just feel like there wasn't enough time to monitor and make sure I am OK before sending me home." "I feel badly, because is a new protocols and people don't stay in the hospital as long as they used to before COVID. Is like you had a baby, are you feeling good? Okay time for you to go home, I feel like I should have stayed longer, but I didn't. I feel like I was failed honestly because first of all, they didn't tell me that my blood pressure was high, or what signs to look out for if I need to come back or call, and you know something like that they didn't educate me on it." "I will give it a 7 over 10 because I think they could do better with follow up. It was just two postpartum follow-ups."
Uncertainty and fear about coronavirus	"I was nervous. I think spend the first three to four months within, unless it was a doctor appointment, because I was afraid of the COVID." "Umm it was scary, there was lot of uncertainties if I want to deliver in the hospital, so there was like my anxiety level high at sometimes." "I am always scared of getting sick, so it won't affect my baby, I try to stay six feet away from people." "Not wanting to get COVID-19, there was like a barrier to not want to go out or not want to go see the doctor because other people may be sick." "Hmm ... It was it was scary because you know. It was something new and unfounded and I especially had concerns because, you know being pregnant, even though there was a vaccine, I chose not to take the vaccine, because I did, there was no research on you know the impact of it on pregnant women or the baby." "There were some scary parts like getting COVID and all that, which made me to miss some of my doctor's appointment you know." "Somehow stressed, emotional stress of thinking of the uncertainty of what the virus would do to the child."
COVID-19 mitigation strategies-associated poor maternal health outcome	"Um I think that's where my postpartum depression came from, because you know, for a while you can't leave the house and I actually have a baby, and it was just weird because it felt like this is how is going to be every single day and I barely go to anywhere anyway, because I was still terrified of COVID." "I was breastfeeding also in pain after given birth I have forgotten what is called, it had to enter my body for 24 h, so I couldn't get up for 24 h, it was miserable. I did experience postpartum depression." "I had bad postpartum depression, so I was put on some different meds to help with that. I was on Zoloft for a little short period. I was just frustrated at that time because I had to take care of my newborn and my other two children myself." "My care was a bit quick they somehow rushed me out of the hospital because of COVID. I was admitted again to the hospital, and I was told that I developed preeclampsia, so I had to stay in hospital for three days, because my blood pressure was extremely high."

3.2.1. Theme 1: Stress Related to COVID-19

Postpartum women reported feelings of stress during the COVID-19 pandemic with experiences in prenatal, delivery, and postpartum care. Participants reported they had been stressed and frustrated to have to take care of their newborn by themselves. The fact that hospitals limited family members and spouses from attending prenatal, delivery, and postpartum visits was distressing for women and affected their emotional state of mind. Participants also indicated physical stress and discomfort from wearing face masks. The following selected quotes support the theme that emerged.

"Somehow stressed, emotional stress of thinking of the uncertainty of what the virus would do to the child."

"It was tough, even though I enjoyed lockdown but just being confined to the house with a newborn Umm and still having to like work from home, it was tough. There was moment of frustrations."

"The COVID-19 restrictions when going to the hospital, it was a little bit stressful."

"I was kind of nervous about everything," "it was a little bit stressful."

"It was a bit stressful you know with the sleepless nights and then trying to get better take care of the baby and do everything by yourself without people around, It was a little you know exhausting."

"I think it was a little more stressful because I had three kids to take care of, and the mask I was wearing also made it stressful. Very uncomfortable and stressful because at every point in time, we also have to mask up, you're sleeping and somebody comes into your room, you have to wake up and mask up."

"Umm stressful, anxious and frustrated and I was moody, very moody but not a bad temper but kind of snappy."

"Frustrated and stressed and COVID was around and I had to deliver during COVID and I had to dislike wearing face mask."

"Wearing masks are stressful and uncomfortable and when you're pregnant, especially when you start getting to the second and third trimester it's very, when walking you know, sometimes you feel breathless."

3.2.2. Theme 2: Disruption of Social Life/Support

Participants indicated that they were not being sufficiently supported during the COVID-19 pandemic due to the mitigation strategies. They complained of lack of support from family and friends. The fact that hospitals restricted family members and spouses from attending prenatal, delivery, and postpartum visits was distressing for the participants and affected their emotional state of mind.

"They had to limit people coming into the room to just one person to know like I know before the pandemic, you will have your maybe your parents your spouse, but you just have to have only one person present. It was out, personally I wasn't happy with it because you Know, I like that experience I wanted family and my spouse to be present but it just had to it was one or the other."

"It was bad to not have, like in during pre-COVID you could have as many people in the room as you want to, but during the COVID I am with one person and you know not having your mom or sister around when you deliver was kind of tough."

"I feel very much separated, being away from family and friends."

"I didn't like the experience that much people where not allow to be with me during delivery, I actually wanted my step mom to be with me because this is my first child."

"I felt a little I guess alone because people didn't visit that much and I couldn't visit as well."

"I could only choose one person to be with me, but when I delivered him, it was his dad and my mom. It was just weird because I just remember everything, even my friends who have kids you know before COVID, everybody was just in the hospital, you know

celebrating the baby and stuff, mine was just so different because you know you can't invite people because of COVID."

"Umm not being able to go anywhere and not being able to have anyone come around, and whenever somebody kind of bring something they would leave it on the doorstep, so I feel like I have to play by yourself and like people had to avoid me at all costs, so I felt very isolated."

"It was a little sad, because due to social distancing I couldn't go visit people and that made me sad."

"At home, I felt a little I guess alone because people didn't visit that much."

"I feel very much separated, being away from family and friends."

3.2.3. Theme 3: Disruption of Expected Healthcare Services

Postpartum women mentioned some disruptions in receiving healthcare services in the beginnings of the pandemic such as cancellation of pregnancy-related appointments, the wait times to see a doctor and for visits in the hospital, delay in labor induction, and hospitalization stay after delivery was shortened.

"I like the way they handle their social distancing procedures but the waiting period was a long one."

"What I can say is that they won't allow you to have your baby until like 39 weeks. They stopped inducing; before COVID-19 they can induce people Okay, but now because of COVID-19, they do not induce people; they want you to get ready, maybe baby almost you know. they will want you to come to the hospital for delivery when you are sure is your due day. This was because they don't want too much people to be in the hospital at the same time."

"It was a long wait, the doctor I was seeing had a lot of patients, a patient was about to have a baby so he had to go there, so I either wait or reschedule."

"They made it in way that once you put to birth within 24 h you are to leave for another person to come in. It was a really tough one."

"They limit their appointment time or the number of people who are present during each appointment. Just to reduce like exposure to other people may have COVID."

"I guess unavailability of scheduling by not been able to get a visit within the week I needed to come because of the COVID it may have been delayed, so I will be coming two weeks after."

"So, I was really concern I don't want to get COVID while pregnant. My prenatal appointment was cancelled by the Doctor and rescheduled for another date."

"It was just really the delivery part and about like being sent home too early, because of COVID guidelines. I came to the hospital on 25th night, gave birth to my child on the 26th and I was back home on the 27th. I just feel like there wasn't enough time to monitor and make sure I am OK before sending me home."

"I feel badly, because is a new protocols and people don't stay in the hospital as long as they used to before COVID. Is like you had a baby, are you feeling good? Okay time for you to go home, I feel like I should have stayed longer, but I didn't. I feel like I was failed honestly because first of all, they didn't tell me that my blood pressure was high, or what signs to look out for if I need to come back or call, and you know something like that they didn't educate me on it."

"I will give it a 7 over 10 because I think they could do better with follow-up. It was just two postpartum follow-ups."

3.2.4. Theme 4: Uncertainty and Fear about Coronavirus

Most of the participants were worried and scared about the risk of getting infected by COVID-19 and how pregnant women are more vulnerable to COVID-19 compared to non-pregnant women. Some of the participants' responses were:

"I was nervous. I think spend the first three to four months within, unless it was a doctor appointment, because I was afraid of the COVID."

"Umm it was scary, there was lot of uncertainties if I want to deliver in the hospital, so there was like my anxiety level high at sometimes."

"I am always scared of getting sick, so it won't affect my baby, I try to stay six feet away from people."

"Not wanting to get COVID-19, there was like a barrier to not want to go out or not want to go see the doctor because other people may be sick."

"Hmm . . . It was it was scary because you know. It was something new and unfounded and I especially had concerns because, you know being pregnant, even though there was a vaccine, I chose not to take the vaccine, because I did, there was no research on you know the impact of it on pregnant women or the baby."

"There were some scary parts like getting COVID and all that, which made me to miss some of my doctor's appointment you know."

"Somehow stressed, emotional stress of thinking of the uncertainty of what the virus would do to the child."

3.2.5. Theme 5: COVID-19 Mitigation Strategies-Associated Poor Maternal Health Outcome

Participants explained the challenges they faced post-delivery due to the social distance measure enforced to curb the spread of COVID-19. Participants reported significant reduction in postpartum follow-ups and lack of social support from family and friends, which resulted in poor maternal health outcomes such as postpartum depression and preeclampsia.

"Um I think that's where my postpartum depression came from, because you know, for a while you can't leave the house and I actually have a baby, and it was just weird because it felt like this is how is going to be every single day and I barely go to anywhere anyway, because I was still terrified of COVID."

"I was breastfeeding also in pain after given birth I have forgotten what is called, it had to enter my body for 24 h, so I couldn't get up for 24 h, it was miserable. I did experience postpartum depression."

"I had bad postpartum depression, so I was put on some different meds to help with that. I was on Zoloft for a little short period. I was just frustrated at that time because I had to take care of my newborn and my other two children myself."

"My care was a bit quick they somehow rushed me out of the hospital because of COVID. I was admitted again to the hospital, and I was told that I developed preeclampsia, so I had to stay in hospital for three days, because my blood pressure was extremely high."

In addition, participants recommended proactiveness from care providers during crises, doctors should provide sufficient sources of information, increasing the number of healthcare providers/facilities to accommodate pregnant women in times of crisis, quality health insurance by improving welfare packages during crises, providing mental health support services for pregnant women during crises, improving on doctor–patient relationships during crises, and care providers should have action plans during crises to prevent delays in services among pregnant women. Some of the participants' responses were:

"We should be more proactive with public health; a lot of misinformation that is available so. clinicians should be in the habit of you know. Advising their patients on the truth about COVID. Because there's a lot of people who still believe that it's a myth or it's real."

"They need to increase the number of hospitals and also the number of healthcare providers. They should improve on the welfare package for insurance."

"They dig deeper to connect women to the support services that they may be in the future so that whenever you do feel lonely and isolated or frustrated you do not only have people in place to talk to, but you also have access to tools and resources that you may need to help get you through those tough times."

"Doctors should try and get closer to their patients, try to know them one on one and also try to impact positively in their life."

4. Discussion

In this exploratory study, the researcher examined pregnancy experiences (prenatal care, delivery care, and postpartum support care) among Black women who were pregnant, delivered, and/or were postpartum during the first year of COVID-19. Interviews were conducted until data saturation occurred (the extent to which no new code could be extracted) from the data. In this study, data saturation was reached with 10 postpartum women. The study findings provide significant insight into Black postpartum women's lived experiences during the COVID-19 pandemic. Postpartum women (who received prenatal, delivery, or postpartum care during the period March 2020–March 2021) described how the COVID-19 pandemic unexpectedly changed the standards of care processes for prenatal, delivery, and postpartum care support. Emotional/physical stress, disruption of social life/support, disruption of expected healthcare services, uncertainty and fear about coronavirus, COVID-19 mitigation strategies associated with poor maternal health outcomes, feelings of depression, and loneliness were common among postpartum women during the COVID-19 pandemic. Most of the women in this study expressed that they could not keep up with their old social lifestyle because the pandemic disrupted their social lives and support. Socially isolating themselves at home and not having visitors during delivery and the postpartum period led to feelings of loneliness. These findings are like results reported by [22–25]. The current study corroborates the emerging evidence that the COVID-19 mitigation strategies exacerbated maternity stress and levels of depression among pregnant and postpartum women, including Black women who are disproportionately impacted by maternity stressors.

Furthermore, postpartum women reported limited social interaction with other pregnant women during prenatal care visits and how social distancing made them feel isolated, which resulted in loneliness. Postpartum women felt that they were not sufficiently supported during prenatal care because they were not allowed to have their spouses or family members attend prenatal visits. Moreover, in another study women reported a sense of loneliness and lack of support [26]. The findings are similar to what women reported in this study.

The study participants reported feelings of stress or they felt stress related to the COVID-19 pandemic. The study revealed how postpartum women were constantly stressed and nervous about everything; participants reported that they were emotionally stressed and had high anxiety. Emotional stress from participants resulted from mood swings and frustration that resulted from a sense of helplessness. Anxiety, a kind of psychological stress that triggers a physiological state and causes a decrease in immunity and increases the production of stress hormones [27]. Study findings also show that postpartum women reported physical stress and discomfort; difficulty in breathing, were frustrated, inconvenienced, and were uncomfortable wearing masks during pregnancy—perhaps causing anxiety symptoms. The participant responses were similar to what was reported by other groups in the general public (non-pregnant people).

The findings of this study show that the COVID-19 mitigation strategies that were enforced to curb the spread of the virus, led to disruption of social life/support for the postpartum women. Overall, participants felt unsupported, lonely, and abandoned due to a perceived lack of family/friends' support. The participants in this study reported their experiences during delivery care. The most common response about the lived experiences with delivery care was about the limited number of persons such as spouses, friends, and family members in the delivery or patient room during the COVID-19 pandemic. Postpartum women explained that they were concerned and worried about spouses not being allowed into the labor room. This finding is like the results of [24]. Participants further explained that they felt lonely and isolated at some point in the delivery room due to the limited number of persons for visitations.

During the postpartum period, women explained that social isolation mitigation strategies resulted in either a complete lack of support from community and family or a significant reduction in postpartum and social support, findings that are very similar to results reported by [28,29]. The literature provides evidence that postpartum women with low social support had higher chances of developing postpartum depression than those with high social support [30,31]. Social support from family members, friends, or significant others is prominent in reducing stress and preventing depression during the prenatal and postpartum periods [32,33].

During the maternal care period, Black postpartum women expressed their experiences with the delivery of healthcare services during the COVID-19 pandemic. Postpartum women in this study reported long wait times at the doctor's office, limited appointments to see doctors, and cancellations of appointments. These findings are similar to the findings of [25,26], which reported that women experienced a reduction and postponement of prenatal care visits. Additionally, hospitalization stays after delivery were shortened; postpartum women stated that they were sent home 24 h after delivery. The response from postpartum women in this study is similar to the findings from [34], which stated that short birth hospitalization length of stay increased from 28.5% to 43.0% for all births (less than two midnights for vaginal deliveries and less than three midnights for cesarean deliveries) [31]. These expected healthcare changes were reported in a previous study, which included cancellation of appointments and restriction on family/friend support during visits to hospitals.

At the beginning of the COVID-19 pandemic, postpartum women were scared about the virus because of misinformation and how pregnant women were more at risk to be infected by COVID-19 compared to non-pregnant women. Postpartum women were concerned about getting infected with coronavirus and afraid about having a healthy delivery without infecting the fetus. These findings are similar to an earlier study, which reported that pregnant women were scared and worried about delivering in the hospital because of the spread of the virus [34]. These experiences affected pregnant women's choices and created uncertainty and fear about their pregnancy and childbirth care.

Thus, pregnant women who experience high stress are prone to hypertension and other pregnancy complications [5,28]. A previous study reported similar results, showing the effects of the COVID-19 pandemic caused depression, which led to increased anxiety levels among pregnant women [29]. Several participants explained the challenges they have faced post-delivery, such as a limited number of postpartum follow-ups and a lack of support from family members, which resulted in postpartum depression and preeclampsia among some participants (the participant felt she should have been in the hospital for more than 24 h to observe her health because she was diagnosed with high blood pressure. Instead, she was discharged without further observation due to the hospital-imposed COVID-19 restrictions; her blood pressure was elevated, which may have caused her to develop preeclampsia). Other studies reported similar findings, stating that the COVID-19 pandemic caused limited social support and home visitations for women; moreover, pregnant women reported more depressive symptoms in the postpartum period [23,26]. The pandemic exacerbated what were already poor maternal outcomes in the United States.

4.1. Strengths

The study is the first to explore the pregnancy experiences of Black women in Mississippi during a selected period of the COVID-19 crisis. The findings characterized the lived experiences of a convenience sample of Black women who received prenatal, delivery, and postpartum care at a Mississippi Family Health Clinic (FHQC) during March 2020–March 2021, the first year of the pandemic. Results showed that the postpartum women described high levels of emotional stress, anxiety, feelings of isolation, and being cut off from family support and a social life that they deemed essential to their well-being. The participants reported similar experiences regardless of whether they were pregnant for the first time, or they had had previous pregnancies. Although the COVID-19 pandemic has impacted everyone, pregnancy has always been a unique life-altering personal, family, and healthcare experience for women. It is unclear what will be the pandemic's long-term on Black women's health and future pregnancies for women who experienced prenatal, delivery, and postpartum care during the pandemic. What we do know is women had elevated levels of stress, anxiety, depression, and feelings of isolation that could potentially impact future pregnancies and require a more formal process of stress-informed care by women's healthcare providers, inclusive of obstetricians, gynecologists, pediatricians, and other primary care physicians.

4.2. Limitations

Despite the new findings and emerging evidence from other research, this study has some limitations. These include a small sample size that limits generalizability to all postpartum women in Mississippi and beyond. Secondly, this qualitative study only included English-speaking participants. The sample was limited to one Family Health Clinic (FQHC) in Mississippi that serves low-income women. The findings may not be generalizable to women receiving care services through all healthcare facilities in Mississippi. Moreover, the use of convenience sampling may introduce a high level of bias and inability to generalize findings. The researchers also observed that the participants turned off their video cameras during virtual interviews. It took much work for the interviewer and observer to ascertain nonverbal gestures and expressions that can be invaluable in qualitative research. Moreover, the follow-up probes did not specifically address the perceived quality of care postpartum women received from the healthcare providers. Omitting quality of care questions is a limitation because the literature documents that it is a factor that often influences how women characterize their care experiences with a healthcare provider or facility.

5. Conclusions

The COVID-19 pandemic exacerbated normal maternity-related stress. The COVID-19 mitigation strategies/behaviors that were mandated to curb the spread of COVID-19 posed challenges for postpartum women such as stress related to COVID-19, disruption of social life/support, disruption of expected healthcare services, uncertainty and fear about coronavirus, and poor maternal health outcome. Postpartum women reported increased anxiety, fear, frustration, lack of social support, long wait times to see the doctor, and shortened hospitalization after delivery. As we emerge from the COVID-19 pandemic or as COVID-19 prevention/mitigation strategies are lifted, there are many questions that continue to emerge related to maternal experiences, outcomes, and future directions for pregnancy care. In the aftermath of a global pandemic that challenged the public health workforce, healthcare systems, delivery of mental health services, and the freedoms and rights that we enjoy, there are many research questions and complex problems to address. The current study sought to better understand one aspect of maternal health in Mississippi. The lack of social support during pandemics like COVID-19 necessitates support groups in healthcare facilities to alleviate maternal healthcare difficulties.

Author Contributions: P.E.T.: conceptualization, design, data collection, execution, and drafting and revision of the manuscript. M.S.-R.: Dissertation chair and co-conceptualization of the study; and review of the manuscript. G.C.-S., S.M., N.A. and R.B.: Dissertation committees, and review of the manuscript. All authors have read and agreed to the published version of the manuscript.

Funding: This research received no external funding.

Institutional Review Board Statement: Jackson State University's Institutional Review Board for ethical approval (0039-22) in accordance with the guidelines of the protection of human Participants as stipulated by the Federal government.

Informed Consent Statement: Informed consent was obtained from all subjects involved in the study.

Data Availability Statement: The data presented in this study are available on request from the corresponding author.

Acknowledgments: I am thankful to Mary Ridley-Shaw for her dedication and guidance in completing my dissertation and serving as the dissertation chair. I also extend thanks to Sheila Mckinney, Nelson Atehortua, Russell Bennett, and Gerri Cannon-Smith for serving as committee members. Additionally, I am grateful for Kyskie Bolton and G.A. Carmichael Family Health Center for permitting access to postpartum women who received services from the healthcare facility. Moreover, thanks to my family and friends for social support. I am extremely grateful for all the women who participated in the study because without them none of this work would have been possible.

Conflicts of Interest: The authors declare no conflict of interest.

References

1. Davis-Floyd, R.; Gutschow, K.; Schwartz, D.A. Pregnancy, Birth and the COVID-19 Pandemic in the United States. *Med. Anthropol.* **2020**, *39*, 413–427. [CrossRef] [PubMed]
2. Eligon, J.; Burch, A.D.; Searcey, D.; Oppel, R.A., Jr. Black Americans face alarming rates of coronavirus infection in some states. *N. Y. Times* **2020**, *7*. Available online: https://www.nytimes.com/2020/04/07/us/coronavirus-race.html (accessed on 7 April 2020).
3. Center for Disease Control and Prevention. Depression among Women. 2020. Available online: https://www.cdc.gov/reproductivehealth/depression/index.htm (accessed on 23 May 2020).
4. Murray, R.; Frank, G. Black Pregnant and COVID-19 Positive. 2020. Available online: https://www.today.com/health/how-coronavirus-affects-black-pregnant-women-t185645 (accessed on 30 June 2020).
5. Centers for Disease Control and Prevention (2021). Trends in Out-Of-Hospital Births in the United States, 1990–2012 (No. 2014). US Department of Health and Human Services, National Center for Health Statistics. Available online: https://www.cdc.gov/nchs/products/databriefs/db144.htm (accessed on 6 March 2014).
6. Lemke, M.K.; Brown, K.K. Syndemic Perspectives to Guide Black Maternal Health Research and Prevention During the COVID-19 Pandemic. *Matern. Child Health J.* **2020**, *24*, 1093–1098. [CrossRef]
7. Knight, M.; Bunch, K.; Vousden, N.; Morris, E.; Simpson, N.; Gale, C.; O'Brien, P.; Quigley, C.; Brocklehurst, P.; Kurinczuk, J.J.; et al. Characteristics and outcomes of pregnant women admitted to hospital with confirmed SARS-CoV-2 infection in UK: National population-based cohort study. *BMJ* **2020**, *369*, m2107. [CrossRef]
8. Dashraath, P.; Jeslyn, W.J.L.; Karen, L.M.X.; Min, L.L.; Sarah, L.; Biswas, A.; Choolani, M.; Mattar, C.; Lin, S.L. Coronavirus disease 2019 (COVID-19) pandemic and pregnancy. *Am. J. Obstet. Gynecol.* **2020**, *222*, 521–531. [CrossRef]
9. Mein, S.A. COVID-19 and Health Disparities: The reality of "The Great Equalizer". *J. Gen. Intern. Med.* **2020**, *35*, 2439–2440. [CrossRef]
10. Masjoudi, M.; Aslani, A.; Khazaeian, S.; Fathnezhad-Kazemi, A. Explaining the experience of prenatal care and investigating the association between psychological factors with self-care in pregnant women during COVID-19 pandemic: A mixed method study protocol. *Reprod. Health* **2020**, *17*, 1–7. [CrossRef]
11. Ashokka, B.; Loh, M.H.; Tan, C.H.; Su, L.L.; Young, B.E.; Lye, D.C.; Biswas, A.; Illanes, E.S.; Choolani, M. Care of the pregnant woman with coronavirus disease 2019 in labor and delivery: Anesthesia, emergency cesarean delivery, differential diagnosis in the acutely ill parturient, care of the newborn, and protection of the healthcare personnel. *Am. J. Obstet. Gynecol.* **2020**, *223*, 66–74. [CrossRef]
12. Schwartz, D.A. An analysis of 38 pregnant women with COVID-19, their newborn infants, and maternal-fetal transmission of SARS-CoV-2: Maternal coronavirus infections and pregnancy outcomes. *Arch. Pathol. Lab. Med.* **2020**, *144*, 799–805. [CrossRef]
13. Metz, T.D. LB02 Maternal and neonatal outcomes of pregnant patients with coronavirus disease 2019 (COVID-19): A multistate cohort. *Am. J. Obstet. Gynecol.* **2021**, *224*, S722. [CrossRef]
14. Chen, Y.; Liu, J.; Zhang, C.; Duan, C.; Zhang, H.; Mol, B.W.; Dennis, C.L.; Yin, T.; Yang, J.; Huang, H. Coronavirus disease 2019 among pregnant Chinese women: Case series data on the safety of vaginal birth and breastfeeding. *BJOG Int. J. Obstet. Gynaecol.* **2020**. [CrossRef]
15. Mississippi State Department of Health. Mississippi Maternal Mortality Report 2013–2016. 2019. Available online: https://msdh.ms.gov/msdhsite/_static/resources/8127.pdf (accessed on 1 April 2019).
16. Wagner, E.H. Chronic disease management: What will it take to improve care for chronic illness? *Eff. Clin. Pract.* **1998**, *1*, 2–4. [PubMed]

7. Gomez, H.M.; Mejia Arbelaez, C.; Ocampo Cañas, J.A. A qualitative study of the experiences of pregnant women in accessing healthcare services during the Zika virus epidemic in Villavicencio, Colombia, 2015–2016. *Int. J. Gynecol. Obstet.* **2020**, *148*, 29–35. [CrossRef] [PubMed]
8. Viaux, S.; Maurice, P.; Cohen, D.; Jouannic, J.M. Giving birth under lockdown during the COVID-19 epidemic. *J. Gynecol. Obstet. Hum. Reprod.* **2020**, *49*, 101785. [CrossRef] [PubMed]
9. Bertaux, D. From the life-history approach to the transformation of sociological practice. In *Biography and Society: The Life History Approach in the Social Sciences*; Sage: London, UK, 1981; pp. 29–45.
10. Creswell, J.W. *Qualitative Inquiry and Research Design: Choosing among Five Approaches*; Sage: Thousand Oaks, CA, USA, 1998; p. 135.
11. Blaylock, R.; Trickey, H.; Sanders, J.; Murphy, C. WRISK voices: A mixed-methods study of women's experiences of pregnancy-related public health advice and risk messages in the UK. *Midwifery* **2022**, *113*, 103433. [CrossRef] [PubMed]
12. Aydin, R.; Aktaş, S. An investigation of women's pregnancy experiences during the COVID-19 pandemic: A qualitative study. *Int. J. Clin. Pract.* **2021**, *75*, e14418. [CrossRef] [PubMed]
13. Berthelot, N.; Lemieux, R.; Garon-Bissonnette, J.; Drouin-Maziade, C.; Martel, É.; Maziade, M. Uptrend in distress and psychiatric symptomatology in pregnant women during the coronavirus disease 2019 pandemic. *Acta Obstet. Gynecol. Scand.* **2020**, *99*, 848–855. [CrossRef]
14. Karavadra, B.; Stockl, A.; Prosser-Snelling, E.; Simpson, P.; Morris, E. Women's perceptions of COVID-19 and their healthcare experiences: A qualitative thematic analysis of a national survey of pregnant women in the United Kingdom. *BMC Pregnancy Childbirth* **2020**, *20*, 1–8. [CrossRef]
15. Sahin, B.M.; Kabakci, E.N. The experiences of pregnant women during the COVID-19 pandemic in Turkey: A qualitative study. *Women Birth* **2021**, *34*, 162–169. [CrossRef]
16. Kotlar, B.; Gerson, E.; Petrillo, S.; Langer, A.; Tiemeier, H. The impact of the COVID-19 pandemic on maternal and perinatal health: A scoping review. *Reprod. Health* **2021**, *18*, 1–39. [CrossRef]
17. Zainiyah, Z.; Susanti, E. Anxiety in Pregnant Women during Coronavirus (COVID-19) Pandemic in East Java, Indonesia. *Maj. Kedokt. Bdg.* **2020**, *52*, 149–153. [CrossRef]
18. Villar, J.; Ariff, S.; Gunier, R.B.; Thiruvengadam, R.; Rauch, S.; Kholin, A.; Ikenoue, S.; Aminu, M.B.; Vecciarelli, C.; Papageorghiou, A.T.; et al. Maternal and neonatal morbidity and mortality among pregnant women with and without COVID-19 infection: The INTERCOVID multinational cohort study. *JAMA Paediatr.* **2021**, *175*, 817–826. [CrossRef] [PubMed]
19. Durankuş, F.; Aksu, E. Effects of the COVID-19 pandemic on anxiety and depressive symptoms in pregnant women: A preliminary study. *J. Matern. Fetal Neonatal Med.* **2022**, *35*, 205–211. [CrossRef] [PubMed]
20. Mortazavi, F.; Ghardashi, F. The lived experiences of pregnant women during COVID-19 pandemic: A descriptive phenomenological study. *BMC Pregnancy Childbirth* **2021**, *21*, 1–10. [CrossRef] [PubMed]
21. Leung, B.M.; Letourneau, N.L.; Giesbrecht, G.F.; Ntanda, H.; Hart, M. Predictors of postpartum depression in partnered mothers and fathers from a longitudinal cohort. *Community Ment. Health J.* **2017**, *53*, 420–431. [CrossRef]
22. Pao, C.; Guintivano, J.; Santos, H.; Meltzer-Brody, S. Postpartum depression and social support in a racially and ethnically diverse population of women. *Arch. Women's Ment. Health* **2019**, *22*, 105–114. [CrossRef]
23. McLeish, J.; Redshaw, M. Mothers' accounts of the impact on emotional wellbeing of organised peer support in pregnancy and early parenthood: A qualitative study. *BMC Pregnancy Childbirth* **2017**, *17*, 1–14. [CrossRef]
24. Handley, S.C.; Gallagher, K.; Breden, A.; Lindgren, E.; Lo, J.Y.; Son, M.; Murosko, D.; Dysart, K.; Lorch, S.A.; Burris, H.H.; et al. Birth hospital length of stay and rehospitalization during COVID-19. *Pediatrics* **2022**, *149*, e2021053498. [CrossRef]

Disclaimer/Publisher's Note: The statements, opinions and data contained in all publications are solely those of the individual author(s) and contributor(s) and not of MDPI and/or the editor(s). MDPI and/or the editor(s) disclaim responsibility for any injury to people or property resulting from any ideas, methods, instructions or products referred to in the content.

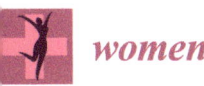

Article

Clinical Equipment as a Potential Impediment to Optimal Intrapartum Monitoring and Delivery for Pregnant Women in South Africa

Kgaladi Mpule Mohlala, Livhuwani Muthelo *, Mpho Gift Mathebula, Masenyani Oupa Mbombi, Tshepo Albert Ntho and Thabo Arthur Phukubye

Department of Nursing Science, Faculty of Health Science, University of Limpopo, Private Bag X1106, Sovenga 0727, South Africa; mpho.mathebula@ul.ac.za (M.G.M.); masenyani.mbombi@ul.ac.za (M.O.M.); tshepo.ntho@ul.ac.za (T.A.N.); arthur.phukubye@ul.ac.za (T.A.P.)
* Correspondence: livhuwani.muthelo@ul.ac.za

Citation: Mohlala, K.M.; Muthelo, L.; Mathebula, M.G.; Mbombi, M.O.; Ntho, T.A.; Phukubye, T.A. Clinical Equipment as a Potential Impediment to Optimal Intrapartum Monitoring and Delivery for Pregnant Women in South Africa. *Women* 2023, *3*, 335–347. https://doi.org/10.3390/women3020025

Academic Editors: Claudio Costantino and Maiorana Antonio

Received: 24 April 2023
Revised: 3 June 2023
Accepted: 8 June 2023
Published: 15 June 2023

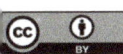

Copyright: © 2023 by the authors. Licensee MDPI, Basel, Switzerland. This article is an open access article distributed under the terms and conditions of the Creative Commons Attribution (CC BY) license (https://creativecommons.org/licenses/by/4.0/).

Abstract: Clinical equipment is essential in a labour unit to assess, monitor, diagnose, and prevent complications during labour. The availability of good working equipment in the labour unit is needed to enhance optimal intrapartum monitoring and delivery for pregnant women. Thus, this paper employed a cross-sectional descriptive design using a quantitative research approach to ascertain how equipment impedes optimal intrapartum monitoring and delivery for pregnant women. A total of 59 midwives were recruited to participate in the study. Data collected using an electronic structured questionnaire were analysed with descriptive statistics using Statistical Package for Social Sciences (SPSS) version 25.0. The study reported that most midwives (68%) in labour units experienced barriers to using equipment when administering care to pregnant women. The barriers were perpetuated by various factors, such as bed capacity, in meeting patient demands, including examination lights, overhead radiant warmers, and examination weighing scales for newborns. Incorporating mandatory computerized maintenance management software is recommended to improve the quality of maternity equipment. In addition, there is a need for regular equipment inspections and maintenance by skilled technicians in selected hospitals of Limpopo Province, South Africa.

Keywords: clinical; equipment; impediment; optimal; intrapartum; monitoring; delivery; pregnant women; midwives

1. Introduction

Equipment is an essential clinical tool in the labour unit to assess, monitor, diagnose and prevent complications during labour. Labour units must be well equipped with exceptionally functional equipment to monitor and help pregnant women deliver to achieve positive birth outcomes [1]. Childbirth should be a safe and rewarding experience for women and their families [2]. Therefore, it is vital to have available equipment in the labour unit that ensures a physiologically safe birth and a positive childbirth experience [3].

The World Health Organisation reports that it is a requirement that basic essential equipment is always available in sufficient quantities in maternity units for utilisation during labour and childbirth [4]. However, midwives in sub-Saharan Africa experience difficulties providing optimum care to pregnant women and their babies, mainly challenged by increasing deliveries with a lack of essential resources in labour units [5–7]. Similarly, in the Philippines, midwives reported that essential routines, monitoring and assessment during labour were not sufficiently conducted due to being compounded by inappropriate infrastructure and supplies [8]. Therefore, the mentioned authors demonstrate that, although the use of equipment is significant during intrapartum monitoring and delivery for a pregnant woman, sufficient allocation and the effective utilisation of equipment by midwives remain barriers to achieving quality care during labour.

Facility midwifery care services need to improve by providing equipment and supplies to increase satisfaction with services received during the intrapartum stage of pregnant women [9]. A study in Sierra Leone indicated that the checklist entries for labour regarding delivery equipment could improve optimum care during intrapartum monitoring and delivery for pregnant women [10]. Significantly, the maintenance of equipment should be prioritised to achieve optimum monitoring and delivery for a pregnant woman effectively [10]. High-quality care is needed during labour. Therefore, improving accessibility to adequately available and functional equipment during labour promotes health and enhances good healthcare services, including quality management for pregnant women and their babies.

A shortage of medical equipment because of either unavailability or non-functioning is a barrier to the ability of the health system to deliver quality health services in South Africa [11]. South African Nursing Council (SANC) Regulation R.2488 (1990 as amended) stipulates conditions under which a registered midwife or accoucheur may carry out her profession. The regulation indicates that a registered midwife or accoucheur shall always have available equipment and the materials required to help pregnant women deliver in the labour unit [12]. This equipment includes the material necessary to perform an episiotomy and suture an episiotomy or a first/second-degree perineum tear. Therefore, there is a need for accessible, functional equipment to ensure the provision of high-quality care during the intrapartum stage to minimize substandard care practices, thereby reducing risks of preventable mortality and morbidity in mothers and newborn babies.

Since 1997, the National Committee on Confidential Enquiries into Maternal Deaths (NCCEMD) has meticulously recorded and analysed all maternal deaths within institutions [13]. They have produced seven comprehensive reports on this issue in South Africa. The reports provide detailed information about the extent of maternal deaths, the types of diseases that cause them and the factors contributing to these deaths, including missed opportunities and inadequate healthcare. Limpopo Province had a maternal mortality rate of 165.16 per 100,000 live births according to the latest NCCEMD report published in January 2018, despite implementing the Saving Mothers and Babies Report 2017–2019 recommendations [14,15].

The current paper aims to ascertain how equipment impedes optimal intrapartum monitoring and delivery for pregnant women in labour units in four selected hospitals in the Sekhukhune District of Limpopo Province, South Africa. The study findings will contribute to the body of knowledge in achieving the objective of the South African Department of Health National Strategy, which aims to improve timeliness, coverage, and quality of antenatal care; manage high-risk pregnancies; and achieve optimal intrapartum monitoring and delivery of pregnant women. In addition, we highlight the status quo of the Sustainable Development Agenda, to be realised by 2030, in terms of Goal 3, which seeks to ensure healthy lives and promote well-being for all ages by reducing the global maternal mortality ratio to less than 70 per 100,000 live births.

2. Material and Methods

2.1. Study Site

A quantitative cross-sectional research design was used to identify and ascertain equipment that may impede quality intrapartum monitoring and delivery for pregnant women in the labour unit. The study was conducted in the labour units of four selected hospitals of Limpopo Province in the Sekhukhune Health District. Limpopo is the fifth largest province of nine in South Africa, covering 10.3% of South Africa's total land area. The province borders neighbouring countries such as Botswana to the west, Zimbabwe to the north, and Mozambique to the east. The province comprises five district hospitals, all rendering intrapartum and delivery care services to pregnant women. Sekhukhune Health District has a capacity of 998 approved beds and 679 actual usable beds, with most labour units having an average bed occupancy of 28–30. These four rural-based hospitals offer maternity health services to pregnant women from rural communities in the Sekhukhune District of Limpopo Province, South Africa.

2.2. Population and Sampling

The study's target population was midwives working in the labour units of the four selected hospitals in Sekhukhune District, who provide care to pregnant women during the intrapartum stage. These midwives were appropriate for this study because they monitor pregnant women during the intrapartum stage and conduct deliveries for pregnant women. Non-probability total sampling was used in the study to select midwives that were interested in taking part in the study. A total population sample of 59 midwives was used because of the small number of midwives working in the selected hospitals' labour units.

2.3. Data Collection

Data was collected by the primary researcher using self-developed questionnaires to determine the equipment that may be likely to impede optimal intrapartum care and delivery for pregnant women in labour units. Data collection was conducted after obtaining ethical clearance from the Turfloop Research Ethical Committee (TREC/82/2021: PG). Subsequently, the study sought permission from the Limpopo health department, the Director of Sekhukhune district hospitals, the chief executive officers of the selected hospitals in the Sekhukhune district, and unit managers of labour units. Permission was also obtained from midwives working in labour units who voluntarily participated in the study.

The questionnaires were formulated after reviewing the literature and validated with Cronbach's alpha (697). The final questionnaires were presented to the supervisor, co-supervisor, and data statistician and were restructured in line with the study objectives. A pilot study was conducted using a sample of seven midwives to assess the readability of the questions, the difficulty, and the time it took to complete the questionnaires. The primary author collected data from February to April 2022 using a self-administered questionnaire. A total of 59 self-administered English-written questionnaires consisting of 4 sections were distributed, with a response rate of 100%. Significantly, the questionnaire used a Likert scale with scores ranging from one to five. The options were Strongly Agree (SA), Agree (A), Strongly Disagree (SD), Disagree (D), and Uncertain (U).

The sections were as follows: Section A: Demographic Data; Section B: The Nurse's Role in the Use of Equipment; Section C: Equipment availability, effectiveness, and maintenance during the intrapartum stage; Section D: Delivery packs. The researcher approached midwives when they had no patients in labour and during their lunch breaks with their agreement to complete the questionnaire, which took 20–30 min.

2.4. Data Analysis

The completed questionnaires were extracted, coded, and captured using the Microsoft Excel programme (2016) and imported into the IBM Statistical Package for Social Science (SSPS) program, version 25.0, for analysis. Descriptive statistics were used to describe and facilitate the interpretation of the findings. Categorical variables were presented as numbers and percentages. Continued variables were presented as mean standard deviations.

2.5. Reliability and Validity of the Study

Reliability in this study was ensured by conducting a pre-test on 10% (7) of the study population in the labour unit. The pilot or pre-test assessed whether the questionnaires measured what they intended to measure and if the time allocated was adequate. Midwives and accoucheurs in labour units were given instructions before completing the questionnaires. Notably, the hospital used for the pilot study was not one of the selected hospitals. Notably, the small-scale study did not change the primary data collection tool.

The content validity of the questionnaires was ensured by performing an in-depth literature review to evaluate if the content of the questionnaires could achieve the study's objectives and by providing a questionnaire to a researcher with expertise in quantitative research. The questionnaires were also submitted to the supervisor, co-supervisor, and statistician for review, and changes were made in accordance with biostatistician recommendations.

3. Presentation of the Study Findings

3.1. Section A: Demographic Profile of the Participants

The demographic profile of participants is presented according to age distribution, gender, qualifications, years of working experience, and qualification distribution as depicted in Figures 1 and 2 below. As illustrated in Figure 1, the total number of midwives who participated in this study was 59, with the age distributions of the midwives ranging from 20 to 59 years, and a majority of the respondents in this study were female (91%). Furthermore, in this study, most midwives possessed registered midwifery qualifications (95%). In addition, most midwives had five years or more of working experience (49%), and most midwives were working day duty (74%).

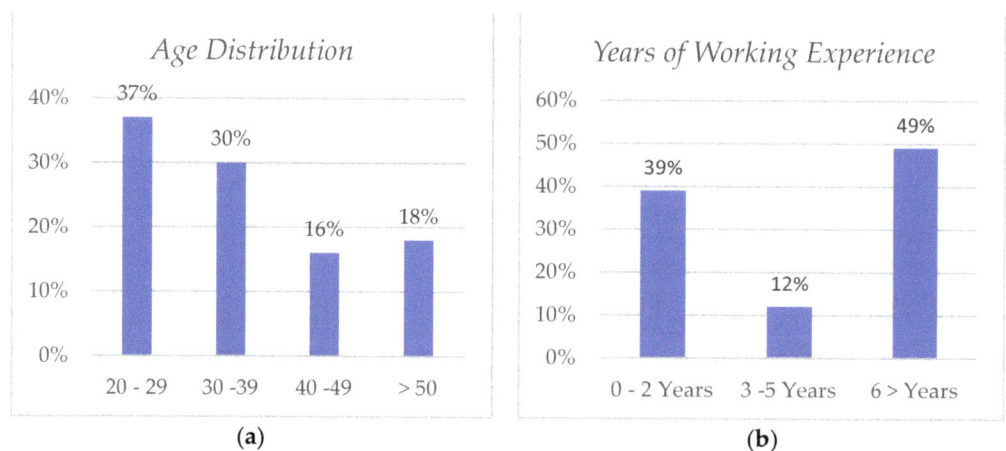

Figure 1. Age (**a**) and years of working experience (**b**).

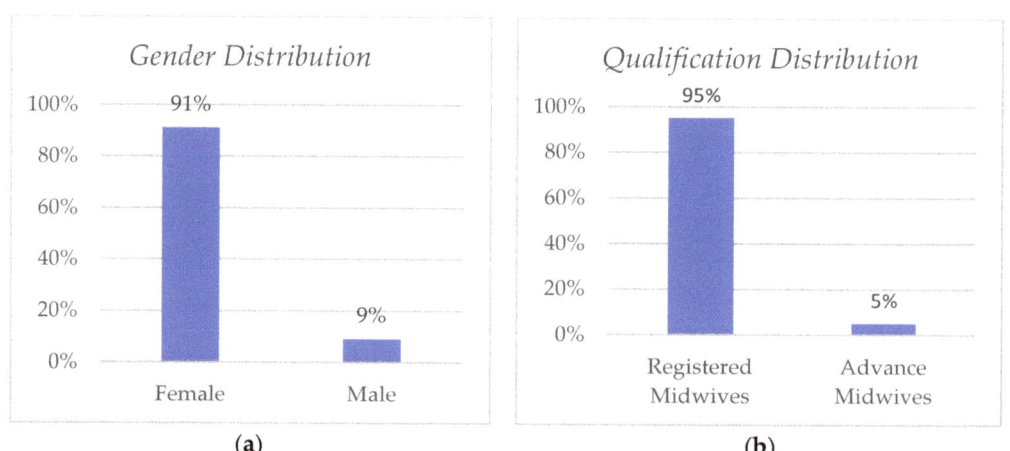

Figure 2. Gender (**a**) and qualification distribution (**b**).

3.2. Section B: Midwives' Roles Regarding the Use of Equipment

As depicted in Figure 3, 100% of respondents (57) knew their roles regarding the use of equipment in the labour unit, 68% (39) experienced barriers with the use of equipment when administering care to pregnant women, 81% (46) indicated that equipment used in the labour unit needed improvement, and 70% (40) indicated that reported non-functional equipment was not attended to promptly. However, 74% (42) indicated that there were quality care practices for pregnant women with the use of equipment in the labour unit.

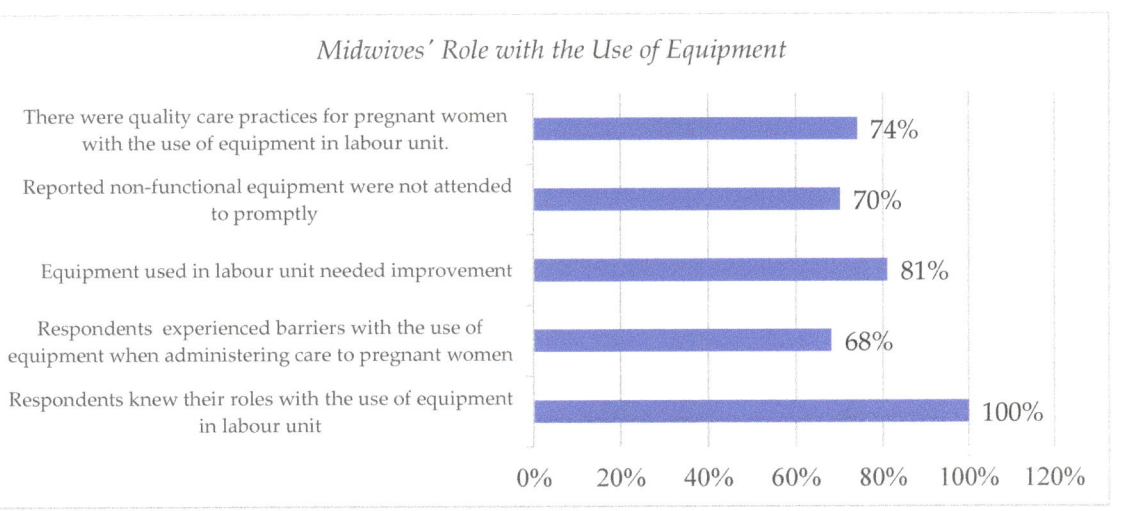

Figure 3. Midwives' roles regarding the use of equipment.

3.3. Section C: Equipment Availability, Effectiveness, and Maintenance during the Intrapartum Stage

As depicted in Table 1, 61% of midwives (35) strongly agreed that the blood pressure (BP) machine was available, and 49% (28) indicated that the BP machine was fully functional. However, 37% (21) of respondents strongly disagreed that BP machines in the labour unit adequately monitor all women during the intrapartum stage and labour. In total, 41% (24) midwives strongly agreed that only one BP machine is used for all pregnant women in the labour unit. Shockingly, 32% (18) of respondents strongly disagreed that BP machines undergo routine maintenance or service.

About 68% (39) of the respondents indicated that a CTG machine was available. Majority of the respondents agreed that CTG machine was functional. Close to half (45% (31)) of the respondents strongly agreed that CTG paper stripes were always available. In addition to equipment availability, effectiveness, and maintenance during the intrapartum stage, 68% of the midwives (39) indicated that they knew the benefits of using a CTG machine, and 44% (25) of midwives also agreed that they could interpret the CTG results. The study results revealed that 49% (28) indicated that a foetal heart rate (FHR) monitor was available and also that 51% (29) of the respondents agreed that the FHR monitor used in the labour unit provides accurate results. However, 43% of midwives (24) strongly felt that the FHR monitor needed improvement.

Table 1. Equipment availability, effectiveness, and maintenance during the intrapartum stage.

Equipment Used during the Intrapartum Stage	SA % (n)	A % (n)	SD % (n)	D % (n)	U % (n)
BP machine is available	61% (35)	37% (21)	0% (0)	2% (1)	0% (0)
BP machine is fully functional (give correct readings)	49% (28)	43% (25)	4% (2)	0% (0)	4% (2)
BP machines available are adequate to monitor all women during the intrapartum stage and labour	28% (16)	9% (5)	37% (21)	24% (14)	2% (1)
Routine maintenance or service of BP machines is performed	24% (14)	23% (13)	32% (18)	17% (10)	4% (2)
Only one BP machine is used for all pregnant women in the labour unit	41% (24)	18% (10)	29% (17)	12% (6)	0% (0)
CTG machine is available	68% (39)	32% (18)	0% (0)	0% (0)	0% (0)
CTG machine is functioning well	47% (27)	38% (22)	9% (5)	4% (2)	2% (1)
CTG paper rolls are always available	45% (31)	30% (17)	12% (7)	4% (2)	0% (0)
I know the benefits of using CTG during the intrapartum stage	68% (39)	32% (18)	0% (0)	0% (0)	0% (0)
I can interpret CTG results	44% (25)	35% (20)	12% (7)	4% (2)	5% (3)
FHR monitor is available	49% (28)	45% (26)	2% (1)	2% (1)	2% (1)
Equipment for monitoring FHR provides accurate readings	35% (20)	51% (29)	5% (3)	4% (2)	5% (3)
There is a need to improve the equipment used for monitoring FHR	43% (24)	29% (17)	11% (6)	16% (9)	2% (1)
The bed capacity is enough to meet the patient demand	19% (11)	18% (10)	28% (16)	35% (20)	0% (0)
Examination lights are available in each delivery room	21% (12)	32% (18)	24% (14)	23% (13)	0% (0)
Examination lights are functioning well in each delivery room	21% (12)	19% (11)	32% (18)	28% (16)	0% (0)
Overhead radiant warmer is available in each delivery room	18% (10)	19% (11)	37% (21)	26% (15)	0% (0)
Overhead radiant warmers are fully functional in each delivery room	19% (11)	14% (8)	51% (29)	16% (9)	0% (0)
Overhead radiant warmers are adequate to meet newborn demands	18% (10)	16% (9)	44% (25)	22% (13)	0% (0)
Examination scales for newborns are available in each delivery room	19% (11)	23% (13)	32% (18)	26% (15)	0% (0)
Examination scales for newborns are functioning well	6% (3)	9% (5)	54% (31)	31% (18)	0% (0)

According to this study, 35% (20) of the participants disagreed that the capacity of beds is sufficient to cater to the needs of patients. In addition, 32% of the respondents (18) agreed that examination lights were available in each delivery room. However, 32% (18) of the midwives strongly disagreed that the examination lights were functioning well. Furthermore, in this study, 37% (21) of the midwives strongly disagreed that an overhead radiant warmer was available in each delivery room, and the majority, 51% (29), strongly disagreed that the radiant warmer was fully functional in each delivery room. In addition, 44% (25) of respondents indicated that the overhead radiant warmer was inadequate to meet newborn demands. In addition to the equipment used during the intrapartum stage, 31% (18) of respondents strongly disagreed that newborn examination scales are available in each delivery room. Equally, the majority, 54% (31), strongly disagreed that examination scales for newborns were functioning well.

3.4. Section D: Delivery Packs

As depicted in Table 2, most of the respondents, 63% (37), strongly agreed that delivery packs were available, and 35% (20) strongly agreed that delivery packs were always complete inside. In addition, this study's findings suggest that most of the midwives, 51% (29), agreed that arterial forceps were available in each delivery pack, and 38% of respondents (21) agreed that arterial forceps were functioning well. Regarding the availability of needle holders, 38% of respondents (22) agreed that they were available in all delivery packs. However, 40% (23) of respondents strongly disagreed that needle holders in each delivery pack were functioning well.

Table 2. Delivery Packs.

Delivery Packs	SA % (n)	A % (n)	SD % (n)	D % (n)	U % (n)
Delivery packs are available	63% (37)	37% (20)	0 (0%)	0 (0%)	0 (0%)
Delivery packs are always complete inside	35% (20)	26% (15)	26% (15)	13% (7)	0 (0%)
Arterial forceps are available in each delivery pack	42% (24)	51% (29)	5% (3)	2% (1)	0 (0%)
Arterial forceps in each delivery pack are functioning well	35% (20)	38% (21)	19% (11)	5% (3)	3% (2)
Needle holder is available in all delivery packs	37% (21)	38% (22)	21% (12)	4% (2)	0% (0)
Needle holder in each delivery pack is functioning well	17% (10)	32% (18)	40% (23)	9% (5)	2% (1)
Some midwives do not use needle holders but instead use their own hands when suturing tears and episiotomy cuts	9% (5)	25% (14)	29% (17)	35% (20)	2% (1)
Umbilical cord scissors are available in each delivery pack	34% (19)	49% (27)	19% (11)	0% (0)	0% (0)
Some umbilical cord scissors are blunt (cannot cut)	38% (22)	46% (26)	7% (4)	9% (5)	0% (0)
I utilise a razor blade for cutting the umbilical cord in the absence of functional umbilical cord scissors	37% (21)	50% (29)	2% (1)	11% (6)	0% (0)
Episiotomy scissors are available in each delivery pack	26% (15)	51% (29)	16% (9)	7% (4)	0% (0)
Some episiotomy scissors are blunt	57% (33)	32% (18)	2% (1)	9% (5)	0% (0)
I utilise a razor blade for cutting episiotomies in the absence of functional episiotomy scissors	35% (20)	41% (23)	5% (3)	19% (11)	0% (0)

A total of 35% (20) of the respondents agreed that some midwives do not use needle holders but instead use their hands when suturing perineal tears and episiotomy cuts. In total, 49% (27) of the midwives in this study agreed that cord scissors were available in each delivery pack. Despite the availability of cord scissors, 46% of respondents (26) agreed that the umbilical cord scissors were blunt, and 50% (29) respondents agreed that they utilized a razor blade for cutting the umbilical cord in the absence of functional umbilical cord scissors. Most respondents, 51% (29), agreed that episiotomy scissors were available in each delivery pack. However, 57% (33) of respondents strongly agreed that episiotomy scissors were blunt, and 41% (23) agreed that razor blades were utilized in the absence of functional episiotomy scissors.

4. Discussion of Research Results

4.1. Demographic Profile of the Respondents

The study aimed to ascertain how equipment impedes optimal intrapartum monitoring and delivery for pregnant women in selected hospitals of Limpopo Province, South Africa. The respondents' demographic data provides information about the characteristics of the population who participated in the study.

Most of the respondents in this study were female (91%), compared with male respondents (9%). This discrepancy might be perpetuated for various reasons, such as cultural, religious, and gender stereotypes that men are not allowed to practice midwifery in some African contexts and pregnant women's beliefs that men are not allowed in maternity units [16]. Furthermore, midwifery care has historically been a female domain, owing to the widely held belief that midwifery is about a female relationship. Of the respondents, 37% were between the age of 20 and 29%, while those aged between 30 and 39% were represented by 30%. Nearly half (49%) of the respondents had six or more years of experience in labour unit. The findings of this study are consistent with those of a study conducted in maternity units at a public hospital in KwaZulu-Natal, where most participants were between 20 and 40 years of age, with an average of 12 years of working experience [17]. Furthermore, in this study, most midwives possessed registered midwifery qualifications (95%), and most midwives (74%) worked the day shift. By contrast, in Western Cape, a study conducted had 93 midwives who participated, and the night shift comprised 57 midwives, while the day shift had only 36 midwives [18].

4.2. Nurse's Role Regarding the Use of Equipment

A midwife or accoucheur is a person who has met the prescribed education requirements for registration as a midwife or accoucheur and who can assume responsibility and accountability for such practices [19]. In this study, all midwives (100%) knew their roles regarding the use of equipment when attending pregnant women in the selected hospitals in Limpopo Province. However, 68% of the respondents experienced challenges with using equipment when administering care to pregnant women, and that is because the non-functional equipment was not attended to promptly, as reported by most of the respondents (70%) in this study; equally, most of the midwives (81%) indicated that equipment used in the labour unit needed improvement. The literature corroborates the results of this study in that there is a challenge with the use of equipment in maternity units in Limpopo Province. For example, a qualitative study conducted in KwaZulu-Natal revealed that midwives found it challenging to perform their duties because of either faulty or unavailable equipment and materials, especially in public hospitals [20]. This implies that a lack of healthcare equipment impedes optimal intrapartum monitoring and delivery for pregnant women. Therefore, by addressing these challenges, the quality of nursing care provided to pregnant women during intrapartum monitoring and delivery can be improved, ultimately reducing complications that may arise from equipment shortages or malfunctioning.

4.3. Equipment Availability, Effectiveness, and Maintenance during the Intrapartum Stage

The current study looked at the equipment used during the intrapartum stage. More than half (61%) of the respondents agreed that BP machines were available. About 49% of the respondents believed that the BP machines were functional. However, the findings of this study revealed that, in the labour units of the selected hospitals, 37% (21) of respondents strongly disagreed that BP machines were adequate to monitor all pregnant women during the intrapartum period. In addition, a plurality (41%) strongly agreed that only one BP machine was used for all admitted pregnant women in the labour unit. The findings of this study are consistent with those of a quantitative study conducted in Limpopo Province in which most respondents (55%) reported that BP machines were functional in the labour room but were not adequate to cater to admitted pregnant women [6].

Concerning equipment for monitoring FHR in labour units, most respondents (51%) agreed that the FHR monitor in the labour unit provides accurate readings. However, most midwives (43%) strongly agreed that there is a need to improve the equipment used for monitoring FHR in the labour units. Moreover, most of the respondents (68%) in this study reported the availability of the CTG machine and its benefits during the intrapartum stage in the labour unit of the selected hospitals in Limpopo Province. In addition, 44% of the midwives knew how to interpret CTG results. The findings of this study are in contrast with the findings of a quantitative study, which revealed that midwives in KwaZulu-Natal public hospitals were clinically lacking in knowledge of CTG [21]. It is noteworthy to mention that the CTG machine is vital to monitor foetal well-being during the intrapartum stage. Thus, the World Health Organization emphasises that CTG knowledge is necessary for critical decision-making during intrapartum monitoring activities [22].

However, in the context of this study, caring for pregnant women during labour following maternity guidelines may not be the case in the selected hospitals in Limpopo

Province because of a lack of BP machines. For example, a guideline for maternity care in Guidelines for Maternity Care in South Africa requires midwives to monitor the blood pressure of pregnant women in labour upon admission; every four hours at the latent phase of labour; hourly at the active phase of labour and after the delivery of the placenta; and one post-delivery [23]. Supporting this assertion, a qualitative study conducted in Kenya, which had a similar rural setting background, revealed that a lack of essential equipment and commodities hindered the provision of standard maternity care [24]. Therefore, for midwives to provide quality maternity care, authorities must ensure that essential equipment and commodities are available in public hospitals.

High-quality intrapartum care is critical to the survival of the mother and the newborn [25]. However, the lack of essential equipment in this study was reported to be a potential impediment to the provision of quality care for pregnant women in the labour units of the selected hospitals. In total, 35% of midwives in this study disagreed that bed capacity is enough to meet patient demands. The findings of this study are consistent with those of studies conducted in various African regions. For example, a study in Kenya in Eastern Africa found that maternity units were overcrowded, resulting in some patients being discharged early to make room for others or even having to sleep on the floor because of a shortage of beds [26]. Similar results were observed in other African regions, such as the Southern African Developing Countries. In Gauteng Province, South Africa, midwives had to improvise to provide midwifery care because of a lack of bed capacity for pregnant women [27]. Notably, the lack of bed capacity to care for patients may be because of various reasons, including an influx of migrant and refugee patients from neighbouring countries, such as Zimbabwe and Mozambique [28,29]. Lack of adequate beds in the labour unit affects the quality of care for pregnant women, compromises their comfort, and impedes the quality of management given to pregnant women in labour.

Examination lights are essential during observations, as they provide suitable visibility and authentic images. However, in this study, examination lights were not all functioning well, as 28% of the respondents disagreed that examination lights functioned well in each delivery room. A qualitative study in Uganda found that poor infrastructure at maternity facilities frustrated health workers and made them feel they could not offer quality care to patients [30]. Adequate infrastructure with electricity and lighting is critical to health workers in rural areas such as Limpopo Province in providing quality healthcare. Shockingly, in this study, 37% of respondents agreed that overhead radiant warmers were available in each delivery room. However, 51% of respondents disagreed that overhead radiant were functioning well. In addition, they were not adequate to meet newborn demands, which affected the quality of care. The World Health Organization Practical Guide for the Thermal Control of the Newborn emphasises that the risk of neonatal hypothermia is significantly increased in labour units where policies, procedures, and equipment for maintaining an optimal thermal environment for the newborn are lacking [31]. The findings of this study suggest that there is a lack of implementation of policies that intend to ensure that quality healthcare is provided. As a result, newborns in labour units are exposed to hypothermia, a potentially dangerous drop in body temperature in newborn babies that causes complications [32].

Moreover, 32% of respondents strongly disagreed that examination scales were available in each labour unit. Similar findings were reported in a qualitative study conducted in Tanzania, where midwives reported a lack of sufficient and suitable weighing scales for newborns, which impedes the healthcare services of newborns [33]. Providing infants with holistic and comprehensive healthcare, such as calculating appropriate medication doses, fluids, and the early diagnosis of developmental defects, depends mainly on accurate birth weight [33,34]. Initiatives such as the Ideal Clinic programme are recommended to address the shortage of essential equipment in labour units. The "Ideal Clinic" is a healthcare facility with good infrastructure and adequate staff, medicine, and supplies of crucial health equipment, including partner and stakeholder support, thus ensuring quality healthcare services [35,36]. A lack of and malfunctions in medical equipment during labour can impact nursing care quality, hindering assessment, diagnosis, and the prevention of complications. Addressing issues related to malfunctioning equipment is imperative to achieve the objectives of Sustainable Development Goal 3, especially in rural areas where people have limited access to private healthcare practitioners because of their low socio-economic status.

4.4. The Delivery Packs

Concerning the equipment used during delivery in the selected hospitals in Limpopo Province, most respondents (63%) strongly agreed that delivery packs were available. In total, 35% of midwives strongly agreed that delivery packs are always complete inside. The findings of this study are in contrast with those of a mixed-method study conducted in four labour units in Zanzibar revealed that delivery packs were often incomplete [37]. In our study, most respondents (51%) agreed that arterial forceps were available in each delivery pack. In addition, 38% of respondents agreed that these arterial forceps were functioning well. The findings of this study also revealed that needle holders were available in all prepared delivery packs, as 38% of respondents agreed.

Despite the availability, 40% of midwives disagreed that the needle holders in each delivery pack were functioning well. In addition, 35% of respondents disagreed that some midwives do not use needle holders but instead use their hands when suturing tears and episiotomy cuts in delivery. Furthermore, 49% of respondents agreed that umbilical cord scissors are available in each delivery pack. However, 46% of midwives also reported that some umbilical cord scissors were blunt (they cannot cut). In addition, half of the respondents (50%) agreed that they used razor blades to cut umbilical cords when there were no functional scissors. The findings of this study are consistent with those of a quality assurance sampling survey conducted in two states of Nigeria, in which new razor blades were used to cut the newborn umbilical cord in about 75% of the deliveries in Bauchi and over 80% in Sokoto States [38]. Although a razor blade is not recommended to cut a newborn's umbilical cord, it is essential to mention that, during emergencies, using a sterile razor blade in practice is an appropriate alternative for cutting the umbilical cord.

Most respondents (51%) in this study agreed that episiotomy scissors were available in each delivery pack. However, 57% of respondents strongly agreed that some episiotomy scissors were blunt. TThus, in this study, 41% of midwives reported that razor blades were used for cutting episiotomies in cases where sharp or functional episiotomy scissors were unavailable. This study's findings contrast with the Guideline for Maternity Care in South Africa, in which episiotomy scissors are listed as essential equipment for maternal healthcare services [22]. Therefore, it is vital to incorporate mandatory computerised maintenance management software to improve the quality of maternity equipment in the labour unit [39]. The study results have significant implications. Using blunt scissors might contribute to serious birth injuries, and, more importantly, it can also increase the risk of perineal tears. Addressing this challenge to mitigate associated risks and enhance the quality of midwifery care provided during labour is highly recommended.

4.5. Limitations of the Study

Even though the study provides insight into equipment as a potential impediment to optimal intrapartum monitoring and delivery for pregnant women, the study results only provide a view of respondents from the selected hospitals in one district of Limpopo Province. Therefore, the study results cannot be generalized to other district hospitals or other hospitals in South Africa. The study was limited to a small population; other researchers can conduct studies that will include more hospitals in South Africa, hence more respondents, to gain more perspectives or views on the study topic, venturing into qualitative research to explore more opinions about the topic.

5. Conclusions

In conclusion, pregnant women face obstacles in receiving optimal intrapartum monitoring and delivery care due to insufficient equipment and inadequate maintenance. High-quality care is needed during labour to enhance positive birth outcomes. Therefore, it is recommended that the employer, the Department of Health, provide the required equipment to labour units and prioritize improving the equipment utilized in labour units with annual budgets by ensuring accessibility to available, adequate, and functional equipment and improving infrastructure. Incorporating mandatory computerized maintenance management software is recommended to improve the quality of maternity equipment. In addition, there is a need for regular equipment inspections and maintenance by skilled technicians in the selected hospitals of Limpopo Province, South Africa.

Author Contributions: Conceptualization, K.M.M., L.M. and M.G.M.; methodology, K.M.M. and M.O.M.; formal analysis, M.O.M. and T.A.P.; investigation, K.M.M.; data curation, K.M.M.; writing—original draft preparation, K.M.M. and T.A.N.; writing—review and editing, K.M.M. and T.A.N.; visualization, T.A.P.; supervision, L.M. and M.G.M. All authors have read and agreed to the published version of the manuscript.

Funding: This research received no external funding.

Institutional Review Board Statement: This study was conducted in accordance with the Declaration of Helsinki, and ethical clearance was obtained from the University of Turfloop Research Ethics Committee (TREC/82/2021: PG). Permission to conduct the study was obtained from the Limpopo Department of Health.

Informed Consent Statement: Informed consent was obtained from all subjects involved in the study.

Data Availability Statement: The data are not shared because of privacy and ethical restrictions.

Acknowledgments: The authors would like to thank the participants who gave consent to participate for their cooperation during the research process.

Conflicts of Interest: The authors declare no conflict of interest.

References

1. Masaba, B.B.; Mmusi-Phetoe, R. A Strategy for Reducing Maternal Mortality in Rural Kenya. *Int. J. Women's Health* **2023**, *31*, 487–498. [CrossRef] [PubMed]
2. Chandraharan, E.; Arulkumaran, S. *Obstetric and Intrapartum Emergencies*; Cambridge University Press: New York, NY, USA, 2021.
3. Cheyne, H.; Duff, M. *Anatomy and Physiology of Labour and Associated Behavioural Clues*; Squaring the Circle, Pinter & Martin: London, UK, 2019.
4. World Health Organization. *Standards for Improving Quality of Maternal and Newborn Care in Health Facilities*; WHO: Geneva, Switzerland, 2016.
5. Bradley, S.; McCourt, C.; Rayment, J.; Parmar, D. Midwives' perspectives on (dis) respectful intrapartum care during facility-based delivery in sub-Saharan Africa: A qualitative systematic review and meta-synthesis. *Reprod. Health* **2019**, *16*, 116. [CrossRef] [PubMed]
6. Ramavhoya, I.T.; Maputle, M.S.; Ramathuba, D.U.; Lebese, R.T.; Netshikweta, L.M. Managers' support on implementation of maternal guidelines, Limpopo province, South Africa. *Curationis* **2020**, *43*, e1–e9. [CrossRef] [PubMed]
7. Adams, T.; Mason, D.; Gebhardt, G.S. Moderate to severe neonatal encephalopathy with suspected hypoxic-ischaemic encephalopathy in cooled term infants born in Tygerberg Academic Hospital: Characteristics of fetal monitoring and modifiable factors. *S. Afr. J. Child Health* **2022**, *16*, 83–88. [CrossRef]
8. Masuda, C.; Ferolin, S.K.; Masuda, K.; Smith, C.; Matsui, M. Evidence-based intrapartum practice and its associated factors at a tertiary teaching hospital in the Philippines, a descriptive mixed-methods study. *BMC Pregnancy Childbirth* **2020**, *20*, 78. [CrossRef]
9. Sigalla, G.N.; Bakar, R.R.; Manongi, R.N. Experiences of facility-based delivery services among women of reproductive age in Unguja Island, Zanzibar: A Qualitative Study. *J. Fam. Med.* **2018**, *5*, 1149.
10. Koroma, M.M.; Kamara, M.A.; Keita, N.; Lokossou, V.K.; Sundufu, A.J.; Jacobsen, K.H. Access to Essential Medications and Equipment for Obstetric and Neonatal Primary Care in Bombali District, Sierra Leone. *World Med. Health Policy* **2019**, *11*, 8–23. [CrossRef]
11. Moyimane, M.B.; Matlala, S.F.; Kekana, M.P. Experiences of nurses on the critical shortage of medical equipment at a rural district hospital in South Africa: A qualitative study. *Pan Afr. Med. J.* **2017**, *28*, 157. [CrossRef]

12. South African Nursing Council. *Regulations Relating to the Conditions under Which Registered Midwives and Enrolled Midwives May Carry on Their Profession*; Regulation R. 2488; SANC: Pretoria, South Africa, 1990.
13. National Committee on Confidential Enquiries into Maternal Deaths. *Saving Mothers 2014–2016: Seventh Triennial Report on Confidential Enquiries into Maternal Deaths in South Africa*; National Department of Health South Africa: Pretoria, South Africa, 2018.
14. Bomela, N.J. Maternal mortality by socio-demographic characteristics and cause of death in South Africa: 2007–2015. *BMC Public Health* **2020**, *20*, 157. [CrossRef]
15. Mothapo, K.E.; Maputle, M.S.; Shilubane, H.N.; Netshikweta, L. Challenges Midwives in Limpopo Province Encounter when Implementing Saving Mothers Recommendations. *Open Nurs. J.* **2020**, *14*, 292–299. [CrossRef]
16. Madlala, S.T.; Ngxongo, T.S.; Sibiya, M.N. Perceptions of pregnant women regarding student accoucheurs' involvement in maternal health care in the Free State Province. *Int. J. Afr. Nurs. Sci.* **2020**, *13*, 100255. [CrossRef]
17. Mhlongo, N.M. Experiences of Midwives Regarding Practice Breakdown in Maternity Units at a Public Hospital in KwaZulu-Natal. Master's Thesis, Durban University of Technology, Durban, South Africa, 2016.
18. Phiri, L.P.; Draper, C.E.; Lambert, E.V.; Kolbe-Alexander, T.L. Nurses' lifestyle behaviours, health priorities and barriers to living a healthy lifestyle: A qualitative descriptive study. *BMC Nurs.* **2014**, *13*, 38. [CrossRef] [PubMed]
19. Martin, S. Quality care during childbirth at a midwife obstetric unit in Cape Town, Western Cape: Women and Midwives' perceptions. Master's Thesis, University of Western Cape, Western Cape, South Africa, 2018.
20. Mhlongo, N.M.; Sibiya, M.N.; Miya, R.M. Experiences of midwives regarding nursing practice breakdown in maternity units at a selected public hospital in KwaZula-Natal. *Afr. J. Nurs. Midwifery* **2016**, *18*, 162–178. [CrossRef]
21. James, S.; Maduna, N.E.; Morton, D.G. Knowledge levels of midwives regarding the interpretation of cardiotocographs at labour units in KwaZulu-Natal public hospitals. *Curationis* **2019**, *42*, 1–7. [CrossRef]
22. World Health Organization. *WHO Recommendations on Intrapartum Care for a Positive Childbirth Experience*; World Health Organization: Geneva, Switzerland, 2018.
23. National Department of Health, South Africa. Guidelines for Maternity Care in South Africa. In *A Manual for Clinics, Community Health Centres and District Hospitals*, 4th ed.; NDoH: Pretoria, South Africa, 2015; Volume 172.
24. Lusambili, A.; Wisofschi, S.; Shumba, C.; Obure, J.; Mulama, K.; Nyaga, L.; Wade, T.J.; Temmerman, M. Health Care Workers' Perspectives of the Influences of Disrespectful Maternity Care in Rural Kenya. *Int. J. Environ. Res. Public Health* **2020**, *17*, 8218. [CrossRef] [PubMed]
25. Brenner, S.; Madhavan, S.; Nseya, C.K.; Sese, C.; Fink, G.; Shapira, G. Competent and deficient provision of childbirth services: A descriptive observational study assessing the quality of intrapartum care in two provinces of the Democratic Republic of the Congo. *BMC Health Serv. Res.* **2022**, *22*, 551. [CrossRef]
26. Gitobu, C.M.; Gichangi, P.B.; Mwanda, W.O. Satisfaction with delivery services offered under the free maternal healthcare policy in Kenyan public health facilities. *J. Environ. Public Health* **2018**, *2018*, 4902864. [CrossRef]
27. Lumadi, T.G.; Matlala, M.S. Perceptions of midwives on shortage and retention of staff at a public hospital in Tshwane District. *Curationis* **2019**, *42*, 1–10.
28. Mutambara, V.M.; Naidu, M. Probing the Context of Vulnerability: Zimbabwean Migrant Women's Experiences of Accessing Public Health Care in South Africa. *Afr. Hum. Mobil. Rev.* **2021**, *7*, 1. [CrossRef]
29. Chekero, T.; Ross, F.C. "On paper" and "having papers": Zimbabwean migrant women's experiences in accessing healthcare in Giyani, Limpopo province, South Africa. *Anthropol. South. Afr.* **2018**, *41*, 41–54. [CrossRef]
30. Munabi-Babigumira, S.; Glenton, C.; Willcox, M.; Nabudere, H. Ugandan health workers' and mothers' views and experiences of the quality of maternity care and the use of informal solutions: A qualitative study. *PLoS ONE* **2019**, *14*, e0213511. [CrossRef]
31. World Health Organization. *Thermal Control of the Newborn: A Practical Guide*; Maternal Health and Safe Motherhood Programme, Division of Family Health; WHO: Geneva, Switzerland, 1993.
32. Dey, K.; Deb, U.K. Modeling and simulation of heat transfer phenomenon from infant radiant warmer for a newborn baby. *Open J. Model. Simul.* **2021**, *9*, 111. [CrossRef]
33. Gladstone, M.E.; Salim, N.; Ogillo, K.; Shamba, D.; Gore-Langton, G.R.; Day, L.T.; Blencowe, H.; Lawn, J.E. Birthweight measurement processes and perceived value: Qualitative research in one EN-BIRTH study hospital in Tanzania. *BMC Pregnancy Childbirth* **2021**, *21*, 232. [CrossRef] [PubMed]
34. Weres, A.; Baran, J.; Czenczek-Lewandowska, E.; Leszczak, J.; Mazur, A. Impact of Birth Weight and Length on Primary Hypertension in Children. *Int. J. Environ. Res. Public Health* **2019**, *16*, 4649. [CrossRef]
35. Ideal Clinic Manual. Ideal Clinic Definitions, Components and Checklists. National Department of Health. Version.19. 2020. Available online: https://www.knowledgehub.org.za/elibrary/ideal (accessed on 9 April 2023).
36. Muthelo, L.; Moradi, F.; Phukubye, T.A.; Mbombi, M.O.; Malema, R.N.; Mabila, L.N. Implementing the ideal clinic program at selected primary healthcare facilities in South Africa. *Int. J. Environ. Res. Public Health* **2021**, *18*, 7762. [CrossRef] [PubMed]
37. De Barra, M.; Gon, G.; Woodd, S.; Graham, W.J.; de Bruin, M.; Kahabuka, C.; Williams, A.J.; Konate, K.; Ali, S.M.; Said, R.; et al. Understanding infection prevention behaviour in maternity wards: A mixed-methods analysis of hand hygiene in Zanzibar. *Soc. Sci. Med.* **2021**, *272*, 113543. [CrossRef] [PubMed]

38. Abegunde, D.; Orobaton, N.; Beal, K.; Bassi, A.; Bamidele, M.; Akomolafe, T.; Ohanyido, F.; Umar-Farouk, O.; Danladi, S.A. Trends in newborn umbilical cord care practices in Sokoto and Bauchi States of Nigeria: The where, who, how, what and the ubiquitous role of traditional birth attendants: A lot quality assurance sampling survey. *BMC Pregnancy Childbirth* **2017**, *17*, 368. [CrossRef]
39. Mkalaf, K.; Gibson, P.; Flanagan, J. A study of current maintenance strategies and the reliability of critical medical equipment in hospitals in relation to patient outcomes. *Int. J. Manag.* **2013**, *7*, 15–28.

Disclaimer/Publisher's Note: The statements, opinions and data contained in all publications are solely those of the individual author(s) and contributor(s) and not of MDPI and/or the editor(s). MDPI and/or the editor(s) disclaim responsibility for any injury to people or property resulting from any ideas, methods, instructions or products referred to in the content.

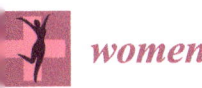 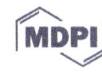

Article

Knowledge, Propensity and Hesitancy among Pregnant Women in the Post-Pandemic Phase Regarding COVID-19 Vaccination: A Prevalence Survey in Southern Italy

Cristina Genovese *,†, Carmela Alessia Biondo †, Caterina Rizzo †, Rosaria Cortese, Isabella La Spina, Paola Tripodi, Bruno Romeo, Vincenza La Fauci, Giuseppe Trimarchi, Vanessa Lo Prete and Raffaele Squeri

Department of Biomedical and Dental Sciences and Morphofunctional Imaging, University of Messina, 98125 Messina, Italy
* Correspondence: cristinagenovese86@gmail.com; Tel.: +39-3240523204
† These authors contributed equally to this work.

Abstract: The vaccination of pregnant women against influenza and COVID-19 may reduce the risk of severe illness in both the women of this population and their babies. Although the risks of non-vaccination are more serious than the side effects, maternal immunization is still the least-used method of prevention due to a lack of information leading to concerns about the safety and efficacy of vaccines, resulting in a low prevalence rate among pregnant individuals. Our study investigates vaccination coverage and the knowledge, attitudes and perceptions of COVID-19 in pregnant women at a university hospital. A questionnaire was created with the following three scores: a vaccination propensity score, a knowledge score and a hesitancy score. The first observation in the results was the very low number of immunized women (only 4.7% received their first dose). The main barrier towards vaccination was found to be fear of adverse events. We noticed a low percentage of influenza and diphtheria tetanus pertussis vaccination compared to other studies. Vaccination propensity was higher when healthcare workers educated their patients. As immunization is a crucial part of public health policy, measuring coverage to identify gaps and monitor trends, especially for individuals considered at high risk, and developing new strategies in order to increase awareness of vaccination during pregnancy is particularly timely and relevant.

Keywords: socioeconomic factors; knowledge; propensity

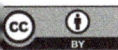

1. Introduction

Vaccination hesitancy is a known phenomenon among various population groups and several socio-cultural contexts [1–4], and it is defined as a delay in accepting or a total refusal of vaccination despite the availability of vaccination services related to information and administration. A particular group for whom hesitancy might be higher is pregnant women. Pregnancy is a particular moment in a woman's lifetime, as she can be exposed to several pathogens affecting both the mother's and the fetus' health, resulting in an increased risk of developing severe disease or complications [5]. Several studies have shown the potential benefits of maternal immunization, mainly related to protection against harmful effects that could be caused by infection such as miscarriage, preterm birth, emergency cesarean section or low birth weight; this protection is effected by inducing the production and transfer of immunoglobulin G through the placenta, as well as expressing secretory antibodies in breast milk [6]. The course of the COVID-19 pandemic, the rapid development of vaccines and a strict immunization campaign have paradoxically led to conflicting opinions, with the end result that acceptance and its predictors among women vary globally [5]. In early 2021, the European Medicines Agency (EMA) approved the following five COVID-19 vaccines: two of them were mRNA vaccines (Pfizer-BioNTech and Moderna), two were viral vector-based vaccines (Oxford-AstraZeneca and Janssen), and one was a protein subunit vaccine (Novavax) [7]. None of them were tested on pregnant women in preclinical trials or pre-marketing clinical trials [7]. Consequently, the main data for their use in pregnancy come from post-marketing surveillance [8]. Due to a lack of knowledge regarding the safety of vaccines, immunization coverage among pregnant women is low despite the existence of solid scientific data to support its effectiveness and safety [9]. This implies that pregnant women only have the following two options: trust science, family, or any other available source of information and receive the vaccine, even with limited data; or skip the vaccine, leaving themselves and their babies vulnerable to adverse events or severe disease caused by COVID-19. Furthermore, common side effects of the Pfizer-BioNTech vaccination were reported by pregnant [10] and non-pregnant women in similar percentages and the administration of the vaccine is not linked with harmful effects. Few cases of gestational hypertension, childbirth issues, miscarriage and premature birth after receiving the Pfizer-BioNTech vaccine have been reported [10]. The indications for vaccination in pregnant women come from the Obstetrics and Gynecology Societies, which suggest that pregnant women choose whether or not to be vaccinated after consulting with their gynecologists and evaluating the risks and benefits [11].

Although the risks of non-vaccination are more serious than the side effects [7], only 11 of the 20 major countries affected by COVID-19 offer free vaccination to pregnant women. [8]

A meta-analysis conducted on the "Consequences and Implications of Coronavirus Disease (COVID-19) on pregnancy and infants" found that the most common symptoms in pregnant women were fever, cough, chest pain, dyspnea and fatigue. Most newborns were delivered preterm and by cesarean section, which sometimes led to abortion. Neonatal outcomes included fetal suffering, low birth weight, APGAR < 7, hospitalization in the neonatal intensive care unit and fetal mortality [11,12]. In Italy, starting in January 2021, artificial immunization with mRNA vaccines was recommended for pregnant women with comorbidities or an increased risk of disease (i.e., healthcare workers) from the second trimester of pregnancy onwards [13]. Moreover, since the beginning of the pandemic, the Italian Obstetric Surveillance System (ItOSS), directed by the Istituto Superiore di Sanità (Italian National Institute of Health, INIH), launched a national survey to identify the effect of COVID-19 on pregnancy [14]. Vaccinating pregnant women with the flu (influenza) vaccine, tetanus toxoid, reduced diphtheria toxoid, acellular pertussis vaccine (DTaP) and COVID-19 vaccine may reduce their risk and their babies' risk of developing severe illness or complications from these infections. The Advisory Committee on Immunization Practices (ACIP) recommends that all pregnant or suspected pregnant women receive the flu vaccine during flu season, which can be given at any time during pregnancy [15]. The ACIP also recommends that women receive DTaP during each pregnancy, preferably in the third trimester, between 28 and 32 weeks of gestation [16]. Increasing awareness among pregnant women [15] about vaccinations that can be administered during pregnancy greatly reduces the risk of the mother and child developing not only the acute form of the disease but also its complications. Given the greater likelihood of developing gestational and/or postpartum complications, in Italy, flu vaccination is strongly recommended in pregnant women regardless of trimester [16], as also affirmed by the Ministerial Circular "Prevention and control of flu: recommendations for season 2022–2023".

Vaccination coverage for COVID-19 is very low in pregnant women; a study conducted in Scotland showed that in the general female population of 18–44 years, only 32.3% of pregnant women had two doses of the vaccine, compared to 77.4% of all women [17]. Moreover, in an American study, only 11.1% of women had completed vaccinations during pregnancy, with differences across age and race. [18]

In a UK study, data were available for 1328 pregnant women, of whom 140 received at least one dose of the COVID-19 vaccine before giving birth and 1188 did not; of those vaccinated, 85.7% received their vaccine in the third trimester of pregnancy and 14.3% in their second trimester of pregnancy. Surprisingly, in an Italian study, vaccination coverage was reported to be equal between pregnant and non-pregnant women for 80% of the sample [19]. The aims of this study are as follows: a) to investigate COVID-19 vaccination coverage in pregnant women attending prepartum programs, ambulatorial visits or routine visits in the province of Messina at a university hospital; b) to evaluate the knowledge of attitudes towards and perceptions of COVID-19 vaccines in pregnant women and the main drivers that motivate or delay vaccination.

2. Materials and Methods

This study was conducted from November 2022 to December 2022, during the anti-flu vaccination campaign, through an ad hoc survey; it was administered using a computer-assisted web interview technique (via Google® forms) to all pregnant women attending prepartum programs, ambulatorial visits or routine visits in the Gynecology and Obstetrics ward of the Polyclinic G. Martino di Messina. All the investigated women chose to participate in the interview (response rate 100%).

The questionnaire had five sections (see Supplementary Material) and was created ad hoc. The first section collected information about socio-demographic status; willingness to undergo recommended vaccinations during pregnancy, such as for DTaP and flu; previous infection with COVID-19; concomitant pathologies; possible drug therapies. The second part was then focused on elements related to knowledge of the vaccine, such as how many doses comprised the primary cycle and knowledge about the possibility of receiving the vaccine during pregnancy and lactation; following this, the third part investigated the most commonly used information sources. In the fourth part, attitude regarding vaccination against COVID-19 was evaluated via short form utilizing the 6-item anti-vaccine scale, which was prepared as a 5-point Likert scale [17]. Women who wanted to receive vaccination or who had already been vaccinated were asked questions regarding their motivations for doing so; women who were not yet vaccinated or unwilling to do so were instead asked questions about their reasons or possible obstacles. A final section gave the opportunity to receive further information on the subject by submitting a telephone number.

The following three scores were designated based on the items posed on the survey: (a) the vaccination propensity score, (b) the vaccine knowledge score and (c) the vaccine hesitancy score.

The vaccine propensity score (VPS) evaluates the propensity and adherence to vaccination using 11 items on the Likert scale. The following scores were assigned based on the given answer: 0 points for disagreement; 1 for a neutral response; 2 for agreement.

The same method was used for the 9 questions asked to create the vaccine hesitancy score (VHS). This score and the corresponding questions were directed at pregnant women who did not receive vaccination for COVID-19.

Regarding the knowledge score (KS), 4 multiple choice questions were constructed where basic knowledge about the COVID-19 vaccine was evaluated. Zero points were given to incorrect or negative answers and one point was given to correct or positive answers.

Statistical Analysis

The median and IQR were calculated for the quantitative variables (age and score), while the absolute and relative frequencies were obtained for the categorical data (vaccination status).

All possible associations between score and the collected data were investigated.

Scores were assessed by evaluating normality verifications through the Shapiro–Wilk test, which allowed us to ascertain the non-normality of the three scores. Comparisons between covariates with two encodings were assessed using the Mann–Whitney test; for covariates with three factors (age and gestational period), comparisons were performed using the Kruskal–Wallis test and its post hoc nonparametric (Conover's test). The threshold for statistical significance was set at $p = 0.050$; p-values of less than 0.050 on two-tailed tests were considered statistically significant. The summary and inferential statistics were analyzed using R software.

3. Results

The sample consisted of 127 women with a mean age of 30.91 ± SD 5.42. The main socio-demographic data are represented in Table 1.

Table 1. Distribution of the study sample according to sociodemographic data.

	N	%
Mean age± SD	30.91 ± SD 5.42	
Employment		
Public employee	21	16.5
Private Employee	48	37.8
Housewife	33	26
Other	4	3.1
Freelance	21	16.5
Educational attainment		
Less than 8 years	14	11
More than 8 years	113	89
Living in ...		
Suburbs	81	63.8
Center	46	36.2
Gestational age		
1st	12	9.6
2nd	28	22.4
3rd	85	68
Level of COVID-19 vaccine received		
No doses	14	11
1st dose	6	4.7
2nd dose	49	38.6
3rd dose	58	45.7

In our sample, 11% of the pregnant women did not undergo vaccination and 4.7% were partially artificially immunized. In our sample, the percentage of vaccinated subjects was higher in the healthy group (72.8%) than in the sick one (5.6%), with significant statistical differences ($p < 0.05$). Moreover, the uptake of flu (28.4%) and DTaP (27.2%) vaccinations among pregnant women was investigated, and among the not-vaccinated group, only 16.5% ($n = 17$) wanted to receive the flu vaccine and 31.1% ($n = 28$) wanted to receive the DTaP vaccine.

Based on education level and age, the occurrence of statistically significant differences in COVID-19 vaccination status was examined. Significant associations were found between the level of education and patient adherence to vaccinations, with a greater number of vaccinated persons with higher levels of education ($p < 0.01$).

The main information sources used were radio and television ($n = 69$; 54.3%), followed by official sources such as the Ministry of Health ($n = 14$; 11%) and healthcare workers (i.e., obstetricians, gynecologists, general practitioners and hygienists) ($n = 35$; 31.59%).

Another emerging trend was the presence of a correlation between the sources of information and the propensity for vaccination as follows: a greater number of unvaccinated pregnant women were informed by the media ($p < 0.01$), while the main source of information for vaccinated subjects was healthcare workers. Regarding knowledge about vaccination, most of the subjects (73.8%) did not know the correct schedule for the COVID-19 vaccine. That being said, most of the interviewees recognized its value and the importance of receiving the vaccination during pregnancy and breastfeeding.

The analysis of the data showed that the motivational factors comprise the geographical accessibility and availability of vaccination centers (70.5%) and willingness to pay or the presence of a free vaccination program (69.1%). More than half of the sample considered it essential to protect themselves from infection (58.1%) and then transmit immunity to the child (60.1%). In addition, in more than 70% of cases, there was a strong recommendation from the gynecologist and midwife. Additionally, 69.9% of the sample recommended vaccination to friends and relatives (Table 2).

Regarding the factors hindering vaccination in women who were not immunized, there was a willingness to await data concerning the effects of vaccination on pregnant and breastfeeding women (70.5%). In particular, 47.4% referred to the lack of data on the effects of COVID-19 vaccination in pregnant women. As observed in another Italian study [18], 70.1% of the unvaccinated pregnant sample would prefer to immunize themselves naturally via COVID-19 infection instead of by vaccination. Accessibility to vaccination centers was not an impeding factor in 75% of the unvaccinated women examined, demonstrating that the main factor of vaccination hesitancy is not a lack of accessibility due to logistical or physical difficulties but rather concerns regarding the long-term effects of vaccination (Table 3).

Table 2. Motivators to receive vaccination from interviews with immunized subjects. ^: the sum of the numbers does not correspond to the sample total due to the absence of some answers.

	Certainly Not % (n)	Probably No % (n)	Maybe Yes Maybe No % (n)	Probably Yes % (n)	Yes of Course % (n)
Protect myself from infection	9.2 (11)	14.1 (17)	13.3 (16)	27.3 (33)	30.8 (37)
Transmission of maternal immunity to my children	5.7 (7)	16.9 (21)	16.3 (20)	21.1 (26)	39 (48)
Availability of free vaccination	8.1 (10) ^	7.4 (9)	15.4 (19)	36.6 (45)	32.5 (40)
Accessibility of vaccination center to get vaccine	4.1 (5)	15.6 (19)	9.8 (12)	24.6 (30)	45.9 (56)
Recommendation from my own gynecologist	1.8 (2)	5.3 (6)	15.9 (18)	40.7 (46)	36.3 (41)
Recommendation from my own obstetric	4.5 (5)	3.6 (4)	20.5 (23)	39.3 (44)	32.1 (36)
It gives more benefits rather than risk	1.8 (2)	4.4 (5)	29.2 (33)	30.1 (34)	34.5 (39)
It is a social liability	1.8 (2)	1.8 (2)	22.1 (25)	28.3 (32)	46 (52)
I would like to get COVID-19 vaccine	9.2 (11)	14.1 (17)	13.3 (16)	27.3 (33)	30.8 (37)
I would like propose vaccination to my friends and relatives	8.1 (10) ^	7.4 (9)	15.4 (19)	36.6 (45)	32.5 (40)

Table 3. Obstacles to receiving vaccination from interviews with non-immunized subjects. ^: the sum of the numbers does not correspond to the sample total due to the absence of some answers.

	Certainly Not % (n)	Probably No % (n)	Maybe Yes Maybe No % (n)	Probably Yes % (n)	Yes of Course % (n)
I am in the 1st trimester of pregnancy ^	39.4 (13)	30.3 (10)	3 (1)	21.2 (7)	6.1 (2)
Difficult access to vaccination center ^	33.3 (12)	41.7 (15)	16.7 (6)	5.6 (2)	2.8 (1)

Table 3. Cont.

	Certainly Not % (n)	Probably No % (n)	Maybe Yes Maybe No % (n)	Probably Yes % (n)	Yes of Course % (n)
Inefficacy or defective of vaccine ^	21.1 (8)	18.4 (7)	21.1 (8)	23.7 (9)	15.8 (6)
The clinical trials did not include pregnant and breastfeeding women ^	5.3 (2)	21.1 (8)	26.3 (10)	26.3 (10)	21.1 (8)
I think that there is an effect on my own child through breastfeeding ^	7.9 (3)	31.6 (12)	18.4 (7)	28.9 (11)	13.2 (5)
The vaccine was promoted for financial reasons by pharmaceutical companies ^	27 (10)	18.9 (7)	13.5 (5)	18.9 (7)	21.6 (8)
I prefer to get natural immunity rather than to get vaccine ^	5.7 (7)	16.9 (21)	16.3 (20)	21.1 (26)	39 (48)
I would like to get vaccine after the evaluation of side effects in pregnancy women and breastfeeding ^	4.1 (5)	15.6 (19)	9.8 (12)	24.6 (30)	45.9 (56)

Further data were obtained by comparing the knowledge score and the propensity score (Table 4). Uncovering a trend of increasing value with increasing age. It also emerged that the propensity score increased for older subjects with a higher level of education (more than 8 years of study). The hesitation score was only highly associated with COVID-19 vaccination status ($p < 0.001$) in non-vaccinated subjects.

Table 4. Knowledge, propensity and hesitancy scores (median, 25° percentile and 75° percentile) by age, educational degree, COVID-19 status, gestational age and comorbidities.

	Age			p Value
	18–24	25–34	>35	
Knowledge Score	1 (1;1)	3 (1;3)	3 (2;3)	0.001
Propensity Score	12 (10;16)	19 (11;21)	20 (17;22)	0.003
Hesitancy Score	4 (4;8)	4 (2;4)	4 (1;4)	0.073
	Educational degree			
	Less than 8 years		More than 8 years	
Knowledge Score	1 (1;2)		3 (1;3)	0.005
Propensity Score	11 (2;12)		20 (14;21)	0.001
Hesitancy Score	6 (3;14)		4 (2;4)	0.066
	COVID-19 vaccination status			
	Vaccinated		Not vaccinated	
Knowledge Score	1 (1;2)		4 (2;4)	0.001
Propensity Score	20 (16;21)		3.5 (0.5;6.5)	0.001
Hesitancy Score	4 (2;4)		11.5 (6;14)	0.001
	Gestational age			
	1st trimester	2nd trimester	3rd trimester	
Knowledge Score	3 (1;3.50)	3 (1;3)	2 (1;3)	0.664
Propensity Score	15.50 (11;19.50)	20 (11;21)	19 (11;21)	0.535
Hesitancy Score	4 (2;6)	4 (1;10)	4 (3;4)	0.823
	Comorbidities			
	Yes		No	
Knowledge Score	3 (1;3)		3 (1;3)	0.847
Propensity Score	18 (10.50;20)		20 (12;21)	0.401
Hesitancy Score	3 (2;4)		4 (3;4)	0.172

4. Discussion

Maternal immunization and the cocooning strategy are fundamental tools used to protect newborns from vaccine-preventable infections. However, not all healthcare workers and people who take care of newborns recommend immunization for these "at-risk categories". This is reflected in the low prevalence of COVID-19 vaccination among pregnant women observed worldwide [1].

This study was planned to assess (a) the rate of COVID-19 vaccination among pregnant women and (b) the knowledge, attitudes, perceptions and concerns of pregnant women about COVID-19 vaccination.

This survey provides insight into the coverage, hesitancy and willingness to receive the COVID-19 vaccination among pregnant women in Italy and also identifies the factors that are related to an individual's decision.

A first observation in the results of this study was the very low number of women (11%) who claimed that they received at least one dose of the COVID-19 vaccine. Moreover, 4.7% of the sample had received only one shot. These data are similar to those of a systematic review that reported vaccine acceptance rates ranging between 3% and 65%. Studies conducted before the COVID-19 vaccine became available in the United States showed that 41% to 47.80% of pregnant people would be interested in receiving the vaccine [19]. However, after vaccination became available, the rates of acceptance decreased or remained equal [20]. Despite the decreased rate of acceptance, most of the interviewees recognized the value and importance of vaccination [21,22]. Our results show a high vaccination rate, reaching 90%, most likely derived from the distribution of the sample. In fact, we found that educational degree and age had a high impact on the acceptance of vaccination, as indicated by Del Giudice et al. [23], and similar to another study, our sample was predominantly composed of people with higher educational attainment compared to those with medium-low instruction levels [24].

Ethnic discrepancies are clearly influenced by socioeconomic level because it affects a person's ability to pay for and receive vaccinations [25]. Moreover, we noticed among pregnant women a low percentage of flu and DTaP vaccine uptake compared to other studies. In fact, according to data from the CDC, flu and DTaP vaccination coverage was highest among women who reported receiving a provider offer or referral for vaccination (63.5% and 62.2%, respectively) [14–16].

Factors that could influence vaccine uptake are socio-demographic factors, individual factors (personal beliefs, political views and risk perception), and finally, social or organizational factors such as social media [26].

Our study also highlights that women with comorbidities, despite being more vulnerable to disease, have a lower vaccination rate, similar to the data obtained by Snajider et al. [24]. We also evaluated the role of information sources related to active immunization and found that HCWs played a large part in the empowerment and adherence of pregnant women with higher vaccination coverage, as indicated in other studies [27].

Overall, the biggest barrier to vaccination was represented by the fear of adverse effects in women who preferred to acquire disease rather than receive the vaccine. We must remember that there are records in VAERS, the Yellow Card Reporting System, and other official databases of adverse events following immunization (AEFIs), both in the general population and in pregnant women. In particular, a study reported that among 1,315,315 Individual Case Safety Reports (ICSRs) related to COVID-19 vaccines, 3252 (0.25%) were related to vaccinations during pregnancy. Although the majority (87.82%) of ICSRs concerned serious AEFIs, their outcomes were mostly favorable. In this study, 85.0% of total ICSRs referred to pregnant women (n = 2764), while 7.9% referred to fetuses/newborns (n = 258). They identified 16,569 AEFIs. Moreover, 55.16% were AEFIs not related to pregnancy (mostly headache, pyrexia and fatigue), while 17.92% were pregnancy-, newborn-or fetus-related AEFIs. The most common type of pregnancy-related AEFI was spontaneous abortion. Messenger RNA (mRNA) vaccines had a lower reported probability of spontaneous abortion than viral-vector-based vaccines (ROR 0.80, 95% CI 0.69–0.93). Moderna and

Oxford-AstraZeneca vaccines had a higher reported probability of spontaneous abortion (ROR 1.2, 95% CI 1.05–1.38 and ROR 1.26, 95% CI 1.08–1.47, respectively), while a lower reported probability was found for the Pfizer-BioNTech vaccine compared with all other COVID-19 vaccines (ROR 0.73, 95% CI 0.64–0.84) [28].

On the other hand, women who are pregnant or were recently pregnant are at increased risk of severe illness with COVID-19. Severe illness means that a woman might need to be hospitalized, receive intensive care, or be placed on a ventilator to help with breathing. Pregnant women with COVID-19 are also more likely to deliver a baby before the start of the 37th week of pregnancy (premature birth). Pregnant women with COVID-19 might also be at increased risk of problems such as stillbirth and pregnancy loss. Pregnant women who are Black or Hispanic are more likely to be affected by infection with COVID-19. Pregnant women who have other medical conditions, such as diabetes, might be at an even higher risk of severe illness due to COVID-19 [29].

The limitations of our study are its observational nature, the lack of investigation into COVID-19 and the implementation of the study only after the introduction of vaccination for COVID-19. Another limitation of this study is the use of self-reported data that could not be independently verified. The results could be affected by several biases (limited by the online survey), such as selection bias and social desirability bias. Furthermore, we did not evaluate the uptake of a fourth shot of the vaccine.

Another limitation is that the prevalence of COVID-19 vaccination in Italy could be dominated by the mandatory nature of the vaccinations in numerous workplaces, with the result that people's knowledge, hesitancy and barriers do not matter when it comes to the vaccination rate.

5. Conclusions

According to the WHO, vaccination is the primary method for preventing and controlling infectious disease epidemics. As a result, it is crucial to measure vaccination coverage and take population empowerment measures in order to spot any gaps and track trends [14]. Understanding the factors that contribute to the non-adherence and/or refusal of vaccination as well as the deployment of specific monitoring programs is crucial given the significance of primary prevention via vaccination. In particular, the availability of a global pharmacovigilance or post-marketing surveillance network that evaluates the effects of vaccination on pregnant women and newborns in the medium and long term is essential [30–33]. Another possible solution is the presence of a national recommendation approving the administration of the COVID-19 vaccine during pregnancy.

According to the international literature and our findings, vaccination bias is not the result of a single cause but rather the consequence of a complex intersection of several factors, probably as a result of a lengthy and intricate history of vaccine hesitation.

Other studies claim the presence of several risk factors to the development of vaccine hesitancy, with the role of many determinants [34,35]. For this reason, adequate vaccine counseling can be an important building block for increasing trust in the healthcare system, which will be essential in countering disinformation and misinformation about the COVID-19 vaccine for pregnant women [36–44]. Further research is necessary to test our results and explore additional questions.

Supplementary Materials: The following supporting information can be downloaded at: https://www.mdpi.com/article/10.3390/women3030028/s1, Questionnaire S1: Knowledge, attitude and perception of sars cov2 vaccination in pregnant women.

Author Contributions: Conceptualization, C.G.; methodology, C.G. and G.T.; software, G.T.; validation, C.G. and R.S.; formal analysis, G.T. and C.G.; investigation, all authors (C.G., C.R., G.T., R.S., R.C., I.L.S., V.L.F., V.L.P., B.R., P.T.). Resources, all authors; data curation, all authors; writing—original draft preparation, all authors; writing—review and editing, C.A.B., C.G. and C.R.; visualization, R.S.; supervision, C.G.; project administration, C.G. All authors have read and agreed to the published version of the manuscript.

Funding: This research received no external funding.

Institutional Review Board Statement: This study was carried out in accordance with the Declaration of Helsinki's ethical standards. The study needed no formal approval by the local Ethics Committee, though a formal communication of the study start was given (notification with a request for acknowledgement). All the subjects who accepted voluntary participation in the survey provided informed consent. Participation was voluntary and without compensation and the survey was anonymous.

Informed Consent Statement: Informed consent was obtained from all subjects involved in the study.

Data Availability Statement: The data presented in this study are available on request from the corresponding author.

Conflicts of Interest: The authors declare no conflict of interest.

References

1. MacDonald, N.E.; SAGE Working Group on Vaccine Hesitancy. Vaccine hesitancy: Definition, scope and determinants. *Vaccine* **2015**, *33*, 4161–4164. [CrossRef]
2. Mumbai News–Times of India. Only 2% of Maharashtra's 20 L Pregnant Women Jabbed. Available online: https://timesofindia.indiatimes.com/city/mumbai/mumbai-more-data-awareness-canpush-pregnant-women-to-take-shot/articleshow/86153665.cms (accessed on 19 January 2022).
3. Riad, A.; Jouzová, A.; Üstün, B.; Lagová, E.; Hruban, L.; Janků, P.; Pokorná, A.; Klugarová, J.; Koščík, M.; Klugar, M. COVID-19 vaccine acceptance of pregnant and lactating women (PLW) in Czechia: An analytical cross-sectional study. *Int. J. Environ. Res. Public Health* **2021**, *18*, 13373. [CrossRef]
4. Januszek, S.M.; Faryniak-Zuzak, A.; Barnaś, E.; Łoziński, T.; Góra, T.; Siwiec, N.; Szczerba, P.; Januszek, R.; Kluz, T. The Approach of Pregnant Women to Vaccination Based on a COVID-19 Systematic Review. *Medicina* **2021**, *57*, 977. [CrossRef]
5. Skjefte, M.; Ngirbabul, M.; Akeju, O.; Escudero, D.; Hernandez-Diaz, S.; Wyszynski, D.F.; Wu, J.W. COVID-19 vaccine acceptance among pregnant women and mothers of young children: Results of a survey in 16 countries. *Eur. J. Epidemiol.* **2021**, *36*, 197–211. [CrossRef]
6. da Silva, M.C.; da Silva, N.C.H.; Ferreira, A.L.C.G.; Ferreira, F.C.G.; de Melo, M.I.B.; da Silva, L.M.X.; Barbosa, C.R.M.; de Magalhães, J.J.F.; Diniz, G.T.N.; Souza, A.I.; et al. Neutralizing antibodies against SARS-CoV-2 in Brazilian pregnant women vaccinated with one or two doses of BNT162b2 mRNA vaccine (Pfizer/WyethTM). *Front. Public. Health* **2023**, *10*, 1054460. [CrossRef] [PubMed]
7. European Medicines Agency (EMA). COVID-19 Vaccines. 2022. Available online: https://www.ema.europa.eu/en/human-regulatory/overview/public-health-threats/coronavirus-disease-covid-19/treatments-vaccines/covid-19-vaccines (accessed on 13 April 2022).
8. Kadali, R.A.K.; Janagama, R.; Peruru, S.R.; Racherla, S.; Tirumala, R.; Madathala, R.R.; Gajula, V. Adverse effects of COVID-19 messenger RNA vaccines among pregnant women: A cross-sectional study on healthcare workers with detailed self-reported symptoms. *Am. J. Obstet. Gynecol.* **2021**, *225*, 458–460. [CrossRef] [PubMed]
9. Mascolo, A.; di Mauro, G.; Fraenza, F.; Gaio, M.; Zinzi, A.; Pentella, C.; Rossi, F.; Capuano, A.; Sportiello, L. Maternal, fetal and neonatal outcomes among pregnant women receiving COVID-19 vaccination: The preg-co-vax study. *Front. Immunol.* **2022**, *13*, 965171. [CrossRef]
10. Carbone, L.; Mappa, I.; Sirico, A.; Di Girolamo, R.; Saccone, G.; Di Mascio, D.; Donadono, V.; Cuomo, L.; Gabrielli, O.; Migliorini, S.; et al. Pregnant women's perspectives on severe acute respiratory syndrome coronavirus 2 vaccine. *Am. J. Obstet. Gynecol. MFM* **2021**, *3*, 100352. [CrossRef]
11. De Medeiros, K.S.; Sarmento, A.C.A.; Costa, A.P.F.; Macêdo, L.T.A.; da Silva, L.A.S.; de Freitas, C.L.; Simões, A.C.Z.; Gonçalves, A.K. Consequences and implications of the coronavirus disease (COVID-19) on pregnancy and newborns: A comprehensive systematic review and meta-analysis. *Int. J. Gynaecol. Obstet.* **2022**, *156*, 394–405. [CrossRef]
12. Sznajder, K.K.; Kjerulff, K.H.; Wang, M.; Hwang, W.; Ramirez, S.I.; Gandhi, C.K. COVID-19 vaccine acceptance and associated factors among pregnant women in Pennsylvania 2020. *Prev. Med. Rep.* **2022**, *26*, 101713. [CrossRef]
13. Italian Ministry of Health. Raccomandazioni Sulla Vaccinazione Anti SARS-CoV-2/COVID-19 in Gravidanza e Allattamento. Available online: https://www.trovanorme.salute.gov.it/norme/renderNormsanPdf?anno=2021&codLeg=82930&parte=1%20&serie=null (accessed on 8 November 2022). (In Italian)
14. Donati, S.; Corsi, E.; Maraschini, A.; Salvatore, M.A. It OSS-COVID-19 Working Group SARS-CoV-2 infection among hospitalised pregnant women and impact of different viral strains on COVID-19 severity in Italy: A national prospective population-based cohort study. *BJOG* **2022**, *129*, 221–231. [CrossRef] [PubMed]
15. CDC. COVID-19 ACIP Vaccine Recommendations. 2022. Available online: https://www.cdc.gov/vaccines/hcp/acip-recs/vacc-specific/covid-19.html (accessed on 7 July 2020).

16. Havers, F.P.; Moro, P.L.; Hunter, P.; Hariri, S.; Bernstein, H. Use of Tetanus Toxoid, Reduced Diphtheria Toxoid, and Acellular Pertussis Vaccines: Updated Recommendations of the Advisory Committee on Immunization Practices–United States, 2019. *MMWR Morb. Mortal. Wkly. Rep.* **2020**, *69*, 77–83. [CrossRef]
17. Stock, S.J.; Carruthers, J.; Calvert, C.; Denny, C.; Donaghy, J.; Goulding, A.; Hopcroft, L.E.M.; Hopkins, L.; McLaughlin, T.; Pan, J.; et al. SARS-CoV-2 infection and COVID-19 vaccination rates in pregnant women in Scotland. *Nat. Med.* **2022**, *28*, 504–512. [CrossRef]
18. Razzaghi, H.; Meghani, M.; Pingali, C.; Crane, B.; Naleway, A.; Weintraub, E.; Kenigsberg, T.A.; Lamias, M.J.; Irving, S.A.; Kauffman, T.L.; et al. COVID-19 Vaccination Coverage among Pregnant Women During Pregnancy–Eight Integrated Health Care Organizations, United States, December 14, 2020–May 8, 2021. *MMWR Morb. Mortal. Wkly. Rep.* **2021**, *70*, 895–899. [CrossRef]
19. Cetin, I.; Mandalari, M.; Cesari, E.; Borriello, C.R.; Ercolanoni, M.; Preziosi, G. SARS-CoV-2 Vaccine Uptake during Pregnancy in Regione Lombardia, Italy: A Population-Based Study of 122,942 Pregnant Women. *Vaccines* **2022**, *10*, 1369. [CrossRef] [PubMed]
20. Sezerol, M.A.; Davun, S. COVID-19 Vaccine Hesitancy and Related Factors among Unvaccinated Pregnant Women during the Pandemic Period in Turkey. *Vaccines* **2023**, *11*, 132. [CrossRef]
21. Lubrano, C.; Vilca, L.M.; Coco, C.; Schirripa, I.; Zuliani, P.L.; Corneo, R.; Pavone, G.; Pellegrino, A.; Vignali, M.; Savasi, V.; et al. Pregnant women's acceptance and views on COVID-19 vaccine in Northern Italy. *J. Obstet. Gynaecol.* **2023**, *43*, 2139596. [PubMed]
22. Levy, A.T.; Singh, S.; Riley, L.E.; Prabhu, M. Acceptance of COVID-19 vaccination in pregnancy: A survey study. *Am. J. Obstet. Gynecol. MFM* **2021**, *3*, 100399. [CrossRef] [PubMed]
23. Pingali, C.; Meghani, M.; Razzaghi, H.; Lamias, M.J.; Weintraub, E.; Kenigsberg, T.A.; Klein, N.P.; Lewis, N.; Fireman, B.; Zerbo, O.; et al. COVID-19 Vaccination Coverage Among Insured Persons Aged ≥16 Years, by Race/Ethnicity and Other Selected Characteristics—Eight Integrated Health Care Organizations, United States, December 14, 2020–May 15, 2021. *MMWR Morb Mortal Wkly Rep.* **2021**, *70*, 985–990. [CrossRef]
24. Mannocci, A.; Scaglione, C.; Casella, G.; Lanzone, A.; La Torre, G. COVID-19 in Pregnancy: Knowledge about the Vaccine and the Effect of the Virus. Reliability and Results of the MAMA-19 Questionnaire. *Int. J. Environ. Res. Public. Health* **2022**, *19*, 14886. [CrossRef] [PubMed]
25. Skirrow, H.; Barnett, S.; Bell, S.; Riaposova, L.; Mounier-Jack, S.; Kampmann, B.; Holder, B. Women's views on accepting COVID-19 vaccination in and after pregnancy, and for their babies: A multi-methods study in the UK. *BMC Pregnancy Childbirth* **2022**, *22*, 33. [CrossRef] [PubMed]
26. Miraglia Del Giudice, G.; Folcarelli, L.; Napoli, A.; Corea, F.; Angelillo, I.F.; Collaborative Working Group. COVID-19 vaccination hesitancy and willingness among pregnant women in Italy. *Front. Public Health* **2022**, *10*, 995382. [CrossRef]
27. Chang, Y.W.; Tsai, S.M.; Lin, P.C.; Chou, F.H. Willingness to receive influenza vaccination during pregnancy and associated factors among pregnant women in Taiwan. *Public Health Nurs.* **2019**, *36*, 284–295. [CrossRef]
28. Ruggiero, R.; Balzano, N.; Di Napoli, R.; Mascolo, A.; Berrino, P.M.; Rafaniello, C.; Sportiello, L.; Rossi, F.; Capuano, A. Capillary leak syndrome following COVID-19 vaccination: Data from the European pharmacovigilance database Eudravigilance. *Front. Immunol.* **2022**, *13*, 956825. [CrossRef]
29. Pregnancy and COVID-19: What Are the Risk? Available online: https://www.mayoclinic.org/diseases-conditions/coronavirus/in-depth/pregnancy-and-covid-19/art-20482639#:~:text=Risks%20during%20pregnancy&text=Pregnant%20women%20with%20COVID%2D19,as%20stillbirth%20and%20pregnancy%20loss (accessed on 7 July 2023).
30. Willing, E. Hitting the target without missing the point: New Zealand's immunisation health target for two year olds. *Policy Stud.* **2016**, *37*, 535–550. [CrossRef]
31. Azami, M.; Nasirkandy, M.P.; Esmaeili Gouvarchin Ghaleh, H.; Ranjbar, R. COVID-19 vaccine acceptance among pregnant women worldwide: A systematic review and meta-analysis. *PLoS ONE* **2022**, *17*, e0272273. [CrossRef]
32. Maher, L.; Hope, K.; Torvaldsen, S.; Lawrence, G.; Dawson, A.; Wiley, K.; Thomson, D.; Hayen, A.; Conaty, S. Influenza vaccination during pregnancy: Coverage rates and influencing factors in two urban districts in Sydney. *Vaccine* **2013**, *31*, 5557–5564. [CrossRef]
33. Del Riccio, M.; Bechini, A.; Buscemi, P.; Bonanni, P.; On Behalf of The Working Group Dhs; Boccalini, S. Reasons for the Intention to Refuse COVID-19 Vaccination and Their Association with Preferred Sources of Information in a Nationwide, Population-Based Sample in Italy, before COVID-19 Vaccines Roll Out. *Vaccines* **2022**, *10*, 913. [CrossRef]
34. Zarbo, C.; Candini, V.; Ferrari, C.; d'Addazio, M.; Calamandrei, G.; Starace, F.; Caserotti, M.; Gavaruzzi, T.; Lotto, L.; Tasso, A.; et al. COVID-19 Vaccine Hesitancy in Italy: Predictors of Acceptance, Fence Sitting and Refusal of the COVID-19 Vaccination. *Front. Public Health* **2022**, *10*, 873098. [CrossRef]
35. Gauld, N.; Martin, S.; Sinclair, O.; Petousis-Harris, H.; Dumble, F.; Grant, C.C. Influences on Pregnant Women's and Health Care Professionals' Behaviour Regarding Maternal Vaccinations: A Qualitative Interview Study. *Vaccines* **2022**, *10*, 76. [CrossRef]
36. Hill, L.; Burrell, B.; Walls, T. Factors influencing women's decisions about having the pertussis-containing vaccine during pregnancy. *J. Prim. Health Care* **2018**, *10*, 62. [CrossRef] [PubMed]
37. Howe, A.S.; Pointon, L.; Gauld, N.; Paynter, J.; Willing, E.; Turner, N. Pertussis and Influenza immunisation coverage of pregnant women in New Zealand. *Vaccine* **2020**, *38*, 6766–6776. [CrossRef]
38. Sarwal, Y.; Sarwal, R. COVID-19 Vaccination in Pregnancy–Need for Global Pharmaco-Vigilance. *Int. J. Gynaecol. Obstet.* **2023**, *162*, 24–28. [CrossRef] [PubMed]

39. Karafillakis, E.; Francis, M.R.; Paterson, P.; Larson, H.J. Trust, emotions and risks: Pregnant women's perceptions, confidence and decision-making practices around maternal vaccination in France. *Vaccine* **2021**, *39*, 4117–4125. [CrossRef] [PubMed]
40. Verger, P.; Dubé, E. Restoring confidence in vaccines in the COVID-19 era. *Expert. Rev. Vaccines* **2020**, *19*, 991–993. [CrossRef]
41. Bert, F.; Olivero, E.; Rossello, P.; Gualano, M.R.; Castaldi, S.; Damiani, G.; D'Errico, M.M.; Di Giovanni, P.; Fantini, M.P.; Fabiani, L.; et al. Knowledge and beliefs on vaccines among a sample of Italian pregnant women: Results from the NAVIDAD study. *Eur. J. Public Health* **2020**, *30*, 286–292. [CrossRef]
42. La Fauci, V.; Squeri, R.; Genovese, C.; Alessi, V.; Facciolà, A. Pregnant women and risk factors: A cross-sectional study. *Eur. J. Public Health* **2020**, *30* (Suppl. S5), ckaa166.916. [CrossRef]
43. Facciolà, A.; Squeri, R.; Genovese, C.; Alessi, V.; La Fauci, V. Perception of rubella risk in pregnancy: An epidemiological survey on a sample of pregnant women. *Ann. Ig.* **2019**, *31* (Suppl. S1), 65–71. [CrossRef]
44. Ferrera, G.; Squeri, R.; Genovese, C. The evolution of vaccines for early childhood: The MMRV. *Ann. Ig.* **2018**, *30* (Suppl. S1), 33–37. [CrossRef]

Disclaimer/Publisher's Note: The statements, opinions and data contained in all publications are solely those of the individual author(s) and contributor(s) and not of MDPI and/or the editor(s). MDPI and/or the editor(s) disclaim responsibility for any injury to people or property resulting from any ideas, methods, instructions or products referred to in the content.

MDPI
St. Alban-Anlage 66
4052 Basel
Switzerland
www.mdpi.com

Women Editorial Office
E-mail: women@mdpi.com
www.mdpi.com/journal/women

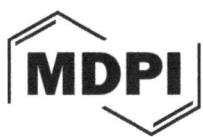

Disclaimer/Publisher's Note: The statements, opinions and data contained in all publications are solely those of the individual author(s) and contributor(s) and not of MDPI and/or the editor(s). MDPI and/or the editor(s) disclaim responsibility for any injury to people or property resulting from any ideas, methods, instructions or products referred to in the content.